CRISIS MANAGEMENT LEADERSHIP:

TEAM TRAINING TO SURVIVE THE CRITICAL MOMENT

5th Edition

Kenneth A. Lipshy, M.D., F.A.C.S.

CRISIS MANAGEMENT
LEADERSHIP

www.CrisisManagementLeadership.com

All photographs by Kenneth A. Lipshy unless otherwise noted.

Text adapted from:
CRISIS MANAGEMENT LEADERSHIP IN THE OPERATING ROOM:
prepare your team to survive any crisis © Dec 23 2013, ISBN: 978-0-9897975-4-2
CRISIS MANAGEMENT LEADERSHIP:
Team Training Guide
© March 13 2014 ISBN: 978-0-615-98976-1
CRISIS MANAGEMENT LEADERSHIP:
Training to Survive the Critical Moment
1st ED. © March 27th 2015. ISBN: 978-0-692-41728-7
2nd ED. © May 30th 2016 ISBN: 978-0-692-72859-8
3rd ED. © Jan 2018 ISBN-10: 0-692-94773-6 ISBN-13: 978-0-692-94773-9
4th ED. © Sept 2021 ISBN: 978-0-578-98323-3
5th ED. © Oct 2025 EPUB ISBN: ISBN: 979-8-218-94084-3; PRINT ISBN: 979-8-218-94097-3

References, permissions, endorsements and acknowledgements are located towards the end of this book and also available in the full text version of *Crisis Management Leadership in the Operating Room: prepare your team to survive any crisis*.

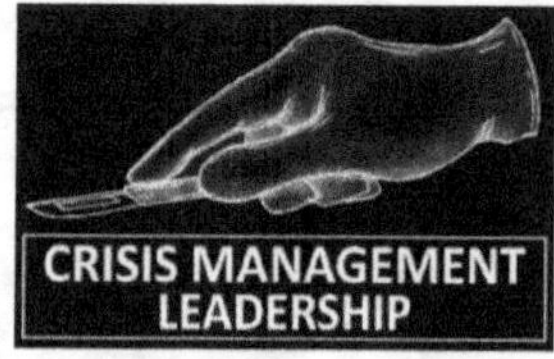

Logo by Bradley Lipshy

WWW.Crisismanagementleadership.com

TABLE OF CONTENTS

ENDORSEMENTS:

Ken Lipshy's *"Crisis Management Leadership in the Operating Room"* is an important contribution for those desiring to apply a scholarly appreciation of both effective management and leadership principles into a vital healthcare context. He promotes an important distinction between management and leadership, which have overlapping but separate attributes — management is about data, process & complexity, while leadership is about establishing a vision, removing obstacles and inspiring success. He does not rest his insights solely to anecdote or limited experience but takes a scholarly approach, focusing on measurable and outcomes-guided leadership. He does so through references to some of the important leaders building scholarly frameworks and proven means of responding to crises, as described by Tom Kolditz and the USUHS Leader-Follower Framework.

~ Lt Gen Eric B. Schoomaker - *United States Army lieutenant general Retired*
Former 42nd Surgeon General of the United States Army and Commanding General, United States Army Medical Command, Commanding General, North Atlantic Regional Medical Command and Walter Reed Army Medical Center.

◆

Crisis Management Leadership in the Operating Room provides an excellent review of human cognitive errors, causes of errors, role of systems in preventing and mitigating errors, and education and training of surgical teams. Topics of crisis management and effective leadership in the Operating Room environment are handled well. The key messages are succinctly articulated throughout the book. This book should be a valuable resource to surgical leaders, practicing surgeons, surgery residents, and members of surgical teams. It should help in underscoring and extending further national efforts currently underway to deliver surgical care of the highest quality and promote safety.

Ajit K. Sachdeva, M.D., F.R.C.S.C., F.A.C.S.
Director, Division of Education American College of Surgeons
Disclaimer: **The opinions expressed in this Foreword are those of the author and do not necessarily represent the official position of the** American College of Surgeons.

◆

This book is invaluable not only for its content but also for the way it passes the information. I must admit that the book was an eye-opener to me in so many ways.
George C. Velmahos, MD, PhD, MSEd, Chief — *Division of Trauma Massachusetts General Hospital*

◆

Healthcare providers need to improve safety within our healthcare system. This book helps us understand how problems occur in the operating room and suggests methods that can be used to control, mitigate, and possibly avoid these crisis situations. Surgical trainees and teams might consider adding it to their required reading list!
~ **John A. Weigelt**, MD, DVM, MMA, *Trauma Division/CC Medical College of Wisconsin, Editor in Chief, Journal of Surgical Education*

◆

This book provides a fantastic framework for improving clinicians' abilities to act intelligently in crisis situations. I recommend it to anyone involved in direct patient care. A must read.
~ **Jeffrey S. Young**, MD, MBA, *Director, Trauma Center, and Chief Patient Safety Officer, UVA Health System*

In his book *Crisis Management Leadership in the Operating Room — Prepare Your Team to Survive Any Crisis* Dr. Lipshy provides a pathway for teams to apply principles of crew resource management within high-reliability organizations to achieve exceptional leadership, communication, and teamwork during care of the surgical patient, especially during crises. Surgeons will enjoy and benefit from Dr. Lipshy's book. *Crisis Management Leadership in the Operating Room — Prepare Your Team to Survive Any Crisis* is a useful read for all operating room team members (surgeons, anesthesiologists, anesthesia providers, nurses, scrub techs, and others), patient safety officers, risk managers, and health care organizational leaders.

~ **Douglas E. Paull, MD,** *Clinical Adjunct Associate Professor of Medicine, Georgetown University SOM; Executive Masters in Clinical Quality and Safety Leadership (EMCQSL) Program (2018-Current), Former Co-Director of Medical Team Training (2007-2010) and Director of Patient Safety Curriculum and Medical Simulation (2010-2016) VHA National Center for Patient Safety.*

While experience remains the most effective teacher for learning how to manage real-life situations, simulation has emerged as an invaluable alternative that allows trainees to practice responding to events they may rarely — or may never — encounter in reality. Over the past several decades, simulation technology has advanced dramatically and is now considered the standard of practice across many high-risk professions. In surgery, the integration of simulation into traditional training programs improves objective performance in the operating room, including enhanced task completion, shorter operative times, and reduced error rates. Team-based simulation training has similarly improved communication, adherence to best-practice protocols, and overall teamwork. In essence, the way one trains profoundly influences how one performs under pressure.

A key factor in the success of simulation training is its capacity to replicate realistic environments. To foster engagement, simulation has evolved from basic computer-based exercises to hyper-realistic, actor-driven scenarios reminiscent of live-action training used in military team preparation. Alongside these advances has been the introduction of immersion and stress-induction training — methods designed to explore how individuals learn and perform under duress. Memory retention and recognition of successful care patterns are often strengthened when trainees learn under moderate stress or following failure. Such training has also inspired the development of crisis checklists, enabling learners to focus sharply on proven pathways once the likely cause of a problem is identified, ultimately improving the chances of successful outcomes.

However, stress-based training is not without its drawbacks. Excessive mental stress can impair attention, overload cognitive capacity, and reduce situational awareness. Under high stress, participants often fixate on specific tasks while overlooking important contextual information. As stress intensifies, the ability to filter irrelevant data deteriorates, memory for critical details diminishes, and rational decision-making falters. These factors collectively degrade both individual and team performance.

Simulation training typically emphasizes specific scenarios, which can unintentionally reinforce rigid, rule-based responses. While this conditioning enhances reaction speed when similar situations arise, it may prove harmful if applied to the wrong context. The "one-size-fits-all" response can steer teams off course. Effective post-simulation debriefing can mitigate this risk, but such debriefing is not consistently implemented across training programs.

Checklists have undeniably improved team performance in managing known threats. Yet, under uncertain or ambiguous circumstances, heightened anxiety may impair the team's ability to identify which checklist applies, leading to maladaptive behaviors. The challenge, therefore, lies in finding the balance — training methods that enhance memory and performance while managing stress, ensuring that teams maintain adaptability and cohesion even under pressure. While these methods and checklists are highly effective in most situations, they may become dangerous when applied incorrectly, particularly in the heat of crisis.

A notable limitation across most simulation studies is the lack of integration between crisis simulation and pre-emptive crisis management leadership training. Limited data suggest that brief preparatory sessions in coping strategies can modestly reduce self-reported stress during simulations, but there remains a paucity of evidence supporting comprehensive didactic instruction on managing oneself and one's team during crises.

Ask elite athletes how they perform their extraordinary feats, and their answers are often vague — or even inaccurate. The same holds true for many leaders after a medical crisis: when asked to explain their actions, they struggle to articulate the precise steps that led to success. This book aims to demystify that process. It serves as a structured guide to leading during **the critical moment** — that decisive period immediately following the onset of crisis, when leadership can determine whether a team succeeds or fails.

Leadership Decision-making during this critical moment remains one of the least studied elements of crisis management. When confronted with an extreme situation, team members instinctively look to their leader for stability and control. Leaders must project calm and confidence, regardless of their internal state. A failure to do so can quickly undermine team cohesion. In high-risk industries, emotional resilience and composure are prerequisites for leadership; individuals who lack these traits often do not advance. In healthcare, however, such selective filtering is rare. Therefore, crisis management leadership training is essential to prepare medical professionals to manage both their own reactions and their team's performance under pressure. Sweeney PJ, Matthews MD, Lester PB

Although medicine can learn valuable lessons from other high-risk fields, it remains a uniquely demanding profession. Unlike first responders or military personnel, physicians rarely begin their day anticipating catastrophe. Physiologically, stress responses that enhance performance in athletes or soldiers — such as elevated heart rates between 150 and 180 beats per minute — can be detrimental in surgery, where fine motor control and calm precision are essential. In this regard, surgeons are more akin to pilots, for whom anxiety and tachycardia compromise performance. Siddle, Sharp Thus, while we can borrow principles from these fields, training in medicine must be specifically tailored to its unique demands.

Crisis Management Leadership: Training to Survive the Critical Moment explores how crisis leadership principles from high-risk industries can be adapted for medical practice. It aims to prepare healthcare professionals not only to survive the critical moment but to lead their teams through it with confidence, clarity, and composure.

Kenneth A Lipshy MD FACS

KENNETH A. LIPSHY, MD, FACS

Lt General Bob Dees to To Tom Kolditz: "It's not whether bad things happen that makes or breaks a commander, it's what he does with the hand that he's dealt that really matters" Permission from Bob Dees AND Tom Kolditz

<table>
<tr><td>

AS A YOUNG LEADER WHO IS INTERESTED IN LEADERSHIP DEVELOPMENT DID YOU FEEL YOU HAD ADEQUATE FRONT LOADING IN YOUR TRAINING TO BE A SKILLED LEADER?
NO! We definitely did not. We seldom see where places invest adequately in leadership training. Typically, we are thrown into leadership situations. We either succeed or fail! Early on you have to learn as an intern how to manage students, then as a resident, then interns, then as a Chief Resident the other residents, then as an attending the residents…
Leading yourself is the most important. You must control your emotions and your thoughts.
Paula Ferrada, MD VCU

</td></tr>
<tr><td>

Was I ready after my residency?… well let's just say my first case out of residency (with no "attending" in the room) was as a fellow. I was instructed to take over a case across the hall as an attending guiding a Chief Resident thru a Whipple in a patient with a cystic neoplasm and prior cyst-jenunostomy in the community. Seemed like everything just fell into place. I do admit that as residents we had significantly more overall responsibilities for our perioperative care and subsequently much more opportunity to operate more independently that is currently practical in the modern resident training era.

</td></tr>
</table>

- Admi H. Stress intervention. A model of stress inoculation training. J Psychosoc Nurs Ment Health Serv. 1997;35(8):37–41
- Billings CE, Cheaney ES. Information transfer problems in the aviation system, (NASA TP-1875), Moffett Fiedl CA: NASA-Ames Research Center."
- Allan CK, Thiagarajan RR, Beke D, Imprescia A, Kappus LJ, Garden A, et al. Simulation-based training delivered directly to the pediatric cardiac intensive care unit engenders preparedness, comfort, and decreased anxiety among multidisciplinary resuscitation teams. J Thorac Cardiovasc Surg. 2010;140(3):646–52.
- Andreatta PB, Hillard M, Krain LP. The impact of stress factors in simulation-based laparoscopic training. Surgery. 2010;147(5):631–9.
- Bianchin M, Mello e Souza T, Medina JH, Izquierdo I. The amygdala is involved in the modulation of long-term memory, but not in working or short-term memory. Neurobiol Learn Mem. 1999 Mar;71(2):127-31.
- Bong CL, Lightdale JR, Fredette ME, Weinstock P. Effects of simulation versus traditional tutorial-based training on physiologic stress levels among clinicians: a pilot study. Simul Healthc. 2010;5(5):272–8.
- Cahill L, Haier RJ, Fallon J, Alkire MT, Tang C, Keator D, et al. Amygdala activity at encoding correlated with long-term, free recall of emotional information. Proc Natl Acad Sci USA. 1996;93:8016–21.

- Cahill L, Gorski L, Le K. Enhanced human memory consolidation with postlearning stress: interaction with the degree of arousal at encoding. Learn Mem. 2003;10:270-4.
- CHROUSOS, G.P. & P.W. GOLD. 1992. The concepts of stress and stress system disorders. JAMA 267: 1244-1252.
- Collyer S, Malecki G. Tactical decision Making under stress: history and overview. Cannon-Bower J and Salas E. Making Decisions under stress APA 1998.
- DeMaria S, Levine AI. The use of Stress to enrich the simulated environment in *The comprehensive Textbook of Healthcare Simulation*, Springer Science and business media New York pp65-72
- Demaria Jr S, Bryson EO, Mooney TJ, Silverstein JH, Reich DL, Bodian C, et al. Adding emotional stressors to training in simulated cardiopulmonary arrest enhances participant performance. Med Educ. 2010;44(10):1006-15.
- Driskell J, Johnston J. Stress exposure in training. Cannon-bowers J, Salas J *Making decisions under stress*, American psychological association 1999
- Elzinga BM, Bakker A, Bremner JD. Stress-induced cortisol elevations are associated with impaired delayed, but not immediate recall. Psychiatry Res. 2005;134:211-23.
- Flin R. Sitting in the hot seat: leaders and teams for critical incident management. Rhona Flin, John Wiley and Sons. 1996.
- Girzadas Jr DV, Delis S, Bose S, Hall J, Rzechula K, Kulstad EB. Measures of stress and learning seem to be equally affected among all roles in a simulation scenario. Simul Healthc. 2009;4(3):149-54.
- Harvey A, Nathens AB, Bandiera G, Leblanc VR. Threat and challenge: cognitive appraisal and stress responses in simulated trauma resuscitations. Med Educ. 2010;44(6):587-94.
- *Helmrich RL, Foushee HC, Benseon R, Russini R. cockpit management attitudes: exploring the attitude-performance linkage. Aviation, space and environmental medicine. 1986, 57: 1198-2000.*
- HENRY, J.P. 1992. Biological basis of the stress response. Int. Physiol. Behav. Sci. 27: 66-83.
- Het S, Schoofs D, Rohleder N, Wolf OT. Stress-induced cortisol level elevations are associated with reduced negative affect after stress: indications for a mood-buffering cortisol effect. Psychosom Med. 2012 Jan;74(1):23-32.
- Hunziker S, Laschinger L, Portmann-Schwarz S, Semmer NK, Tschan F, Marsch S. Perceived stress and team performance during a simulated resuscitation. Intensive Care Med. 2011;37(9):1473-9.
- Hunziker S, Semmer NK, Tschan F, Schuetz P, Mueller B, Marsch S. Dynamics and association of different acute stress markers with performance during a simulated resuscitation. Resuscitation. 2012;83(5):572-8.
- Joels M, Pu Z, Wiegert O, Oitzl MS, Krugers HJ. Learning under stress: how does it work? Trends Cogn Sci. 2006;10:152-8.
- Joëls M, Fernandez G, Roozendaal B. Stress and emotional memory: a matter of timing. Trends Cogn Sci. 2011;15(6):280-8.
- Keitel A, Ringleb M, Schwartges I, Weik U, Picker O, Stockhorst U, et al. Endocrine and psychological stress responses in a simulated emergency situation. Psychoneuroendocrinology. 2011;36(1):98-108.
- Klein G. The sources of power, how people make decisions. Cambridge: MIT press, 199: 127
- Kudielka BM, Gierens A, Hellhammer DH, Wüst S, Schlotz W. Salivary cortisol in ambulatory assessment--some dos, some don'ts, and some open questions. Psychosom Med. 2012 May;74(4):418-31.
- LeBlanc VR. The effects of acute stress on performance: implications for health professions education. Acad Med. 2009;84(10 Suppl):S25-33.
- Lipshitz R, Shaul OB. 1997. Schemata and mental models in recognition-primed decision making.
- Mattie Tops, Femke T. A. Buisman-Pijlman, Maarten A. S. Boksem, Albertus A. Wijers, and Jakob Korf. Cortisol-Induced Increases of Plasma Oxytocin Levels Predict Decreased Immediate Free Recall of Unpleasant Words Front Psychiatry. 2012; 3: 43.McEwen BS. Definitions and concepts of stress. In: Fink G, editor. Encyclopedia of stress. San Diego: Academic; 2000.McGaugh JL. Memory—a century of consolidation. Science. 2000;287:248-51.
- Meichenbaum D, Deffenbacher JL. Stress inoculation training. The Counseling Psychologist. 1988;16:69-90.
- Miller GA. The magical number seven plus or minus two: some limits on our capacity for processing information. Psychological review 1956. 63:81-97
- Müller MP, Hänsel M, Fichtner A, Hardt F, Weber S, Kirschbaum C, et al. Excellence in performance and stress reduction during two different full scale simulator training courses: a pilot study. Resuscitation. 2009;80(8):919-24.Nater UM, Moor C, Okere U, Stallkamp R, Martin M, Ehlert U, et al. Performance on a declarative memory task is better in high than low cortisol responders to psychosocial stress. Psychoneuroendocrinology. 2007;32:758-63.
- Packard MG, Goodman J. Emotional arousal and multiple memory systems in the mammalian brain. Front Behav Neurosci. 2012;6:14.
- Payne JD, Jackson ED, Ryan L, Hoscheidt S, Jacobs WJ, Nadel L. The impact of stress on neutral and emotional aspects of episodic memory. Memory. 2006;14:1-16.
- Payne JD, Jackson ED, Hoscheidt S, Ryan L, Jacobs WJ, Nadel L.Stress administered prior to encoding impairs neutral but enhances emotional long-term episodic memories. Learn Mem. 2007;14(12):861-8.
- Roozendaal B. Stress and memory: opposing effects of glucocorticoids on memory consolidation and memory retrieval. Neurobiol Learn Mem. 2002;78:578-95.
- Roozendaal B, Quirarte GL, McGaugh JL. Stress-activated hormonal systems and the regulation of memory storage. Ann NY Acad Sci. 1999;821:247-58.
- Roozendaal B. Glucocorticoids and the regulation of memory consolidation. Psychoneuroendocrinology. 2000;25:213-38.

- Rush RM; Simulation in Military and Battlefield Medicine environment in *The comprehensive Textbook of Healthcare Simulation*, Springer Science and business media New York; pp401-413
- Sandi C, Pinelo-Nava MT. Stress and memory: behavioral effects and neurobiological mechanisms. Neural Plast. 2007;2007:78970.
- Sandi C, Pinelo-Nava MT. Stress and memory: behavioral effects and neurobiological mechanisms. Neural Plast. 2007;2007:78970.
- Saunders T, Driskell JE, Johnston JH, Salas E. The effect of stress inoculation training on anxiety and performance. J Occup Health Psychol. 1996 Apr;1(2):170-86.
- Schwabe L, Oitzl MS, Philippsen C, Richter S, Bohringer A; Wippich W, et al. Stress modulates the use of spatial and stimulus–response learning strategies in humans. Learn Mem. 2007;14:109–16.
- Schwabe L, Wolf OT. The context counts: congruent learning and testing environments prevent memory retrieval impairment following stress. Cogn Affect Behav Neurosci. 2009;9(3):229–36.
- Schwabe L, Wolf OT, Oitzl MS. Memory formation under stress: quantity and quality. Neurosci Biobehav Rev. 2010;34:584–91.
- Schwabe L, Wolf OT.Learning under stress impairs memory formation. Neurobiol Learn Mem. 2010 Feb;93(2):183-8
- Schwabe L, Wolf OT.Stress prompts habit behavior in humans. J Neurosci. 2009 Jun 3;29(22):7191-8.
- Saunders T, Driskell JE, Johnston JH, Salas E. The effect of stress inoculation training on anxiety and performance. J Occup Health Psychol. 1996;1(2):170–86.
- Serfaty D, Entin E, J Johnston J. Team coordination training in cannon-bowers J and Salas E. making Decisions under stress APA 1998. P 222.
- schendel JD, Hagman JD. On sustaining procedural skills over a prolonged retention interval. Journal of applied psychology 1982 67:605-610.)
- Serfaty D, Entin EE, Johnston JJ. Team coordination training Cannon-bowers j, Salas J ed. Making decisions under stress, American psychological association, 1999.
- Sharps MJ. *Processing Under Pressure: Stress, Memory and Decision-Making in Law Enforcement*. Flushing, NY: Looseleaf Law Publications; 2010
- Siddle B. *Sharpening the Warriors Edge: The Psychology and Science of Training*. 10th ed. Belleville, IL: PPCT Research publications; 2008.
- Sweeney PJ, Matthews MD, Lester PB. *Leadership in Dangerous Situations*. Annapolis, MD: Naval Institute Press; 2011.
- Spettell CM, Liebert RM. Training for safety in automated person-machine systems. Am Psychol. 1986;41:545–50.
- Wolf O. T. (2009). Stress and memory in humans: twelve years of progress? Brain Res.1293, 142–154.
- Zaambok C, Klein G. Naturalistic decision making. Mahwah NJ Erlbaum 1997 293-304.

I.   INTRODUCTION

STUDENT OBJECTIVES WHEN USING THIS GUIDE:
1. Explain what defines a crisis
2. Recite effective leadership basics
3. Describe how human error contributes to adverse events.
4. Discuss how using the following factors effectively during the CRITICAL MOMENT will allow a team to be successful:
   a. Describe cognitive functions during normal and stressful circumstances.
   b. Demonstrate their control over maladaptive behavior- panic and dissociation- using a **CRITICAL PAUSE**.
   c. Explain how to establish clear lines of leadership and followership.
   d. Describe Effective Communication.
   e. Discuss the process of maintaining situational awareness.
   f. Perform effective risk management strategies.
5. Explain why its critical that we don't work as lone wolves.
6. Describe how system deficiencies can allow simple errors to progress to catastrophes or how the system can be prepared to mitigate a mistake.

KEY CONCEPTS-   LEADERSHIP IN THE MIDST OF A CRISIS:

ERROR: Human behavior is consistently negatively affected by error, which tends to either be a direct or an indirect cause of most disasters. One must understand the origination of errors in order to plan to avoid them during crisis management.

CRISIS MANAGEMENT: In the face of adversity there are two pathways: one leading to success and the other to failure. Successful crisis management depends upon:
1. <u>Problem Recognition.</u>
2. <u>Containment of maladaptive behaviour</u> – such as panic, tunnel vision, dissociation, etc.
3. <u>Establishment of effective leadership - which relies upon:</u>
   a. Leadership skill understanding.
   b. Accurate closed loop communication.
   c. Effective followership.
   d. Shared mental model and effective reconciliation
   e. Mutual Trust
   f. Containment of fixation and other errors.
   g. Maintenance of situational awareness.
   h. Establishment and continual assessment of an effective plan.

SYSTEMS INTERCONNECTIONS: Most disasters are inevitably found to arise from a long chain of intertwined seemingly unrelated events. In many instances, had there been an absence of one or several individual events the outcome may have been more favourable.

At any moment, conditions in a healthcare environment can change abruptly, threatening a patient, the team, or even the provider. A select few individuals seem to possess the innate composure and decisiveness of seasoned military commanders — but most of us do not. Research into these natural leadership qualities remains sparse and imprecise. It is difficult for investigators to define such "gifts" in ways that can be measured, replicated, or taught. Likewise, those who possess these traits often find it challenging to translate them into structured processes that others can learn.

Although stress inoculation training has been shown to reduce anxiety and improve performance when individuals later face similar scenarios, the evidence is less clear regarding whether pre-training briefings or post-training debriefings are more effective at promoting universally applicable coping strategies. What is clear is that stress-adaptation techniques learned before or during simulation enhance learning and decision-making capacity. Yet, full-scale integration of stress-reduction and crisis-decision frameworks into standard training has not been a central focus to date.

Most high-risk industries train explicitly for sudden, high-stakes crises. In contrast, medical education rarely integrates these topics comprehensively within a single curriculum. A **High Reliability Organization (HRO)** is one designed to minimize the impact of adverse events on its system and its people. Ideally, such systems are built with multiple barriers to prevent a single error from escalating into catastrophe. Because it is impossible to predict every potential failure, the key is to understand how resilient — or vulnerable — the organization and its teams are when faced with the unexpected.

Healthcare leaders bear the responsibility for designing safety mechanisms that anticipate complex risks and mitigate harm when crises occur. The aviation industry provides a striking example: during the 1980s, initial pilot resistance to change eventually gave way to a data-driven realization — crisis preparedness training directly reduced accidents and fatalities. Programs designed by aviators for aviators proved most successful and remain foundational in aviation culture. Likewise, training created by healthcare professionals, for healthcare professionals, is likely to yield more meaningful and lasting improvements than externally imposed initiatives.

As Conley, Singer, and Gawande (2011) observed, surgeons are far more likely to follow a trusted surgical leader than to comply with a safety directive introduced by a "quality officer." This underscores a critical truth: cultural change in safety must originate from within the profession itself. Every clinician has witnessed a moment when a colleague — or an entire team — failed to respond adaptively to an unforeseen challenge. Rather than dismissing such events as anomalies, we should instead ask why they do not occur more frequently — and, more importantly, how to prevent them altogether. The principles presented in this text aim to help teams train proactively to avoid disaster following unexpected crises.

Culture of Safety

Safety experts challenge us to reflect on whether we are truly cultivating a *culture* of safety — or merely striving for safe *standard operations*. The difference is profound. The former shapes how we think, speak, and act every day; the latter influences only how we respond in specific situations.

Three concerns persist today (as they did when the Institute of Medicine (IOM) published *To Err Is Human* in 1999 (Kohn):

1. We still have far to go in eliminating sentinel events.
2. Most adverse events stem from human and system-level factors rather than individual negligence.
3. Sustainable progress depends on transforming organizational culture and processes, not merely correcting individual behavior.

Healthcare continues to echo the refrain that "medicine is not safe" and that "we must improve patient safety." The **Manchester Patient Safety Framework (MaPSAF)** developed by Dianne Parker and Darren Ashcroft illustrates the stages through which organizations evolve—from reactive systems to cultures of safety. Achieving cultural safety requires focusing on *how* we operate, not just on *what* we measure. [Ashcroft]

Daved van Stralen, a pioneer in high-reliability thinking, eloquently captures this concept:

"Safety is not the goal; it is embedded in how we operate in adverse or hostile environments—a critical distinction. At one HRO conference, amid widespread publicity about patient deaths from medical errors, nearly every speaker began with statistics about these tragedies and the need for healthcare to be 'more safe.' I cautioned that such statements, though well-intentioned, distract from the more important question of how and what to change. Those of us who studied HROs did not learn them as a means to become safe or resilient—we learned them as the way to operate in time-compressed, hazardous, and unstructured environments. Good operations were inherently safe. The focus was on resolving the event; safety was integral, not separate. If your goal is simply to be safe, then the only sure path is not to engage at all."

This distinction lies at the heart of crisis leadership. High reliability is not achieved through a checklist or a single intervention—it is cultivated through mindset, preparation, and disciplined execution under pressure. True safety is not an endpoint but a byproduct of operational excellence.

IMAGINE THIS SCENARIO:

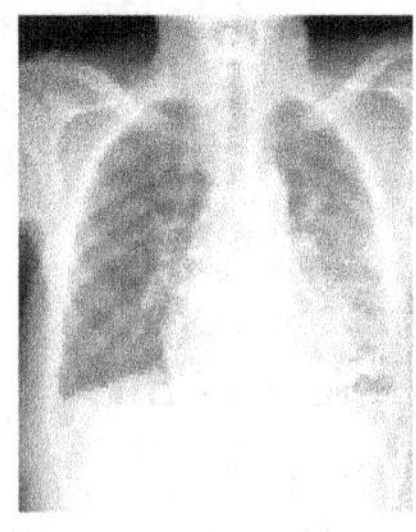

You are called early Monday a.m. by one of the hospitalists to see a patient who had a prior chest tube and pleurodesis. They want to discharge him to an outside community living center, BUT he has had an intermittently high white blood cell count and low-grade fever. A CT scan Friday afternoon revealed a small collection of fluid on the side of the prior chest tube and they would like this aspirated before discharging him. You agree to aspirate it in Radiology under ultrasound guidance between OR cases. You have a dry aspiration and decide to abort the procedure, when all of the sudden the patient coughs violently and begins to spew up cups of blood. After what seems like a long period of time someone finally finds a pulse oximeter and monitor. The patient is rapidly desaturating and his blood pressure is falling fast.........your phone keeps ringing..... the O.R. is waiting on you and wants you now!

HOW WELL WOULD YOU PERFORM IF THIS WAS YOU?

Image from Google Images

Rorke Denver (former head of basic and advanced SEAL training and author of- *DAMN FEW: making the modern day SEAL warrior*) in our conversation about leadership under duress, stated: "Just lead! Your behavior will be mimicked & amplified."

"Calm is contagious. If you keep your head, you keep your head."

"In 14 years of training, I've never seen *'calm is contagious'* proven wrong. Calm is being focused on the job at hand when you need to do it at its most intense moment."

So.... **How *does* one stay calm and lead under pressure?** It is not as instinctual as most try to convince themselves, but can be learned through proper training.

WHAT CHARACTERISTICS ALLOW COMMANDERS TO SUCCEED IN THE MIDST OF UNCERTAIN DANGEROUS SITUATIONS?
1. **INTUITION**: The gift of *Coup d' oeil*=the ability to instantaneously make sense of a seemingly disastrous situation and rapidly envision a course of action. While partly innate, intuition is shaped by prior learning and training.
2. **RESOLVE**: The gift of resolve = carry out a plan in spite of uncertainty.
3. **FLEXIBILITY**: The gift of flexibility = adjust accordingly when the unexpected happens.
Sweeney PJ, Matthews MD, Lester PB. *Leadership in Dangerous Situations.*

IT IS EASY TO RECOGNIZE A DYSFUNCTIONAL TEAM DURING A CRISIS…… BUT CAN YOU DESCRIBE WHAT AN EFFICIENT EFFECTIVE TEAM LOOKS LIKE? HOW LIKELY IS YOUR TEAM TO BE RESILIENT IN THE MIDST OF ITS NEXT CRISIS?

THE CRITICAL PAUSE:
After an adverse event occurs, it is extremely important as a leader to take a brief moment to assess your situation. You need to take a minute or two to analyze what has happened and reorganize your team. Many leaders fail to take advantage of that moment, losing an opportunity to salvage the situation. Col. Patrick Sweeney, Personal com.

"It's like pornography- you know when you see it but can't explain it" JD Richardson (personal communication)

TEAM RESILIENCE
Resilience: the ability to return to baseline following an adversity. Resilience emerges from strengthening team viability through team and individual training.
Viability: ability of a team to function effectively.
Viability is a function of:
   a. Team cohesiveness- willing to serve the team or mission.
   b. Team trust- confidence of skills of team members and in members honoring their commitment.
   c. Collective efficacy- shared belief that the team can work together.
Hardiness: strength in the face of overwhelming odds with sense of control and commitment to the team and mission. Hardiness is highest in those who are strong in terms of optimism and adept at active coping mechanisms (adversity viewed as a challenge as opposed to a threat). Sweeney PJ, Matthews MD, Lester PB. *Leadership in Dangerous Situations.*

"You cannot control *external* chaos but you must control your own *internal* chaos. If your team cannot work together, and all you have is chaos in your team, that just makes everything worse. You must control your team." Sean McCay-**Asymmetric Combat Institute**

While you cannot control particular events, you can control your reaction and response to that event. Training and advanced expectations can prepare you to respond to these unplanned situations. Leaders must remember that people must perceive a sense of control over their destiny. Sweeney PJ, Matthews MD, Lester PB. *Leadership in Dangerous Situations.*

MYTHS REGARDING CAPABILITY OF TEAMS TO HANDLE A CRISIS
1. Only idiots make mistakes!
2. Team training doesn't work!
3. It's the hospital's fault we have these problems!
4. Stop worrying! Crises and errors rarely happen!
5. We are all trained and ready to go!
6. We can handle anything and do not let it affect us when things go wrong!

The Six Myths of Patient Safety

Despite decades of progress, several persistent myths continue to undermine efforts to improve patient safety in healthcare. Recognizing and confronting these misconceptions is essential to developing a truly reliable and resilient safety culture.

Myth 1: "Only incompetent people make mistakes."
Fact: Human error can occur at any time and for a multitude of reasons. Competence does not confer immunity to error. Understanding *how* and *why* mistakes occur is critical so that their consequences can be prevented or mitigated. Safety depends not on perfection, but on systems designed to anticipate and absorb human fallibility.

Myth 2: "Team training and checklists have never been proven to make a real difference."
This argument is often framed as skepticism toward initiatives perceived as bureaucratic or unnecessary: "We see these checklists as a waste of time — tools meant to empower people who don't need to be involved. We want data showing that they actually reduce morbidity and mortality."
Fact: The evidence from both aviation and healthcare literature clearly demonstrates that structured team training and standardized checklists improve safety outcomes. Early resistance in medicine mirrors what aviation faced decades ago — initial disbelief followed by undeniable data showing that communication, coordination, and procedural consistency save lives.

Myth 3: "Patient safety is a leadership issue — it requires hospital administration buy-in, not physician involvement."
"Training programs need organizational leadership to run and maintain them. Surgeons shouldn't have to lead these efforts."
Fact: Physician leadership is indispensable to transforming safety culture. In aviation, pilots were initially resistant to safety mandates, yet after two decades of evidence — and ultimately congressional oversight — they recognized their responsibility in leading cultural change. Likewise, sustainable progress in healthcare requires physicians to be active leaders, not passive participants, in patient safety initiatives.

Myth 4: "We're safe because we never have crises."
"We haven't had an adverse event here in years."
Fact: While fewer than 3–5% of operative cases involve a true crisis, rarity does not equate to readiness. When such events do occur, poor management can rapidly escalate to fatal outcomes. The absence of crises should never be interpreted as the presence of safety — it may instead reflect luck, underreporting, or complacency.

Myth 5: "We're ready for anything — our teams can handle any crisis."
"We've always worked well together. Checklists and team training aren't necessary — we already know how to lead."
Fact: Multiple studies have shown that physicians often overestimate their leadership and communication abilities during crises. Non-physician team members frequently perceive physicians as poor team leaders, particularly under stress. True readiness requires not confidence, but continual training, humility, and reflection.

Myth 6: "We don't let patient care errors affect us — these events don't have personal consequences."
Fact: This belief is dangerously false. Numerous studies demonstrate that involvement in medical errors contributes directly to clinician distress, distraction, and burnout — the so-called "second victim" phenomenon. A culture that ignores these personal impacts risks perpetuating the same conditions that lead to future errors. (modified from Runciman et al)

In Summary

Each of these myths represents a barrier to building a culture of safety grounded in humility, systems thinking, and shared accountability. As history has shown in other high-reliability industries, progress begins only when professionals acknowledge that safety is not a measure of individual perfection but a collective commitment to vigilance, communication, and continuous learning.

> *Heraclitus -"Out of every one hundred men, ten shouldn't even be there, eighty are just targets, nine are the real fighters, and we are lucky to have them, for they make the battle. Ah, but the one, one is a warrior, and he will bring the others back."*

INAPPROPRIATE REACTION FOR A SENIOR ATTENDING:

"As a resident, in the middle of dissecting out a difficult gangrenous gallbladder, the gallbladder just ripped off the patient's common duct. Everything was so friable it was almost impossible to tell what was what. Bile started draining into the wound (and some blood). The attending surgeon just turned white as a ghost and said 'this patient is going to die! We killed this patient!' We could not believe he said that. I quietly turned to the tech and asked for a butterfly needle and some contrast. We shot a cholangiogram after we found a bile containing structure. Using that as a landmark we figured out what was what. To this day I don't understand why he responded that way."

WHY SHOULD WE WORRY ABOUT CRISES IN OUR ENVIRONMENT? BECAUSE:

- Experience does not prevent failure - senior providers consistently make mistakes during crises.
- In 50% of crises, signs are non-specific, with a delay seen in the determination of the cause & appropriate corrective action.
- During complex life-threatening crises, teams are forced to rely upon cognitive tasking far beyond the information processing capacity of the human brain.
- Fewer than 10-20% of humans are capable of effectively responding during a threatening event.

(Runciman, Runciman, Webb, Cooper, Drifts, Clifton, Edwards, Gonzales, Backpacker 2006)

The rarity of critical events, combined with the lack of consistent and formal crisis management training, may explain several concerning findings from anesthesia studies. These studies have demonstrated that:

- **Experience alone does not prevent failure**, and
- **Even senior providers are prone to error during crises.**

This is particularly alarming given that the same research revealed additional insights:

- In nearly **50% of crises**, early warning signs were **non-specific**, leading to delays in identifying the underlying cause and implementing appropriate corrective actions.
- During **complex, life-threatening events**, clinical teams are forced to engage in cognitive processing demands that **exceed the brain's natural information-handling capacity**. Runciman, Runciman, Webb, Cooper, Drifts, Edwards

Despite decades of focus on patient safety, medical errors persist. Furthermore, newer generations of trainees may not be receiving the same depth of preparation for crisis management as their predecessors. This gap underscores the urgent need for healthcare teams to:

- **Deepen their understanding of human factors** contributing to medical error;
- **Strengthen system design** to prevent minor errors from escalating into full-blown crises; and
- **Train deliberately and realistically** to manage crises with composure and coordinated teamwork.

Although there has been encouraging progress in the structured assessment of communication, professionalism, and procedural skill among healthcare providers, **formal team training in crisis intervention remains limited**. When a team lacks effective coping mechanisms under stress, even minor events can spiral into catastrophe.

Ultimately, **robust system design**, when combined with **proactive, simulation-based team training**, offers the best protection against escalation from crisis to **disaster** — defined as the point at which significant, potentially irreversible damage has occurred. (Gaba, Calland, Helmreich, Pizzi, Cooper, Diehl, Arora, Runciman, Runciman, Webb)

For a superb example of leadership under pressure, read Ben Aaron's account of their management of Ronald Reagan in the appendix "**AN INTERVIEW WITH BEN AARON, MD - THE TEAM THAT SAVED RONALD REAGAN.** *Washington DC March 30 1981, 2:27 pm. Thank you Dr. Aaron!*

WHAT DO SURGEONS SAY ABOUT STRATEGIES FOR MANAGING CRISES?

2009 SURVEY OF AUSTRALIAN SURGEONS
"There is no systematic institutional strategy for dealing with stress. "
"High-risk/high reliability industries have introduced stress and crisis-management training to prepare junior trainees to respond effectively and efficiently to on the job stressors." [Arora]

In a 2009 Australian survey, surgeons were asked about particular needs of a crisis training course and they reported the following:

☐ *"The whole persona of a surgeon is somebody who can make quick decisions and cope with anything. Except when things go wrong.... then that same person can't think straight makes mistakes and loses all judgment; everything descends into chaos and patient care is seriously compromised because he just crumbles under stress."*

☐ *"Surgery is a stressful environment. Yet the surgical community seldom acknowledges the stress associated with carrying out surgical procedures, possibly because emphasis on leadership and self-confidence is so high that stress is often perceived as a sign of weakness or failure. There is no systematic institutional strategy for dealing with stress. Consequentially, inexperienced trainers are not explicitly taught how to manage these intraoperative stressors when they occur and learn to cope only through observing their seniors manage similar scenarios or from making their own mistakes."*

☐ *"There is clear evidence that excessive levels of stress have a deleterious effect on performance. As a result, high-risk/high reliability industries have introduced stress and crisis-management training to prepare junior trainees to respond effectively and efficiently to on-the-job stressors."* [Arora]

Additionally, in this 2009 Australian survey, surgeons were asked to describe the coping strategies they employed during a crisis. The survey reflected that surgeons in general have a minimalistic understanding of the various processes involved in preparation for and surviving as a team during a disaster. The expressed vague ideas as to how they prepared and reacted during these situations, but unlike other high-pressured fields, a clear organized process was evidently lacking for surgeons. [Arora]

In a survey of surgical faculty and senior general surgery residents from a single academic center, 96% percent of the surgeons felt confident and would expect to be successful during a crisis situation. While 60% stated they did not find these situations particularly stressful, 40% did. [Wiggins] This was a self-assessment and others have warned about *"optimist bias,"* the well-known attribute of clinicians, in which most individual members of a group view and report their abilities as *better than the average* (also known as Dunning-Kruger effect). [Thomas, Sexton Helmriech, et al, Makary, sexton Freischlag]

An additional dangerous phenomenon is the ability of individuals to rely on their more experienced partner's or superior's ability to handle crises from past experience. These individuals are unlikely to be motivated to spend any time or effort on training. [Runciman]

I asked an experienced surgeon if and why we should attempt to discuss OR crisis management with experienced surgeons and his response was *"b/c the experienced practicing surgeon, has established a flow and sequence that makes it even more rare for these events...in essence makes that MD the LEAST experienced/practiced @ managing that French scenario: "cluesterfuque"!!!! ☻"*

ME TO INTERN: *"so can you think of any time you have had to deal with an unexpected crisis situation?" Intern "well I am an intern so I just call for help". Me "So you never had to work by yourself when a patient was crashing?" Intern "actually we just finished an ablation of an anal condyloma and the patient was in PACU when he suddenly began to cough up blood. It was just me and a nurse, the attending was elsewhere. It was pretty hairy. We intubated him and then others came to help."*

WE DON'T NEED LEADERSHIP TRAINING"!

Recent information regarding physician overconfidence and healthcare professional lack of attentiveness and acceptance of deviance as the normality (highlighted in the box below) is even more alarming

PHYSICIANS APPEAR OVERCONFIDENT IN THEIR PERSONAL LEADERSHIP SKILLS.

- In a large recent simulation study using close to 50 residents during Interdisciplinary Emergent Clinical Scenarios, 75 % felt that the difference between a good and excellent resident was his /her teamwork and team management.
- Study showed significant improvement in leadership skills over the course of the academic year (PGY1 and 2).
- *BUT ONLY 51%* felt the course improved their personal teamwork skills and **42.9%** felt it improved their communication skills (that is, 47.1% felt they were fine to begin with) which is consistent with the Dunning-Kruger effect as seen in most other team training exercises whereby respondents believe their capabiliites supercede their teammates when it comes to teamwork skills.

Nikasa, Stewart with permission Thomas, Sexton, Helmriech.

- 2006 review of 17 papers in the US, Canada, Australia, NZ and UK
- Concluded that physicians have a <u>limited ability to accurately self-assess</u> and that the current processes used to evaluate competence requires more focus on external assessment. Davis et all

"IF ALL ELSE FAILS, I HAVE PLENTY OF SAFETY NETS AROUND ME TO SAVE ME! ....RIGHT??"

CAN WE EMPHATICALLY TRUST THOSE AROUND US?

DO WE HAVE SAFETY NETS?
HEALTHCARE PROFESSIONAL LACK OF ATTENTIVENESS
AND ACCEPTANCE OF DEVIANCE AS THE NORMALITY

- Healthcare staff are frequently inattentive even in the midst of critical phases in events.

"videotaping the OR environment revealed how often individuals were not paying attention, despite their impression otherwise." This attitude appeared to have occurred during critical event phases as well. Bowermaster R, Eghtesady P,

"Egregious violations of standards of practice become normalized in healthcare delivery systems" Banja J,
The Normalization of deviance in Healthcare. With permission

WHEN THE CALL TO LEAD PROVES SUCCCESSFUL:

"As a resident we had a call from the Emergency Room to see an obese patient who had severe abdomen pain and a pulsatile abdominal mass. I entered the room and he was profoundly hypertensive and indeed had a massive pulsatile abdominal mass. I called the attending to tell him this man had a ruptured aneurysm. Before he called us back, the patient's blood pressure rapidly began to fall. The attending finally talked with me and demanded a CT scan. The CT confirmed he had a ruptured aneurysm. After calling the operating room first, I called the attending and told him we were going straight to the operating room. By the time we got into the room, the patient was doing very poorly (he had a barely palpable pulse). I told the staff that we could not wait for the attending and that we had to prep and drape the patient. After looking at me like I was crazy, we did so. The patient's pressure continued to fall and I asked anesthesia if they had blood ready. They confirmed we had blood available so I asked that they induce the patient. I told the nurse to have an aortic compression device ready to go and to hand me a scalpel. As expected, as soon as they induced him, he immediately dropped his blood pressure to just barely palpable (still had a normal rhythm on the monitor though). We opened the patient and I reached up blindly and grabbed his aorta under the diaphragm. I told anesthesia to rescue him and that I could not hold the aorta for too long. By the time the attending arrived, everyone yelled "GO SCRUB!" The patient lived."

For interviews with Carol Moulton on Comfort zones and risk-taking see "Comfort zones and risk taking in surgery" see Appendix C page 184

*For interview with Daniel Kuhn regarding **TRAUMA DECONDITIONING** and its effect oon surgeon post-traumatic stress syndrome secondary to a significant untoward professional or personal event, see "Surgeon Resiliency, Risk Aversion and Performance Concerns" See appendix C Page 185*

WHAT FACTORS MAKE RESPONSE TO A CRISIS CHALLENGING AND WHY ARE WE FREQUENTLY INEFFECTIVE?

Ask a batter to describe in detail about that moment he is standing there at home plate watching the ball clear the fence, just how he knew that was a home run…. the response likely is **"I felt it!"** Some experiences are just too difficult for a professional to describe in detail. The same is very true in the medical profession; it is extremely difficult for successful leaders in medicine to tell exactly how they survive difficult situations. As was noted above, in many cases their self-proclaimed stoic performance may actually have been less decisive than they described. **This guide is an attempt to demystify this process.**

FACTORS PRESENT DURING CRISES WHICH MAKE RESPONSES MORE CHALLENGING		
PRESENCE OF NON-SPECIFIC SIGNS INITIALLY: • **Blood pressure change** • **Pulse Oximetry change** • **Increase in ETCO$_2$**	THE LACK OF SKILLED ASSISTANCE AVAILABLE DURING THE NECESSARY TIME FRAME.	PARTICULAR SET OF CIRCUMSTANCES MAY NEVER HAVE BEEN ENCOUNTERED BEFORE.
<u>RECENTLY INTRODUCED VARIABLES BRING ON UNFORSEEN CONSEQUENCES:</u> • **Processes** • **Staff** • **Equipment**	• INTERACTION OF MULTIPLE COMPLEX ISSUES • LAYERS OF COMPLEXITY ADDED AS PROBLEMS ARISE.	THE NEED TO RESOLVE FACTORS FASTER THAN THE TEAM IS CABABLE OF COMPREHENDING WHAT THE SITUATION IS.
FACTORS RELATING TO INEFFECTIVE PROVIDER RESPONSE DURING A CRISIS		
<u>TRAINED RESPONSE FOR CLINICIANS:</u> ➤ SEARCH FOR MORE COMMON PROBLEMS AND SOLUTIONS. ➤ FOCUS AWAY FROM THE UNUSUAL.	<u>RULE-BASED COGNITIVE REASONING</u> TYPICALLY RESULTS IN USING UP APPLICABLE RULES OR APPLYING THE WRONG PRINCIPLE. (*)	USE OF <u>KNOWLEDGE-BASED DELIBERATIVE REASONING</u> TYPICALLY ENDS UP SLOWER THAN IS ACCEPTABLE FOR THESE SCENARIOS.
CONFIRMATION BIASES AND FIXATION ERRORS ARE RAMPANT.	ANXIETY DEGRADES PERFORMANCE.	MULTICIPLICITY OF TASKS NEEDED SIMULTANEOUSLY DEGRADES PERFORMANCE.
Runciman		

Runciman's group identified that when complex life-threatening crises happen the team is required to rely upon cognitive tasking above and beyond the information processing capacity of the human brain. In their trial 1/8 of the providers were not able to use their checklist effectively. Their work highlighted the facts that **a)** *experience does not prevent failure*, and **b)** *even senior providers make mistakes during crises.* Their conclusion was that in more than *HALF* of the crises, *the signs were non-specific* and *did not result in a rapid conclusion in the cause.* Runciman

SIMILARITIES AND DIFFERENCES BETWEEN AVIATION, THE O.R. AND FIRE-FIGHTING

We are often told that team dynamics in aviation and medicine are strikingly similar and that, therefore, safety principles from the cockpit should be fully integrated into patient safety initiatives. Indeed, the parallels are compelling: both fields operate in high-stakes environments where teamwork, communication, and precision are essential. Consequently, aviation-derived tools such as checklists and team training have successfully translated into healthcare and have markedly improved patient safety.

However, several key differences limit the complete transferability of these models. When patient care proceeds along expected pathways, checklists—much like those used in aviation—work exceptionally well to ensure consistency and reduce the risk of error. Yet that benefit can diminish rapidly once a crisis emerges and uncertainty replaces predictability.

Pilots, for example, are trained to rely on checklists even during emergencies, as demonstrated by Captain Chesley "Sully" Sullenberger during the 2009 US Airways Flight 1549 incident. In the moments following a double engine failure caused by a bird strike, Sullenberger and co-pilot Jeff Skiles methodically worked through several emergency procedures. However, when none of the listed solutions resolved the problem, they were forced to rely on judgment, intuition, and experience. Within three minutes, Sullenberger made the fateful decision to land in the Hudson River rather than attempt a return to LaGuardia Airport—a decision that ultimately saved all 155 lives aboard. ^(Sweeney PJ, Matthews MD, Lester PB)

This example highlights a crucial truth: **checklists provide a foundation, but leadership, situational awareness, and adaptive decision-making determine survival when no checklist fits the situation.**

Medicine mirrors aviation in this respect, but with an important distinction—the human body is far more variable than any aircraft. Principles that apply to one patient may not apply to another. Moreover, pilots rarely choose to fly into hurricanes, while surgeons routinely operate on patients with known high risks and the potential for crisis. Checklists remain highly effective once the problem is identified and the team understands the relevant factors. The challenge lies in the period of ambiguity—when the cause of deterioration is unclear and cognitive overload threatens to paralyze the team. In these moments, **effective leadership** is vital to guide the group through confusion and maladaptive responses toward decisive, coordinated action.

Similar patterns are seen in the fire service, where teams operate under extreme uncertainty and must constantly adapt to rapidly evolving conditions. Fires—like human physiology—are inherently unpredictable. ^{Cooper, Henrickson, Helmreich, Okray, CRM fire service, CRM coast guard, Chopra, Kumar, McDonald, Helmreich} While the majority of aviation events can be managed through adherence to protocol and structured teamwork, true crises demand leadership and cognitive flexibility beyond routine procedures.

Thus, both aviation and healthcare share the same paradox: *STRUCTURED SYSTEMS PREVENT MOST ERRORS, BUT SURVIVAL IN CRISIS DEPENDS ON HUMAN JUDGMENT.* Spontaneous, life-threatening events are rare in both fields, yet when they do occur, success depends less on the presence of a checklist and more on the presence of individuals capable of leading decisively under pressure.

SIMILARITIES - DIFFERENCES IN COCKPITS & OR'S

	COCKPIT	OPERATING ROOM *
SOP'S, RULES AND REGULATIONS	Clear rules and regulations, by SOP's, checklists and manual.	SOP's and checklists in early stages, not accepted and remain variable. Checklists more beneficial in <u>human-machine</u> interfaces, than human-human.
TEAM SIZE	Small team -same organization. Training is consistent. Team stays during mission.	Team construct changes constantly. Not all members work for same employer directly.
INTERACTION WITH OTHER GROUPS	Primary workplace is clearly defined and isolated.	Many subgroups-more fluid and dynamic- without formalized control.
LINES OF AUTHORITY	Clear lines of authority. Captain - ultimate responsibility for decisions and conduct of flight.	Lines of authority with in subgroups, but not overall. Lack of commanding authority invites conflict.
TRAINING, RESEARCH AND INFORMATION SHARING	Shared concern with safety. Organizations open to research to decrease accidents. Archival data available. Regular training in simulators required.	Field is driven by fear of litigation should evidence of substandard practice be revealed. No corporate willingness to share data. Psychological training seen in pilots is rare in medicine.
COMPLEXITY	Opportunities for variation in weather, air-traffic, mechanical problems, require variety of decision-making processes and prioritization among alternatives.	Much more complex environment psychologically than the cockpit.
HUMAN ERROR AS A CAUSE OF ACCIDENTS	1970's research indicates that 70% of crashes are due to human error.	Much more recent data indicates that 75-80% of medical errors are due to human error.

*Same may be true in most other areas of your health-care facility. Cooper, Henrickson, Helmreich, Chopra, Kumar, McDonald, Helmreich

---

"Flying an aircraft is a lot easier than taking out the head of the pancreas. Even in the midst of a crisis, checklists are effective. Captain Sullenberger and Jeff Skiles followed their checklists even to the last second before landing in the Hudson. Checklists are not ingrained in stone and need modifications. They should be concise and easy to use. If they are not working for you, then make them easy to use. They are meant to conform and not restrain."

Richard Karl; retired Chair Dept Surgery USF Tampa; founding medical director of Moffitt Cancer Center; author of the book Across the Red Line: Stories from the Surgical Life. *PERSONAL* COMMUNICATION with permission

Question for LD Britt - is it a misnomer to say we desire an aviation high reliability organization (hro) model in medicine? *"we may not be hitting a home run BUT we need to build upon these results. We need to embrace this and move on! This requires a multidisciplinary attack. Team training is just one of the components. You cannot minimize these results. I know Richard Karl well. So, if he says medicine cannot function in an entirely aviation-based model, you better believe it. He is a pilot, so he should know. I said it before, AVIATION IS NOT THE SAME AS MEDICINE. Medicine is much more complex. Aviation typically has a relatively stable environment when planes are operational. You get a weather report and it changes infrequently. In aviation, you don't have to worry about comorbidities or typically worry about secondary changes. There is no parallel to what we have in medicine. There are always unknowns in medicine. We are just beating ourselves too much over this. We need to move on and build a new model for this new healthcare world. "* Lipshy KA. Britt LD. Bull Am Coll Surg. 2017 Feb;102(2):22-29. With permission from LD Britt

---

PONENTIALLY, AND BY THE TIME YOU RECOGNIZE SOMETHING BAD HAS HAPPENED, YOU ARE DEAD!" Thomas Lubanau II BS; Retired Wyoming Fire Chief; Co-Author *Crew Resource Management for the Fire Service*- PERSONAL COMMUNICATION w/ permission, T. Lubanau.

RESLIENCE: WHAT CAN WE LEARN FROM OTHER HIGH RISK - HIGH RELIABILITY ORGANIZATIONS?

Much of what we know regarding patient safety and crisis management stems from work in other high risk / High Reliability Organizations (HRO).

For instance, have you ever wondered how an aircraft carrier becomes resilient to fatal errors? In a high-risk environment where accidents are considered "normal" (Perrow), it is remarkable that fatal accidents are not more prevalent. HRO's focus on avoiding catastrophic failures – those that could cripple the organization – while functioning at a very high capacity / productivity. (LaPorte, TR, Consolini, PM.) The concept of "High Reliability Organizations" began at the University of California (Todd LaPorte, Gene I Rochlin, Berkley CA) in the 1970's via a joint meeting with PG&E (the largest electrical utilities provider in the country), air traffic control and Rear Admiral Carl Mercer (commander of the USS Carl Vinson) (Rochlin).

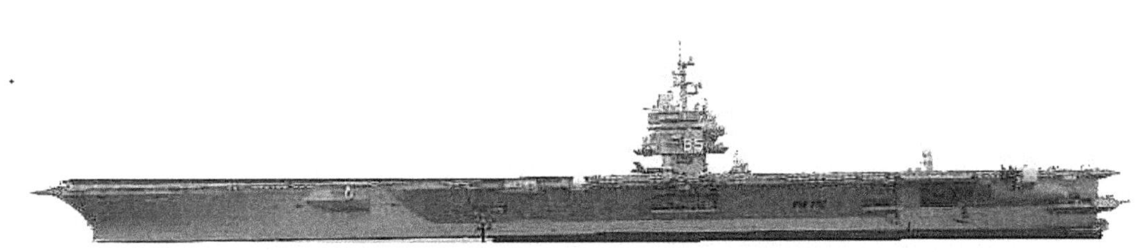

HRO's reduce the likelihood of a serious "fatal" accident via five key principles:
PREOCCUPATION WITH FAILURE!
RELUCTANCE TO SIMPLIFY!
SENSITIVITY TO OPERATIONS!
COMMITMENT TO RESILIENCE!
DEFERENCE TO EXPERTISE!
Wiley; 2007. Photo: Lipshy KA. USS Enterprise in the James River April, 2010.

Aircraft carriers operate in a continued state of readiness and safety, utilizing a crew composed of men and women virtually all less than 20 years of age. The success of these large ships in remaining safe, hinges upon the command's preoccupation with resilience. Leadership is engaged in the constant thinking about potential failure, taking nothing for granted, sensitivity to all levels of operation, and commitment to being resilient. Part of focusing on failure includes constant assessment and rehearsal for those almost never but potentially catastrophic events. Weick

...it is a sign of a great leader who accepts and prepares for the worst-case scenario rather than hoping to avoid a crisis... Thomas Kolditz *PERSONAL* COMMUNICATION

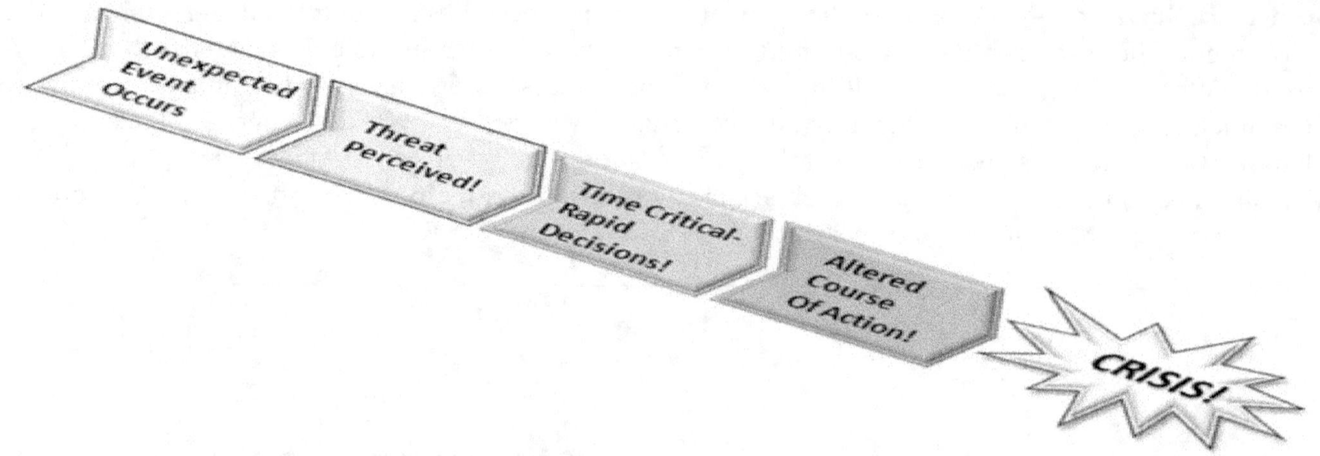

THE FOUR ELEMENTS OF A CRISIS

A critical event (accident, error, or other surprise) may be followed crisis evolution if its unexpected, poses a perceived threat, requires rapid time critical decision making and an alteration of course. Seeger, Venette, Lipshy

One thing is certain: what constitutes a routine day for fire chiefs, police commanders, or special forces officers would likely qualify as a crisis for most healthcare professionals. For these high-risk professionals, such events are part of their operational environment and are often managed without disruption. However, for healthcare providers, situations such as structural fires, mass casualties, or active shooter incidents are unexpected and immediately perceived as threats.

The Four Elements of a Crisis

For an event to evolve into a true *crisis*, four key elements are generally present:

1. **Surprise — the unexpected event.**
   A crisis begins when a team is suddenly confronted with an unanticipated and unfamiliar situation. Most often, the team had been functioning under routine expectations that operations would continue normally. When this unfamiliar event occurs, it disrupts that sense of predictability. The initial response of many leaders is often *minimization* or *denial*, particularly when they are already cognitively or physically engaged in another demanding task. As will be discussed later, successful navigation through this phase requires that someone within the team acknowledges that a significant event has occurred. Recognition is the first critical step toward resolution.

2. **Threat to the organization, team, or mission.**
   In healthcare, the mission is clear: to help patients recover as quickly and safely as possible, ensuring no additional harm is done. During a crisis, this mission is suddenly and visibly jeopardized. The threat manifests as a gap between the *desired state* (a stable, safe patient) and the *current reality* (an unstable, deteriorating situation). The perceived severity of the crisis is directly related to the potential loss — whether to the patient, the team, or the organization's mission.

3. **Time-critical, high-pressure decision-making.**
   By definition, a crisis compresses time. Decisions must be made rapidly to prevent harm. Yet, this same urgency can paradoxically slow or distort performance. Time pressure often induces *decisional paralysis* — an inability to act — or, conversely, impetuous action without sufficient data or analysis. This compression of time makes crisis decision-making especially vulnerable to *cognitive error*, as will be discussed in later sections.

4. **Transformation — the need for change.**
   A crisis demands adaptation. If no change occurs — if the team persists in its usual processes and routines — failure is almost inevitable. Typically, the baseline system becomes overwhelmed: there

are too many variables, too much information, too few resources, and too little time. Success requires transformation—modifying strategies, reallocating tasks, and reimagining the approach to meet the demands of the new reality. Seeger, Venette, Hermann

Any event that is **unexpected**, **threatens the mission**, **compresses decision time**, and **requires transformation** qualifies as a *crisis*. Importantly, what constitutes a crisis for one individual or team may not be a crisis for another. Perception is context-dependent—defined not by the event itself, but by the preparedness, resilience, and adaptability of those who face it.

<table>
<tr><td>

CRITICAL MOMENTS IN BATTLE

What determines if something is a crisis for your team absolutely depends on if that event is a threat to you or your mission and whether you now have to make rapid critical decisions to make a complete change in your original intent.

It is extremely difficult to find examples of this in combat literature. Having said that, one of the best descriptions of an unexpected military crisis is depicted in Marcus Luttrell's real-life memoir, Lone Survivor. His SEAL team finds themselves discovered by locals in hostile terrain (environmentally and militarily). They rapidly come to grips that they must abort their mission and change plans. They have no communication to the outside world and must rely on their existing team infrastructure for decision making processes. As a group they go through their options one by one. The chief does not give his opinion until he has heard from everyone. The Chief explains things as he sees it, then he takes a vote, making a life altering decision. He risks the lives of his SEAL team to spare three Afghan villagers who do not show any appreciation for that act of kindness. In spite of the lethality of the decision, and the hindsight that they made a grave mistake, no one faults their leader. In spite of the fear that grows inside them, no one alters their support of their leader and instead they back up his decision. Marcus Luttrell Lone Survivor

</td></tr>
</table>

Health-care crises are typically patient related. That is, something in the patient's structure or physiology goes awry and the team is expected to respond appropriately. Other times, various unexpected obstacles intervene, shifting a routine health-related treatment pattern to an alternate course of action that can spiral out of control quickly. These events are usually internal to the organization but certainly events unrelated to the health-care center can occur (fire, earthquake, flood, tornado, hurricane, power outage, gunmen, to name a few).

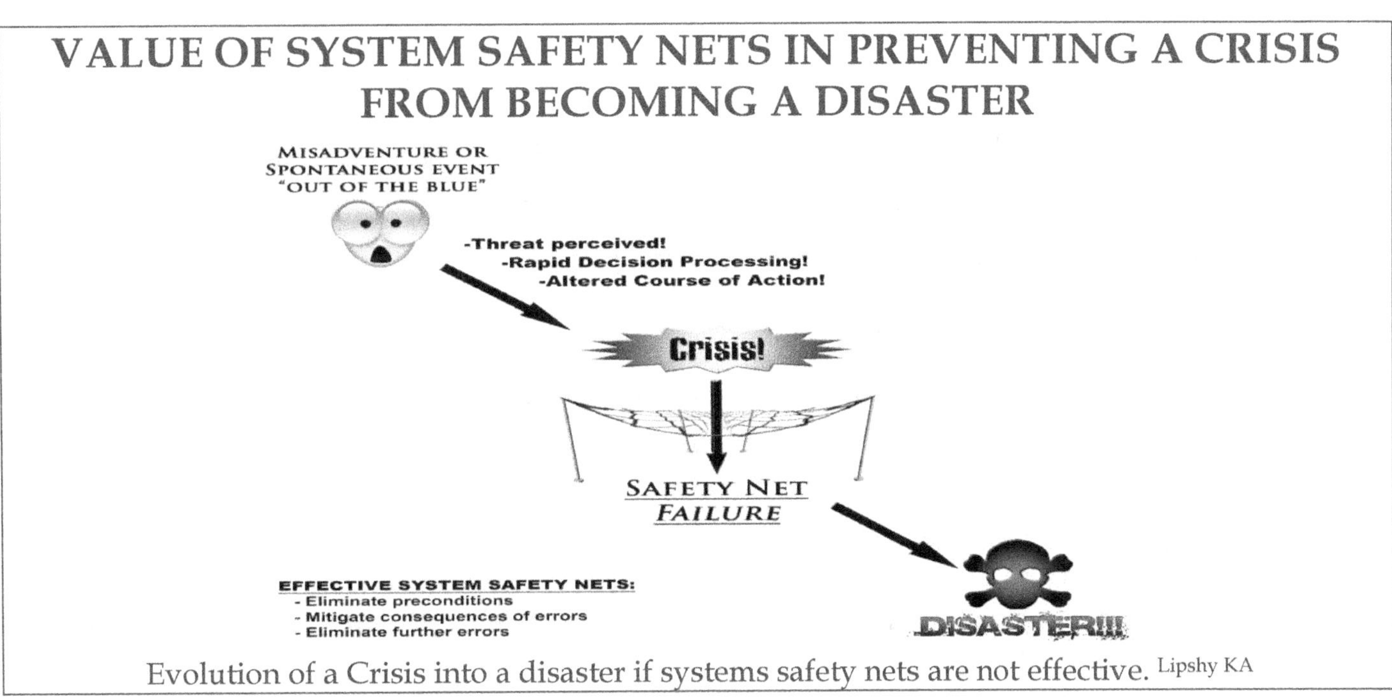

Evolution of a Crisis into a disaster if systems safety nets are not effective. Lipshy KA

Unexpected cognitive errors or spontaneous events from "out-of-the-blue" can rapidly transform a crisis situation into a disaster when pre-existing conditions, imperfect system safety nets, and further errors prevent mitigation at a salvageable state. The time to learn these lessons is *before* they happen. Failure to do so sets your team up for failure.

COMMON ORIGINS OF CRISES:

1. Incremental evolution of smaller adverse events

2. Missing the warning signs of an impending problem

3. Unexpected sudden change in patient condition due to something someone on the team did or inherent patient problem, or equipment/product problem or reaction.

CRISES ARE UNEXPECTED BECAUSE:

1. Something that was supposed to happen didn't.

2. Something that was not supposed to happen did. [Gaba]

> Sometimes you make it through a crisis and survive, but that does not necessarily mean that it all went all that well. Often times in retrospect, when we look back, we were one step away from failure and were just damn lucky we pulled through.

> *".. as we know, there are known knowns; there are things we know we know. We also know there are known unknowns; that is to say we know there are some things we do not know. But there are also unknown unknowns – the ones we don't know we don't know. And if one looks throughout the history of our country and other free countries, it is the latter category that tend to be the difficult ones. "*
> US Sec. of Defense Donald Rumsfeld at a U.S. (DoD news briefing on February 12, 2002

TWO TRAINING CRISIS MANAGEMENT TRAINING CAMPS:

There are potentially two ways to teach crisis management:

1. "MacGyver" Mindset*: Try to improve a person's skill at responding to difficult situations by effecting generalized cognitive enhancement (see section on fluid intelligence for more on this subject); or

2. Improve a person's response to a given situation by presenting him or her with a variant of that specific situation in training before he or she encounters it as a real-world event.

Medical, military and first responder training are typically designed to follow the second pattern.

CAPT Frank K. Butler, Jr., MC USN **Retired** Platoon commander Navy Underwater Demolition and SEAL teams. Lt Col Dave Grosman 'On Combat'

WHY TRAIN?

- Experience is typically the best form of training but life-like simulation is a close second.
- Simulation training affords the opportunity for trainees to experience life-like experiences with the emotional demands they are likely to encounter thereby preparing them with appropriate coping strategies. [Okray]

POTENTIAL TRAINING SCENARIO PITFALLS:

- While constant training and scenarios are important, you can never tell for certain how future incidents will pan out.
- Professionals should be aware that our instinctual responses to perform under pressure will result in our reacting in the same manner we were trained- so be careful how you train. If training is centered around specific details and events, and not on elimination of rigid / inflexible thinking, then the trainee's attitude becomes rigid and inflexible when they encounter situations and they are not able to adapt to a new unfamiliar scenario.
- We have ingrained our responses to specific situations and only learn to use those responses in all situations we face and that response may not only be non-ideal, but could be deadly.
- We must be able to think for ourselves and say: "STOP! This does not apply to this situation. Things have changed too much and they no longer fit. We cannot depend on our prior ingrained responses and must reassess the situation and develop a plan that fits". Ingrained habitual responses can be deadly when the action is applied to the wrong circumstance (read Rorke Denver's book for deadly examples). [Okray]

TRAINING ADAPTIVE TEAMS:

- Tactical Decision Making Under Stress (TADMUS) programs have shown that teams that perform the best under stressful situations are those that adapt their decision-making strategies, coordination strategies and their structure when faced with escalating workload and stress.
- <u>**Adaptive teams are high performers and adaptability is trainable.**</u>
- The team must all have a common mental model of the situation. This requires sharing of information constantly by the leader.
- The team must have a common language of communication.
- The team must develop anticipatory behavior.
- The highest likelihood of developing an adaptable team that performs effectively under stress occurs through assuring that the team trains together under similar conditions.

It is unlikely that a team that has not perfected their ability to perform seamlessly under normal conditions will perform effectively in a crisis. Klein G; Collyer S; Serfaty D; Lipshitz R;

CHAPTER I. INTRODUCTION REFERENCES

- Arora S, Sevdalis N, Nestel D, et al. The impact of stress on surgical performance: a systematic review of the literature. *Surgery.* 2010;147:318–330.
- Ashcroft DM, Morecrof C, Parker D, Noyce PR. Safety culture assessment in community pharmacy: development, face validity and feasibility of the Manchester Patients Safety Assessment Framework. *Qual Saf Health Care.* 2005;14(6):417-21.
- Banja J. The normalization of deviance in healthcare delivery. *Bus Horiz.* 2010 ; 53(2): 139.
- Bowermaster R, Miller M, Ashcraft T, Boyd M, Brar A, Manning P, Eghtesady P. Application of the Aviation Black Box Principle in Pediatric Cardiac Surgery: Tracking All Failures in the Pediatric Cardiac Operating Room. *J Am Coll Surg* 2015;220:149-155.
- Chopra V, Bovill JG, Spierdjk J, Koornneef F. Reported significant observations during anesthesia: a prospective analysis over an 18 year period. *Br J Anaesth.* 1992;68:13-17.
- Clifton BS, Hotten WIT. Deaths associated with anesthesia. Br J Anaesth. 1963:35:250-259.
- Collyer S, Malecki G. *Tactical decision Making under stress: history and overview* in Cannon-Bower J and Salas E. Making Decisions under stress APA 1998.
- Conley DM, Singer SJ, Edmondson L, Berry WR, Gawande AA. Effective Surgical Safety Checklist Implementation. Journal of the American College of Surgeons. 2011; 212(5):873–879.
- Cooper GE, White MD, Lauber JK. Resource management on the flightdeck: proceedings of a NASA/ industry workshop. In: *NASA Conference Publication No. CP-2120.* San Francisco, CA: NASA - Ames Research Center; 1980.
- Cooper JB, Newbower RS, Long CD, McPeek B. Preventable anesthesia mishaps: a study of human factors. Anesthesiology. 1978;49(6):399-406.
- Davis D, Mazmanian P, Fordis M, Van Harrison R, Thorpe KE, Math M; Perrier L. Accuracy of Physician Self-assessment Compared With Observed Measures of Competence A Systematic Review. *JAMA.* 2006;296(9):1094-1102.
- Diehl, A. *"Does cockpit management training reduce aircrew error?"* Proceedings of the Twenty-Second International Seminar of the International Society Of Air Safety Investigators. Canberra, Australia. November 4-7, 1991. *ISASI Forum.*1991;24(4):46.
- Dripps RD, Lamont A, Eckenhoff JE. The role of anesthesia in surgical mortality. JAMA. 1961;178(3):261-266.
- Edwards G, Morton HJV, Pask EA, Wylie WD. Deaths associated with anesthesia: report on 1000 cases. Anaesthesia . 1956;11:194-220.
- Gaba DM, Fish KJ, Howard SK. *Crisis Management in Anesthesiology.* New York, NY: Churchill Livingstone; 1994.
- Gonzales L. *Deep Survival: Who Lives, Who Dies and Why.* New York, NY: WW Norton; 2003
- The survival list: 101 skills guaranteed to get you out of trouble fast. Backpacker Oct 2006;34(244:8):45-53.
- Henrickson SE, Wadhera RK, El Bardissi AW, Wiegmann DA, Sundt TM. Development and pilot evaluation of a preoperative briefing protocol for cardiovascular surgery. *J Am Coll Surg.* 2009;208:1115-1123.
- Helmreich RL, Ashleigh CM, Wilhelm JA. Evolution of CRM training in commercial aviation. *Int J Aviati Psychol.* 1999;9(1):19-32.
- Helmreich RL, Merritt AC. *Culture at Work in Aviation and Medicine.* Aldershot, UK: Ashgate Press; 1998.
- Helmreich RL, Schaefer HG; Team performance in the operating room. In: Bogner MS ed. *Human Error in Medicine.* Hillside, NJ: Lawrence Erlbaum; 1994.
- Institute of Medicine, Committee on Quality Health Care in America. Crossing the Quality Chasm: A new health system for the 21st century. Committee on quality of health care in America. Washington, D.C.: National Academies Press; 2001.
- Klein G. The sources of power, how people make decisions. Cambridge: MIT Press, 1999.
- Klein G. Naturalistic Decision Making. Human Factors: The Journal of the Human Factors and Ergonomics Society. **2008;**50(3):**456-460.**
- **Klein G, Pliske R, Crandall B, Woods DD. Problem Detection. Cogn Tech Work. 2005;7:14-28.**
- Kumar MM, Fish KJ. Anaesthesia crisis resource management training: an intimidating concept, a rewarding experience. *Can J Anaesth.* 1996;43:430-434.
- LaPorte, TR, Consolini, PM. Working in Practice but not in theory: theoretical challenges of "high reliability organizations'. Journal of Public administration research and theory: J-PART 1991 1(1)19-48.
- La Porte, Todd R. "High reliability organizations: Unlikely, demanding and at risk." Journal of contingencies and crisis management 4, no. 2 (1996): 60-71.
- Lipshitz R, Shaul OB. *Schemata and mental models in recognition-primed decision making.* In Zsambok, C. E. & Klein, G., Naturalistic Decision Making. Mahwah. NJ. Lawrence Erlbaum Associates, 1997. 293-304.
- Lipshy KA. Britt LD. How do we improve patient safety? A look at the issues and an interview with Dr. Britt. Bull Am Coll Surg. 2017 Feb;102(2):22-29.

- Luttrel, Marcus *Lone Survivor: The Eyewitness Account of Operation Redwing and the Lost Heroes of SEAL Team 10* (June 2006) Little, Brown and Company
- Makary MA, Sexton JB, Freischlag JA, et al. Operating room teamwork among physicians and nurses: teamwork in the eye of the beholder. *J Am Coll Surg*. 2006; 202:746–752.
- McDonald JS, Peterson S. Lethal errors in anesthesiology. *Anesthesiology*. 1985;63:A497.
- Nicksa G, Anderson C, Fidler R, Stewart L. Innovative Approach Using Interprofessional Simulation to Educate Surgical Residents in Technical and Nontechnical Skills in High-Risk Clinical Scenarios. *JAMA Surg*. 2015;150(3):201-207.
- Perrow, C. Normal Accidents: Living with high risk technologies. Princeton University Press. Princeton NJ 1999.
- Pizzi L, Goldfarb NI, Nash DB, Crew resource management and its applications in medicine. In: Shojania KG, Duncan BW, McDonald KM, Wachter RM, Markowitz AJ eds. *Making Health Care Safer: A Critical Analysis of Patient Safety Practices: Evidence Reports/Technology Assessments, No. 43*. Rockville, MD: Agency for Healthcare Research and Quality; 2001. http://www.ncbi.nlm.nih.gov/books/NBK26999. Accessed December 12, 2012.
- Rochlin GI, LaPorte TR, and Roberts KH. 'The Self-Designing High-Reliability Organization: Aircraft Carrier Flight Operations at Sea', Naval War College Review, 1987 40(4):76–90.
- Rochlin, GI. How to hunt a very reliable organization. Journal of contingencies and crisis management. 2011. 19(1): 14-20.
- Runciman WB, Webb RK, Klepper ID, Lee R, Williamson JA, Barker L. The Australian incident monitoring study: crisis management: validation of an algorithm by analysis of 2000 incident reports. *Anaesthia Intensive Care*. 1993;21:579-592
- Runciman WB, Merry AF. Crises in clinical care: an approach to management. *Qual Saf Health Care*. 2005;14(3):156-163.
- Okray R, Lubnau T. *Crew Resource Management for the Fire Service*. Tulsa, OK: PennWell Press; 2004.
- Schulman, Paul R. "Problems in the organization of organization theory: an essay in honour of Todd LaPorte." Journal of contingencies and crisis management 19, no. 1 (2011): 43-50.
- Serfaty D, Entin E, J Johnston J. *Team coordination training* in Cannon-Bowers J and Salas E. Making Decisions Under Stress APA 1998. P 222.
- Sexton JB, Thomas EJ, Helmrriech RL. Error, stress, and teamwork in medicine and aviation: cross sectional surveys. *BMJ*. March 2000;320(7237):745–749.
- Thomas EJ, Sexton JB, Helmreich RL. Discrepant attitudes about teamwork among critical care nurses and physicians. *Crit Care Med*. 2003;31(3):956–959.
- Sweeney PJ, Matthews MD, Lester PB. *Leadership in Dangerous Situations*. Annapolis, MD: Naval Institute Press; 2011.
- Weick KE, Sutcliffe KM. Managing the unexpected: resilient performance in an age of uncertainty. San Francisco CA: John Wiley; 2007.
- Webb RK, Currie M, Morgan CA, et al. The Australian incident monitoring study: an analysis of 2000 incident reports. *Anaesthia and Intensive Care*. 1993;21:520-528
- Wiggins-Dohlvik K, Stewart RM, Babbitt RJ, Gelfond J, Zarzabal LA, Willis RE. Surgeons' performance during critical situations: competence, confidence, and composure. *Am J Surg*. 2009;198(6):817-823.

II. LEADERSHIP 101: LEADERSHIP IN THE 21st CENTURY. BASIC LEADERSHIP SKILLSETS TO SURVIVE IN A NEW ERA.

A. Introduction
1. Definitions, Roles and Responsibilities. What is leadership?
2. Why bother with leadership training?
3. What was the stereotypic leadership of the 19th-20th century?
4. Times have changed! Why?

B. NEW SKILLS: What new skillsets do modern leaders need to possess?
1. What is the role of the team leader in this new era of leadership?
2. What command structure works best in this new era of leadership?
3. **TRUST!** What modern leaders require to maintain a successful decentralized command!
4. Building morale and gaining influence.
5. How does one know if they have reached the point that they are a successful leader?

C. Putting it all together

OBJECTIVES. LEADERSHIP 101:
FOUNDATIONS IN BASIC LEADERSHIP SKILLS TO SURVIVE IN THE NEW ERA

A. INTRODUCTION
1. DISCUSS THE REAL MEANING OF LEADERSHIP.
2. DISCUSS WHY WE SHOULD BOTHER WITH LEADERSHIP TRAINING.

3. DISCUSS THE DIFFERENCE IN LEADERSHIP IN THE 19TH-20TH CENTURY AND NOW AND WHY THIS HAS CHANGED

B. NEW SKILLS: WHAT NEW SKILLSETS DO MODERN LEADERS NEED TO POSSESS?
1. DISCUSS THE ROLE OF THE TEAM LEADER IN THIS NEW ERA OF LEADERSHIP?
2. DISCUSS THE COMMAND STRUCTURE WORKS BEST IN THIS NEW ERA OF LEADERSHIP?
3. DISCUSS THE KEY FACTOR FOR MODERN LEADERS TO MAINTAIN A SUCCESSFUL DECENTRALIZED COMMAND?
4. DISCUSS TRUST! WHAT IS TRUST AND HOW DO WE GAIN IT?
5. DISCUSS HOW ONE BUILDS MORALE AND GAINS INFLUENCE
6. RESILIENCY: LEADING IN THE MIDST OF CRISIS AND SURVIVING THROUGH FAILURE-
7. TIME MANAGEMENT FOR LEADERS-
8. DISCUSS HOW ONE KNOWS IF THEY HAVE REACHED THE POINT THAT THEY ARE A SUCCESSFUL LEADER

There's an African proverb that says, "If you want to go fast, go alone. If you want to go far, go together"

A. INTRODUCTION: Why Do We Need Leadership Training if We Are "Natural Leaders"?

While many organizations offer leadership programs tailored to their operational environments, most focus narrowly on *task-specific* or *administrative* competencies rather than the broader, human-centered skills that make leaders truly effective. There is an unspoken assumption that those entering such programs are already "natural leaders" who require only role-specific technical instruction. As a result, genuine leadership development—focused on communication, influence, emotional intelligence, and team dynamics—is often neglected.

In reality, most leaders receive little or no formal training in leadership fundamentals. Outside the military and structured organizations like Scouting, leadership skills are often acquired informally — through observation and trial-and-error. Unfortunately, learning by osmosis makes it far easier to pick up *bad habits* than to master effective ones. Once ingrained, these behaviors can be difficult to unlearn.

Another recurring challenge I have observed over the years is a misconception held by many senior administrators: that those who work under them must be "Jack-of-all-trades" — excellent at everything. Performance evaluations often reflect this unrealistic expectation, offering feedback such as:

"He excels at time management but struggles with people skills. I've recommended he attend 'People Skills 101.'"

While self-improvement in weaker areas is always valuable, experience has taught me that striving to be exceptional in every domain is both unrealistic and counterproductive. True leadership requires recognizing one's limitations and surrounding oneself with others whose strengths complement those weaknesses. God bless my patient section leaders for their relentless ability to challenge me when the see a potential flaw in a decision I am making and to ask the bold questions to assure I am fully thinking a problem through from every angle.

Rath and Conchie capture this concept beautifully in *Strengths-Based Leadership*:

"If you spend your life trying to be good at everything, you will never be great at anything. While society encourages us to be well-rounded, this approach inadvertently breeds mediocrity. Perhaps the greatest misconception of all is that of the well-rounded leader.

Organizations seek leaders who are great communicators, visionary thinkers, and reliable executors. All of these qualities are desirable, yet we have never found one individual who excels equally across all areas. Those who strive to be competent in everything often become the least effective leaders."
— *Rath T, Conchie B.*

Thus, the purpose of this chapter — and indeed this book — is not to train readers to be good at everything, but rather to help them become highly effective in the areas where they naturally excel, to acknowledge and understand their weaker areas, and to build teams that fill those gaps.

This chapter provides an overview of foundational leadership principles that are often missing from traditional organizational training. These represent the everyday skills leaders must consciously cultivate to be consistently effective. The nuances of *crisis leadership* — how leadership behaviors shift when routine gives way to chaos — are discussed in detail in Chapter IV.

The intent here is not to provide exhaustive instruction on each leadership component. Entire courses and books exist for that purpose. Instead, the goal is to help readers recognize domains they may not have considered, reflect on their current capabilities, and identify reputable resources for further development (see Index).

As I often remind trainees:

"Everyone expects us to be natural-born leaders. Everyone expects that, no matter the situation, we will manage it. Someone is always watching, looking to you as an example. So put on your best show — because once you display poor leadership, you can't erase that memory. Team morale often depends on how *you* handle the moment."

Neil Grunberg, leadership instructor at the Uniformed Services University, reminds us that physicians consistently rank at the top of the public's most prestigious professions (Harris Poll, September 2014). By default, the public — and our colleagues — expect professionalism and composure at all times. (Callahan & Grunberg, Pollack)

I can personally attest that over the years, I have served as both a good and poor example of leadership. Stress and fatigue inevitably bring out the worst in us. However, like surgical technique or athletic performance, leadership skills improve with consistent, deliberate practice. Those who rehearse these behaviors daily are far more likely to exhibit them naturally when faced with high-stress or crisis situations.

1. DEFINITIONS, ROLES, AND RESPONSIBILITIES

It may seem unnecessary to begin with definitions, but clarity of terminology is essential when teaching and practicing leadership. Common understanding ensures that instruction and discussion are grounded in shared meaning.

What Is Leadership?

Simply put, leadership is the process and skillset by which an individual or organization influences others to achieve a common goal.

Peter Northouse notes that *"the number of definitions of leadership likely equals the number of individuals attempting to define it."* During a Uniformed Services University Bushmasters Course orientation in 2016, Neil Grunberg expanded on this by emphasizing that leadership reflects *"the intersection of experience, beliefs, culture, and the various leadership types within an organization."*

Grunberg defines leadership as:

"The enhancement of behaviors (actions), cognition (thoughts and beliefs), and motivations (reasons for actions and thoughts) to achieve goals that benefit individuals and groups."

He further reminds us that medical leadership, particularly within military or high-stakes healthcare systems, must account for the dynamic interaction between the healthcare team, command structure, and the public. (Grunberg; Northouse)

Leadership: The process by which an individual influences a group to achieve a common goal.

What Is Leading?

Leading is the *act* of providing direction, guidance, and purpose. Without leadership, groups lack coordination, accountability, and vision — conditions that inevitably lead to confusion and failure.

Without leadership, no one is responsible. Without leadership, bad things happen.

What Is a Team?

A team is a group of individuals collaborating toward a shared goal, combining their diverse responsibilities and expertise to achieve outcomes that exceed individual effort.

What Is Teamwork?

Teamwork is the process of effective collaboration within that team — aligning communication, trust, and mutual accountability to accomplish a shared mission.

As a group, we succeed as a team — and we fail as a team.

GO TO CHAPTER **IV.I. FOLLOWERSHIP, TEAMS and TEAMWORK!**

It's not where you go but who you meet along the way! **Genesis Lipshy**
Surgery is a team sport! **Roger Perry, MD**

2. GLOBAL RESPONSIBILITIES OF A LEADER IN ANY SITUATION

While the tone and priorities of leadership may shift depending on the situation — routine operations versus crisis response — the **core responsibilities** of an effective leader remain remarkably consistent.

General Responsibilities of Leadership

In nearly every setting, leadership responsibilities include the following:

- **Understanding and embodying the organizational mission and vision** so thoroughly that the leader can communicate them clearly and convincingly to their own team or unit.

- **Developing and articulating a unit-level mission and vision** aligned with the broader organizational goals. These guiding principles should shape all aspects of operations—from daily workflow and hiring to communication and training practices.
- **Maintaining open communication** within the unit and with upper leadership, especially when actions or decisions begin to stray from the organizational mission or when safety concerns arise.
- **Preserving morale.** Sustained team performance depends on an environment where members feel valued, supported, and engaged.
- **Planning ahead** by fostering strategic forecasting and encouraging professional growth and advancement.
- **Empowering others** to take ownership of their assigned responsibilities while recognizing and rewarding success. Encourage transparent discussion of failures as learning opportunities rather than sources of blame.
- **Ensuring fiscal responsibility.** Effective leaders are stewards of resources, balancing mission needs with sustainability.
- **Promoting and sustaining a culture of safety and accountability** throughout all levels of the organization.

In short, whether in times of calm or chaos, a leader must set direction, communicate purpose, safeguard morale, and uphold integrity.

3. WHEN ARE WE CALLED TO LEAD?

Leaders often emerge under very different circumstances. Some step forward by design, others by necessity.

Situational or Temporary Leadership

At times, leadership is thrust upon us:

- You may assume a **temporary leadership role** during an acute crisis or emergency.
- You may become the de facto leader by virtue of your training or expertise—for example, being the only person present with CPR, ACLS, or ATLS certification.

Long-Term or Formal Leadership

Other leadership roles are more enduring:

- You may have been **elected**, **volunteered**, or **appointed** to a formal leadership position.
- You may be part of a **structured hierarchy** where leadership is positional and clearly delineated, such as in the military, law enforcement, or fire service.
- Alternatively, you may work within a system where leadership is implied but not rigidly enforced—common in many professional or business organizations.

Regardless of the setting, successful leadership generally requires the same fundamental characteristics—**adaptability, communication, accountability, and trust**. The exception occurs during life-threatening events, where leaders may need to temporarily adopt a more **autocratic** approach to ensure survival and order.

Interestingly, as Robert Lim notes in his work on *Surgery in Austere Environments*, even in combat settings, surgical teams often rely on the same collaborative principles they use in peacetime hospitals. Effective leadership principles remain constant, even when the stakes change.

4. WHY BOTHER WITH LEADERSHIP TRAINING?

Times have changed—and this isn't your grandfather's world anymore.

Until recently, physician leadership education focused primarily on administrative and professional issues such as quality improvement, patient advocacy, regulatory oversight, physician autonomy, compensation, litigation, and business practices. Rarely did such programs address the *how* of leadership—how to communicate effectively, build trust, motivate a team, or guide others through change.

This gap likely stemmed from two factors. First, medicine relied heavily on the Halstedian or Socratic apprenticeship model, where leadership was assumed to be learned through mentorship and observation. Second, many physicians viewed leadership instruction as unnecessary or even beneath them—after all, doctors were seen as near-demigods whose authority was rarely questioned. Displaying vulnerability or uncertainty was considered weakness.

Historically, aspiring leaders attached themselves to mentors they admired and simply emulated their behavior—for better or worse. This informal model often perpetuated bad habits and reinforced hierarchical thinking.

The same stagnation occurred in business leadership models throughout much of the 20th century. Employees rarely questioned their superiors—either from fear of reprisal or from lack of education and empowerment. Leadership equated to control; employees were viewed as laborers, not contributors. Even within the federal government, employees lacked protections to report misconduct until the Whistleblower Protection Act of 1989 (Pub. L. 101-12) provided legal safeguards for exposing wrongdoing.

As long as productivity was maintained, organizations clung to rigid, top-down management structures. However, when foreign industries began to surpass U.S. manufacturing productivity in the early 2000s, the limitations of that model became undeniable. The paradigm shifted: innovation and teamwork began to outpace control and compliance. The concept of the "manager" gave way to that of the leader—one who guides teams toward success amid uncertainty. (A. Edmondson - personal correspondence see back of book)

Today's environment demands leaders who can inspire, collaborate, and adapt—not simply manage tasks or enforce order. Leadership training is therefore not a luxury but a necessity.

5. STEREOTYPIC LEADERSHIP

For much of history, the archetype of leadership was shaped by **authority, mystique, and fear.** The classic leader was paternalistic, autocratic, and often revered for charisma, decisiveness, or sheer confidence.

Two decades ago, leadership courses focused primarily on refining those traits—assuming that leadership could not truly be *taught*. The belief was that effective leaders were born, not developed. Followers expected leaders to exude certainty and power; if someone *looked* like a leader, others followed without question.

In business, as in medicine, the hierarchical "boss–employee" or "leader–follower" model dominated. Management by fear was commonplace—a legacy of Machiavellian political strategies that emphasized control over collaboration. When a leader failed, the blame invariably fell on subordinates.

Physician leadership of the 19th and early 20th centuries reflected these same stereotypes.

The Stereotypical Physician Leader (19th–20th Century)
- **Paternalistic:** Male-dominated, hierarchical structure.
- **Autocratic:** Task-oriented and authority-driven.
- **Mystical persona:** Physicians, especially surgeons, were revered as near-divine figures. Limited public access to medical knowledge meant patients depended entirely on their doctor's authority.
- **Followers by faith:** Patients and subordinates accepted leadership decisions without question—trusting in expertise rather than engaging in shared decision-making.

This model of leadership, though effective in its time, is ill-suited to modern healthcare and the interprofessional, transparent culture it demands. Leadership today is defined less by mystique and more by **authenticity, collaboration, and emotional intelligence.**

> "Look I am either in charge or I am not! Which is it going to be? You can't have me in both positions" This is often a typical surgeon response to challenges in the Hospital. We tend to start off cooperative because we assume we are in charge and in control. But as we realize we are not in charge and not in control, we make demands, then loudly express cynicism and frustration. We then make more demands and become more frustrated. Finally, we frequently throw up their hands and dissolve responsibility. In

- ☐ Majority of SUCCESSFUL leaders in the past could get by on their innate leadership qualities: good looks, charisma, eloquence, sharp wit, decisive mind (ability to take risk when others falter), calm under pressure, self-confident, intelligent…
- ☐ Leadership courses geared to teach one how to enhance those traits but not necessarily learn new skills as it was not believed that leadership could be taught.
- ☐ Followers expected these qualities in their leaders.
- ☐ In the past, business leadership such as seen at General Motors, Ford Motors, and virtually every other major business, thrived on the hierarchal boss-employee, leader-follower structure.
- ☐ Machiavellian described principles predominated where fear in management was a staple maneuver to assure success.

6. TIMES HAVE CHANGED — IN BUSINESS, HEALTHCARE... EVERYWHERE

"Trust in me, just in me. Shut your eyes and trust in me." — Ka's Song, *The Jungle Book* (Walt Disney, 1967)

The days of blind trust and leadership by submission are long gone. You can no longer expect your team — or your organization — to "just trust you." Blind loyalty, once a hallmark of traditional leadership, is no longer a reliable currency. To survive and thrive as a leader today, you must adapt. The leadership model has evolved, demanding a new balance between innate traits and learned skills.

Beginning in the late 20th century, seismic shifts in culture, communication, and organizational structure reshaped what it means to lead. Modern leadership is no longer defined by command and control but by connection, collaboration, and competence. In this age, we always should be prepared to explain our actions to any of our team regardless if we believe we made the correct decision.

Why Has the Leadership Model Changed?
-    From Commanders to Collaborators: The Rise of the Team Model

In business, the rigid *managerial* model has given way to a *leadership–team* paradigm that emphasizes shared purpose, trust, and collective intelligence.

In medicine, the transformation is even more striking. The era of the "captain of the ship" is largely over. For decades, surgeons functioned as solitary authorities — personally directing every element of a patient's care, from the ICU ventilator to the operating table. Today's surgeon, however, is a team leader, collaborating with anesthesiologists, intensivists, oncologists, nurses, and advanced practice providers as *co-equals* in the care process.

The modern surgical environment requires leaders who can inspire, coordinate, and empower multidisciplinary teams, not simply issue directives.

-    The Humanization of the Surgeon

Surgical training was once synonymous with endurance: long hours, sleep deprivation, poor nutrition, limited family contact, and frequent exposure to emotionally harsh environments. Few questioned the model — it was assumed that such suffering was essential to developing competence.

Although many surgeons still debate the merits of residency work-hour restrictions, there is no denying that these changes have humanized the profession. Duty-hour limitations opened the door to frank discussions once considered taboo — burnout, mindfulness, mental health, suicide, substance abuse, and disruptive behavior.

This humanization has also contributed to the demystification of the physician's persona. The absolute authority once associated with command-and-control leadership has lost its legitimacy. Outbursts and intimidation no longer inspire respect; they erode credibility.

Today, leadership skills such as communication, emotional intelligence, team building, systems thinking, and change management are not optional — they are core competencies. The Accreditation Council for Graduate Medical Education (ACGME) now explicitly requires these as part of training. (Lobas)

- The Democratization of Information

The world has grown smaller — and far more transparent. Over the last two decades, the explosion of accessible information has permanently changed the physician–patient dynamic.

Where physicians once held near-exclusive knowledge of disease processes, patients now arrive informed — sometimes better informed — about their diagnoses and treatment options. This democratization of information has eroded the mystique of medicine and placed new demands on leaders: humility, active listening, and respect for shared decision-making.

- Generational and Communication Shifts

Communication norms have changed profoundly. Newer generations expect dialogue, not directives. Modern teams — composed of younger professionals and trainees — value transparency, collaboration, and authenticity. They are comfortable challenging authority and questioning established norms. They are also accustomed to multitasking, group learning, and rapid feedback cycles, which contrast sharply with the hierarchical, Socratic "pimping" model of medical education.

These generational shifts demand that leaders adapt their communication style: authority must now be *earned* through respect and example, not presumed by title or experience.

- The Era of Customer Satisfaction and Accountability

We live in an age where customer satisfaction reigns supreme. In healthcare, that "customer" is not only the patient but also the family, the referring physician, and even the institutional partners who assess quality metrics.

Leaders must balance compassion with efficiency, outcomes with empathy, and safety with satisfaction. The margin for arrogance or opacity is gone.

- Toward Equity and Inclusion

Leadership has also been reshaped by the gradual elimination of gender and racial barriers. Diverse teams are more innovative, resilient, and reflective of the populations they serve. Modern leaders must model inclusivity, not as a symbolic gesture but as a strategic advantage grounded in fairness and performance.

- From Innate to Taught: Leadership as a Learnable Discipline

Perhaps the most transformative shift is the recognition that leadership can be taught.

For centuries, leadership was thought to be an inborn quality — bestowed on a few "natural" leaders. Today, research in education, psychology, and organizational science confirms that effective leadership behaviors can be systematically developed through training, reflection, and mentorship. (Pearce)

The modern leader must therefore commit to lifelong learning — refining both the *science* and the *art* of leading.

- In Summary

The 21st-century leader — whether in business, healthcare, or the military — must be agile, emotionally intelligent, and collaborative. Titles no longer guarantee trust. Authority must be earned through credibility, consistency, and care.

We can no longer ask our teams to "shut their eyes and trust in us."
Instead, we must open our eyes — fully — to the evolving expectations, values, and humanity of those we lead.

> "Managers are not confronted with problems that are independent of each other, but with dynamic situations that consist of complex systems of changing problems that interact with each other. I call such situations messes. Problems are abstractions extracted from messes by analysis…. Managers do not solve problems; they manage messes." RL Ackoff 1979

NICE GUYS FINISH FIRST, NOT LAST!

In the past the old adage "nice guys finished last" seemed to hold true. At the American College of Surgeons Clinical Congress 2016, during the panel discussion titled "Principles of leadership for the young surgeon", Ronald V Maier, MD (Seattle Washington) discussed "Leadership in the ACS. how to get involved and how to maintain that involvement over the years". One key leadership pointer he provided us was that "YOU CANNOT BE MEAN! " "You treat people fairly. You are honest. You speak the truth. You are not a thug or a bully."

For those who are in doubt, an opinion in the **Wall Street Journal** *October 20 2016 entitled "Nice people really do have more fun" noted that people who are noted to have nice personalities outperformed jerks 85% of the time (2003 Univ. SC study quoted).*

MEDICAL STUDENT INTERVIEW QUESTIONS HAVE CHANGED FROM 20 YEARS AGO!

Leadership Skills are at the top of the list!

A. Leadership/Team Management questions

§ *Cite an example of where you had a major impact on a group or organization, either by taking initiative, building consensus or solving a problem.*

§ *Cite an example of how you dealt with a minority opinion in a group.*

§ *Explain your role in a teamwork or collegial project, including how you dealt with non-productive or disruptive members.*

Self-Awareness

§ *Cite an example of when you made a mistake and how you dealt with it (willingness to admit mistakes).*

§ *Describe how you have managed demanding and complex situations (time management skill).*

What has changed in these modern leadership aspects?

Successful modern-day leaders comprehend subjects such as ethical leadership, servant leadership, emotional intelligence, transformational leadership, psychological safety, team – communication training and the like. These are now mainstays in the majority of leadership courses.

LEADERSHIP IN THE MODERN ERA REQUIRES INSIGHT INTO:

- ☐ Servant leadership.
- ☐ Transformational Leadership.
- ☐ Crew Resource Management, Team training and NOW TEAMING.
- ☐ Resiliency: Emotional-Lifestyle-Burnout Management, Mindfulness Training and Embracing Failure
- ☐ Ethics, Morals, and Psychological Safety

7. Why Should Physicians Care That Leadership Models Have Changed?

Why would a physician care if leadership models have changed?
Because the landscape of medicine itself has changed — and continues to evolve faster than ever.

To begin with, multiple workforce analyses predict a significant shortfall of physicians, particularly surgeons, within the next decade. As the number of providers decreases and the complexity of healthcare delivery grows, the need for strong, adaptive physician leadership will only become more urgent.

Despite these challenges, the public continues to view the physician as one of society's most prestigious and trusted professions. Until that perception changes, physicians—and healthcare professionals as a whole—will continue to be looked upon as natural leaders, expected to step forward when the situation demands direction.

If physicians and other healthcare professionals do not assume leadership roles, non-clinical administrators and external entities will. Leadership in healthcare will not remain vacant—it will simply be filled by those who show up. To ensure that medicine is guided by those who understand patient care from the inside, clinicians must actively claim their place at the table.

As my colleague John Stewart, MD, often reminds me:
"You're either at the table—or on the menu."
If healthcare professionals wish to shape a safe, ethical, and sustainable healthcare system, they must participate in its leadership rather than surrender that responsibility to others. If you sit back and do nothing, you control nothing.

8. The Shift Toward Non-Technical Competencies

The call for leadership education is not just philosophical—it's embedded in modern medical standards.

In 1999, the Accreditation Council for Graduate Medical Education (ACGME) identified interpersonal and communication skills and professionalism as two of the six core competencies for physician training. These competencies marked a significant departure from the purely technical focus of previous decades.

In 2006, researchers at the University of Aberdeen introduced the concept of Non-Technical Skills for Surgeons (NOTSS)—a framework that delineated behavioral and cognitive skill sets essential for surgical safety and effectiveness. These included situational awareness, decision-making, communication, teamwork, and leadership—skills once dismissed as "soft" but now recognized as vital to patient outcomes. (Flin, ACGME, ACS)

A decade later, at the August 2016 National Surgical Patient Safety Summit convened by the American College of Surgeons (ACS) and the American Academy of Orthopaedic Surgeons (AAOS), leaders from across disciplines reached a decisive conclusion after extensive debate:

NON-TECHNICAL SKILLS ARE EQUALLY AS CRITICAL AS TECHNICAL SKILLS IN SURGERY.

This consensus underscores a new reality: technical excellence alone is not enough. Leadership, communication, emotional intelligence, and teamwork are now recognized as essential components of surgical—and medical—competence.

In Summary

Physicians must care about the evolution of leadership models because **the profession's credibility, autonomy, and future depend on it.** Modern healthcare requires leaders who can manage complexity, inspire collaboration, and advocate for both patients and providers.

To abdicate leadership is to forfeit influence.

To lead with humility, awareness, and purpose is to safeguard the integrity of our profession—and the safety of those we serve.

IN THEIR UNIFORMED SERVICES UNIVERSITY LEAD PROGRAM NEIL GRUNBERG NOTES THE FOLLOWING IMPORTANT TRANSFORMATIONS IN LEADERSHIP OVER THE CENTURIES:

- One of the first portrayals of leadership qualifications is likely noted in Homer's Iliad. In that historical document, leaders were appointed, strong, charismatic, cunning, and loyal. Traditional

leadership traits noted in the Iliad, associated with memorable leaders, were focused on the leaders physical, knowledge, performance and personality strengths.
- One of the first modern portrayal of traditional leadership types was noted by Kurt Lewin (1930s). His works broke leadership into three basic types:
- Authoritarian (leader assumes all control).
  - Democratic (leader works with followers in developing policy and principles).
  - Laissez Faire (leader allows followers to generate rules and regulations).
- In the last couple of decades, leadership focus has shifted away from "who the leader is" towards "what the leaders does". With this shift, Focus is more on strengthening personality, confidence, humility, resilience, emotional intelligence (EQ), followership, communication (clarity and brevity), and experienced based knowledge.
- Compared to the past, modern leaders are expected to emphasis awareness of their environment, context, and relationships. Grunberg,et al

*(According to projections by the Association of American Medical Colleges, the nation will be short more than 90,000 total physicians by 2020 and 130,000 physicians by 2025. General surgery is predicted to be among the hardest hit, with a shortage of 21,400 surgeons by 2020. The number of practicing general surgeons is expected to fall to 30,800 by 2020 from 39,100 in 2000.".   www.beckershospitalreview.com/)

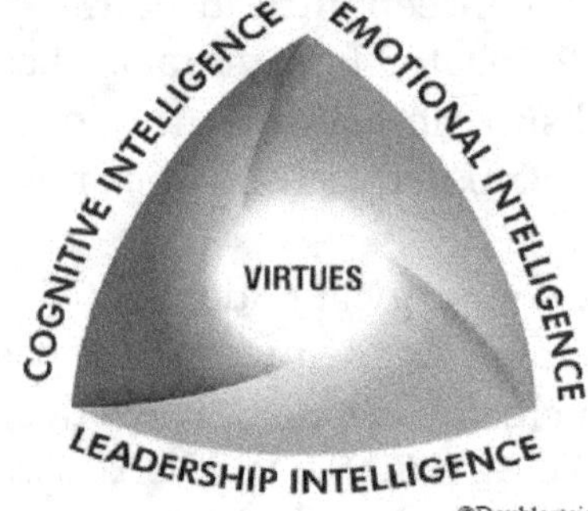

The Professionalism Intelligence Model has three components – the Cognitive Intelligence, Emotional Intelligence, and Leadership Intelligence. The CI is what you know, the EI is managing your own and others' emotions and the LI is knowing how the act.
These three are anchored on a set of virtues. These virtues can either be individually derived or community derived.
The model has a few key aspects as we spoke about. It is a living model- meaning it should grow as the person progresses through professional development. Furthermore, it should be balanced. Meaning – having a high CI is not enough to be a true medical professional.
This model provides a framework for professional identity formation and is complementary to other models of leadership and emotional intelligence.
Developed by Barry Doublestein, Walter Lee and Richard Pfohl with permission

B. NEW SKILLS: WHAT NEW SKILLSETS DO MODERN LEADERS NEED TO POSSESS?

Modern leaders have a much more difficult task - their life is a constant balance act possessing
- Understanding there are no bad teams just bad leaders.
- Discipline with flexibility /adaptability.
- Confidence without cockiness.
- Courage without being reckless /stupid.
- Competitive streak but capable of loss.
- Global awareness but attentive to details.
- Attentiveness without getting lost in the mundane. Adapted from Willink and Babin

"I learned from experienced surgeons that your innate response is to jump back when you encounter a spurting vessel but a trained surgeon learns to move forwards to control the bleeding. That is similar to anyone's response to an unfamiliar threat. You must learn as a leader to move forwards." **Stanley R. Wachs, PhD**

1. WHAT IS THE ROLE OF THE TEAM LEADER IN THIS NEW ERA?

In this new era, to be an effective leader, you must be a TEAM LEADER, not just a boss. **What is a team?** A team is a group of people collaborating while doing their job tending to their responsibilities to be more effective for an improved outcome. **What is teamwork?** Teamwork is the process where a group of individuals (team) collaborate to become more effective at attaining a common mission. Having a unified **MISSION or VISION** is critical for the team. Without a mission, you have a bunch of people just doing their job. The team leader assures that directing the team towards the success of the mission or vision keeps the team focused in the right direction. Without a common vision, individuals quickly become self-focused and discordant. Few if any modern societal advances are made by a single individual or teams without a mission. Without a unified vision, team-member motivation wanes quickly.

By nature, knowingly or not, surgeons, willingly accept the role as leader. We accept responsibility to care for our patients. By default, we must accept that we accept responsibility for the actions and results of our team. Effective leaders take ownership of their team and accept that there are no bad teams just bad leaders. When the team or a member fails the leader looks within themselves first to understand how they could have served the team better. With the right leadership, even the weakest teams will succeed. Not all teams succeed, but leaders harboring the traits herein have a much better chance of success than poor leaders with a strong group of team followers.

MISSIONS, VISIONS, AND VALUES — OH MY!

At the start of most strategic planning meetings, I can still recall the lengthy debates over crafting the organization's *Mission, Vision, and Values.*

To be honest, no one ever told me why these mattered—and as a result, my attention span (and my ADHD) usually took me elsewhere.

At first glance, the exercise can seem tedious or overly corporate. Many leaders quietly wonder why so much time is devoted to a few polished sentences when there's real work to be done. But I've come to realize that developing these three "calling cards" is as essential to leadership as framing is to building a house. Without them, the structure collapses under its own weight.

WHY WE NEED MISSIONS, VISIONS AND VALUES PUBLICIZED

Your Mission:

Your mission defines the *distinctive purpose* of the organization—its reason for existence. It answers: "Why do we exist? What makes us stand out from the rest?"

Your Vision:

Your vision articulates what the organization aspires to become. It's the image of success—the future you hope to achieve. It asks:
"What will we look like when we succeed?"
"What is our hope for the future?"

Your Values:

Your values are the guiding principles that shape every decision within the organization. They answer: "What do we believe in?"

THE REAL VALUE OF MISSION AND VISION STATEMENTS

Mission and vision statements are not corporate ornaments—they are the scaffolding upon which every organizational activity rests. They establish a common purpose, and, as Chester Barnard noted in *The Functions of the Executive,* organizations succeed only when their members share:

1. A willingness to serve,
2. A system of communication, and
3. A common purpose.

Without that shared sense of purpose, organizations easily lose focus in the chaos of complexity. When everyone understands *why* they belong and *what* they are working toward, cohesion and commitment naturally follow.

THE MISSION

Mission statements are intentionally broad and enduring. They are the foundation upon which everything else is built—but they must also be flexible. Over time, the environment changes, and survival requires adaptability.

An effective mission statement should be simple, memorable, and universally understood by every member of the organization. It should be brief enough to recite and meaningful enough to motivate.

At the unit level, a clear mission can unite even small teams.

For example, a surgical service might simply state:

"We strive to return our patients to optimal functional condition, enabling them to resume as normal a life as possible."

That one line can drive purpose, focus, and pride in daily work.

THE VISION

A vision paints the picture of what success looks like—it helps teams visualize the destination before they start the journey. I think of it as a mental map: you are here; your vision is there. To move from point A to point G, you need direction—and occasional reassurance that you're still on course.

When developing a vision, leaders should anticipate a full spectrum of reactions from their team—from enthusiastic support to skepticism or apathy. Effective leaders must balance firmness on core principles with flexibility on execution.

Understanding your "customers" is critical to shaping your vision. In healthcare, who are they? Patients, of course—but also staff, colleagues, investors, and the community we serve. Your vision must align with their needs, not just your aspirations.

If you want people to commit to your vision:

- It must inspire, not just list goals.
- It must be simple and clear.
- It must make sense in the real-world context of your workplace.
- It must serve as a guidepost—your cornerstone reminding you where you began.
- It must provide a scaffold for building achievable, meaningful goals.

A good vision doesn't just describe the future—it motivates the present.

USING MISSION AND VISION FOR TIME MANAGEMENT

Even with the best intentions, it's easy to start the day focused on your mission and end it wondering where your time went. All it takes is one well-placed email, an unexpected comment, or a crisis to derail your focus.

At the end of a busy day, ask yourself:

"What did I accomplish that actually advanced our mission or vision?"

Before engaging in any task, consider:

"Is this critical?"

"Is this mission-critical?"

In healthcare, priorities are sometimes obvious—a deteriorating patient always takes precedence. But competing demands are common. Imagine you have an elective hernia repair scheduled at the same time as a crucial budget meeting. Both are important: one affects patient care, the other sustains your department's future.

In these moments, leadership means delegating wisely. Perhaps a well-prepared business manager can represent you at the budget meeting, or—with the patient's consent—a trusted colleague can handle the procedure.

The key is to ensure that every action, every decision, aligns with the mission—even when you can't do everything yourself.

As Barnard emphasized, successful leaders maintain equilibrium by ensuring that every task contributes to the collective purpose. Without that alignment, the day-to-day grind replaces progress with mere activity.

MISSIONS, VISIONS, AND VALUES SHOULD NOT AND CANNOT BE FORCED UPON ORGANIZATIONAL MEMBERS!

After the 2015 National Surgical Patient Safety Summit (Aug 2016), Richard Karl, MD* reminded me that "you can't just slide a checklist under the operating room door and expect it to work!" Joe Doty wrote in 2009 that "carrying a card printed with Army Values, or being able to recite them, is a far cry from understanding what the words mean, believing in them, internalizing them, and ultimately, embodying the values into one's thoughts, feelings, beliefs and behaviors." (Doty and Sowden p 71)

*Pilot rated to fly Boeing 737's, Captain for JetSuite, Irvine CA, Founder of the Surgical Safety Institute, and Chairman Emeritus of the Dept of Surgery, University of South Florida, Tampa, Fl.

2. WHAT COMMAND STRUCTURE WORKS BEST IN THIS NEW ERA OF LEADERSHIP?

As noted previously, in most situations, the boss-employee, hierarchal structure does not work effectively as it did in the past. Processes are far more complicated, the public has instantaneous access to everything that is going on in your company, markets are in constant flux and workforces must be more fluid than ever. A **DECENTRALIZED COMMAND** works better. ^{Adapted from Willink and Babin}

DECENTRALIZED COMMAND- THE OPPOSITE OF A MANAGERIAL WORKPLACE:

To effectively lead a decentralized command, a leader must simultaneously understand the broader operational picture while maintaining attention to critical details. This requires global awareness without slipping into micromanagement. Leaders often attempt to control complexity by personally directing every task and individual. However, as situations grow more complex, fear of increased responsibility without direct control can overwhelm the command structure. This reaction is counterintuitive. A leader's cognitive capacity, physical presence, and situational knowledge are inherently limited. Attempting to control everything not only exceeds these limits but also bogs down subordinate units, forcing them to focus on constant reporting and awaiting further instructions rather than acting decisively. The more complex the situation, the more essential it becomes to empower subordinate leaders to take charge of their teams—and for those leaders to do the same at every level. When the broader mission and standard operating procedures are clearly understood, subordinates gain the clarity needed to make informed decisions and act independently in support of that mission, within the commander's intent. ^{Adapted from Willink and Babin}

In a personal conversation with me over coffee one weekend, Lieutenant General Paul K. Van Riper (US Marine Corp Ret) described to me his use of **Decentralized Command Structure**. During the *Millennium Challenge 2002 (MC 2002),* held at the Joint Forces Command Center here in Virginia, Van Ripper was the commander of the "Red Team". The aim of the *MC 2002* project was to ascertain the effectiveness of a new direction in warfare tactics. The new direction was an emphasis on technology that allowed more control and communication over weaponry and tactics at command central. Van Riper's command approach was one which utilized less communication and more use of archaic messaging practices (couriers to avoid interception). He explained that by not relying on the outer command structures communicating every single move and / or minor change in plans, they had more opportunity to react to circumstances as they developed. As long as they followed the generalized game plan, they were relatively free to move and attack. The result was that they always appeared to be ahead of the US forces inevitably sinking the US fleet within the first part of the exercise. Van Riper's focus was on less communication and fewer details. The result was that his central command avoided becoming bogged down with the details and allowed the main command structure to focus on the global details. Had they demanded constant knowledge and communication, they would not have been nearly as effective.

HELMUTH VON MOLTKE's DECENTRALIZED COMMAND STRUCTURE:

Chief of Staff von Moltke understood that "No plan of operations extends with certainty beyond the first collision of the main body of the enemy".

Moltke was a German Military leader for thirty years. During his reign, he realized that given the expanding size of their armies, his central leadership could not exercise detailed control over his entire force. He accepted that subordinates would and should use independent judgment during battle. He developed strategies that allowed initiative in taking deviations as long as the officers stayed within the general premises of the mission. ^{Hughes, D}

GLOBAL AWARENESS WITH ATTENTION TO DETAIL

"Don't sweat the small stuff—but make sure you have someone on your team who will. Even small knives can bleed you to death."

Leadership requires a delicate balance: maintaining global awareness while ensuring attention to detail. A leader doesn't need to know every step of every process but must ensure that those responsible for each area are both competent and communicative.

To "see the forest," you must be confident that someone is monitoring the trees—and that at least one of them understands how the *cells* of those trees function. You don't need to track how the mitochondria generate energy or how the tubules carry nutrients, but you must trust that someone on your team does. Successful leadership demands simultaneous strategic vision and operational awareness.

You must understand the major steps required to accomplish your mission or goal, without becoming lost in the minutiae of frontline work. When someone on the front line becomes bogged down, your job is not to take over their task but to know *who* can assist them. Leaders should coordinate recovery and resources—not perform every job themselves. This is never a solo journey but always a group effort… never travel alone

---

Losing the Global Picture

It's easy, especially under stress, for leaders to become consumed by local concerns and lose sight of the bigger picture. In moments of distress, our natural defense mechanism is often distraction by detail—focusing on small, concrete tasks to avoid the overwhelming magnitude of the crisis.

This instinct can be dangerous in leadership. When we feel personally responsible for victims or outcomes, we sometimes step into the action rather than lead from above. Boston Police Chief Dan Linskey described this exact reaction after the 2013 Marathon bombing, when leaders instinctively shifted from command roles to direct intervention. In doing so, they risked losing situational awareness and coordination across the wider response. *(See Linskey's reflections at:* http://crisislead.blogspot.com/2016/05/resiliency-lessons-on-leadership_10.html*)*

Leading Under Stress

In times of crisis, great leaders do not accumulate tasks—they shed them. They delegate decisively, communicate openly, and focus on maintaining team cohesion. Strong leaders keep the big picture in mind while understanding the key requirements of each critical task.

Stress can fracture teams, creating conflict both within units and between them. During those times, leaders must prioritize the greater mission over individual frustrations. When pressure mounts, it's vital to reach out for support, collaborate across boundaries, and remember that leadership is not solitary—it's collective.

Leaders cannot hide behind desks or assign blame from a distance. They must rise to the occasion, engage directly with their teams, and strive to understand what is truly happening on the ground.

At the same time, effective leaders recognize that followers need to vent. When upper command imposes seemingly impossible or illogical demands, frustration is natural. A wise leader listens without judgment, validates those emotions, and ensures that legitimate safety or ethical concerns are communicated upward through proper channels.

Leadership flows in both directions. Just as you must remain situationally aware of your team's challenges, you must also keep upper command situationally aware of realities on the ground. In that exchange lies the essence of resilient leadership: awareness at every level, anchored by trust, communication, and composure.

3. WHAT DO MODERN LEADERS REQUIRE TO MAINTAIN A RESILIENT TEAM AND A SUCCESSFUL DECENTRALIZED COMMAND? TRUST!

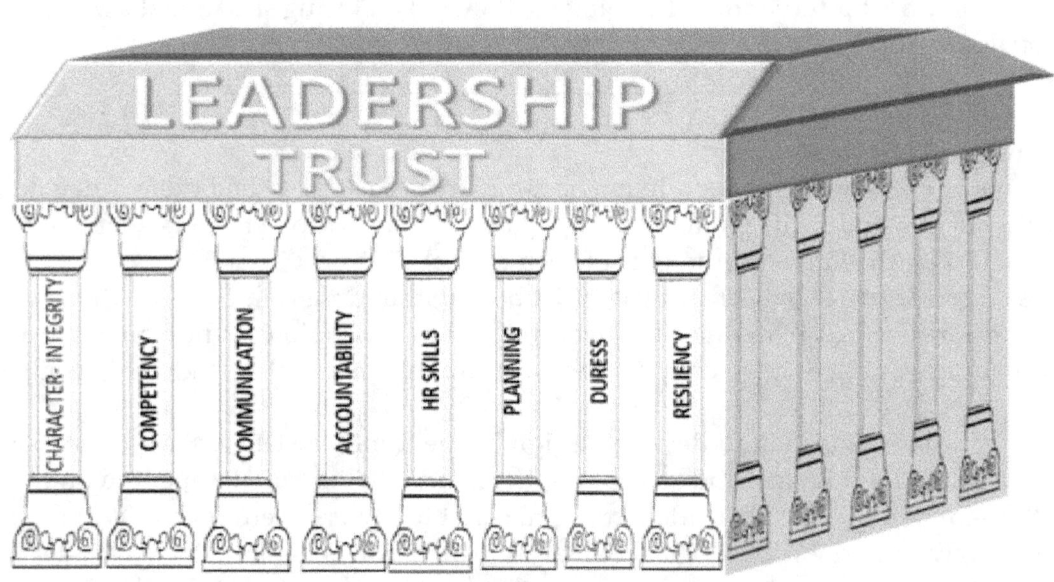

LIPSHY K. CRISIS MANAGEMENT LEADERSHIP: TEAM TRAINING TO SURVIVE THE CRITICAL MOMENT

RESILIENT TEAMS ARE BUILT THRU TRUST AND TRUST DEPENDS UPON LEADERS WHO HAVE:

- <u>Character</u>.
- <u>Competency.</u>
- <u>Quality communication and information sharing skills.</u>
- <u>Responsibility and accountability.</u>
- <u>Human Resource skills.</u>

- **Be Prepared!** Practice and planning.
- **Be Prepared!** Prepare for leadership under duress.
- **Be Prepared!** Focus on their personal resiliency through personal management.

TO BE AN EFFECTIVE, SUCCESSFUL MODERN LEADER, ONE TYPICALLY HAS TO MAINTAIN A CONTINUAL CONFLICT IN CHARACTER. YOU WILL LIKELY NEED TO:

- Assure ownership without being over-controlling allowing subordinates control.
- Discipline with flexibility / adaptability.
- Competitive streak but capable of graciously accepting a loss.
- Humbleness without passivity- great leaders maintain humility and mutual respect. They acknowledge their team's failure as their own but give all credit for success to the team.
- Empathy with staff without being overly emotional- close enough to subordinates to understand their emotions but not be blinded by their personal issues. One person cannot be more important than the mission.
- Aggressiveness without being overbearing.
- Authority figure but encourages psychological trust.
- Consistent and Adaptable at same time but not schizophrenic- can't change rules after every breeze.

Adapted from Willink and Babin

---

a. <u>VIABILITY, RESILIENCE AND TRUST:</u>

Resilient teams are built thru trust!

VIABILITY

Viability refers to a team's ability to sustain itself over time. It is one of the foundational elements of effective team performance. Viable teams not only function efficiently during normal operations but also maintain the capacity to continue performing when circumstances change.

As Sweeney et al. describe in their book and interviews, the foundation of team viability rests on three core components: cohesion, trust, and collective efficacy.

- Cohesion arises from each member's willingness to serve the team and the mission rather than individual interests.
- Trust develops from confidence in one another's competence and the belief that each member will uphold their responsibilities and commitments.
- Collective efficacy is the shared conviction that, together, the team can accomplish more than any one individual could alone.

When these three components are strong, the team becomes self-sustaining. Members believe that their combined effort produces greater success than isolated performance.

In healthcare, this distinction becomes particularly evident. Most operating room teams work well side-by-side, but not always hand-in-hand — and that difference becomes painfully clear when a crisis unfolds.

Teams that are merely co-located can function under routine circumstances; truly viable teams, by contrast, integrate their work, communicate continuously, and share responsibility for outcomes.

RESILIENCE

While viability ensures a team's ability to function over time, resilience determines its ability to recover and perform under stress.

Resilience is the capacity of a team to bounce back to baseline performance after exposure to a disruptive or threatening event. It reflects not just endurance, but the ability to adapt, reorganize, and regain stability.

Resilience depends on three interrelated domains:

- Cognitive resilience — the ability to think clearly and solve problems under pressure.

- Emotional resilience — the ability to regulate emotions and remain composed in the face of stress.
- Social resilience — the strength of interpersonal bonds and support networks within the team.

Unlike viability, which can exist without extensive training, resilience must be built deliberately. Teams operating in high-threat or high-stakes environments—such as surgical, trauma, or emergency response teams—develop resilience through repetitive, realistic rehearsal. Teams that train until they "cannot get it wrong" perform more effectively when the real event occurs. These repeated cognitive, emotional, and social rehearsals strengthen both individual confidence and collective coordination.

A team's resilience is also profoundly influenced by the emotional resilience of its leader. In crises, teams instinctively look to their leader for stability. A leader who remains calm, composed, and decisive under pressure provides psychological safety and steadiness to others.

Ultimately, both viability and resilience depend on trust—trust in the leader, trust among team members, and the leader's trust in their followers. This reciprocal confidence forms the backbone of performance in both ordinary and extraordinary circumstances.

(Sweeney PJ, Matthews MD, Lester PB. See Section: "Resiliency — Leading and Surviving Through a Crisis and Surviving Failure.")

---

b. TRUST:

> **Trust: "a person's willingness to accept (and/or increase) their vulnerability by relying on implicit or explicit information."**
>
> In Trust you are taking on an acceptable degree of uncertainty.
>
> This trust relies upon our "gut feeling" of another person's ability (competence), integrity (benevolence, honesty, truthfulness), reliability (conscientious, predictable), humility (discernment of own limitations and willingness to ask for help). Ten Cate O.

THE TRUST FACTOR — HERDING CATS

In spite of what people may think, a leader **must** be able to *herd cats.*

Cats only follow someone they trust—and even then, they may still bite.

It's a cold fact of leadership that-

- **Followers don't have to love you.**
- They don't even have to like you.
- They won't always agree with you.
- But they *must* trust you—and, ideally, respect you.

As **Sweeney et al.** explain, trust is *"the willingness to assume vulnerability to the actions of another based on a sense of confidence in that member."* In uncertain or high-risk environments—combat, crisis response, or complex healthcare systems—trust is essential. It provides **a sense of psychological security** and establishes the bonds that lead to cooperation, coordination, and ultimately, mission success.

Trust, however, is **a two-way street.**

- Leaders who trust their followers tend to empower them—granting latitude in decision-making, encouraging honest dialogue, and valuing their input.
- Followers who trust their leader are more likely to commit fully to the mission and to persevere under pressure.

As Sweeney and colleagues summarized to me-

"Trust is the adhesive that bonds people, allowing them to work cooperatively to achieve a higher purpose or mission."

How Trust Is Built

Trust does not appear spontaneously—it is **earned and reinforced** through consistent behavior.

Sweeney et al. identify several interdependent sources of trust:

- **Personal attributes:** competence, character, and empathy or genuine care.

- **Relationship factors:** mutual respect, open communication, a shared higher purpose, and the willingness to empower others.
- **Organizational culture:** policies, directives, and practices that promote fairness, transparency, and integrity.
- **Situational context:** temporary teams or shifting dependencies require renewed efforts to establish and maintain trust.

In short, trust is built not only on **what leaders do**, but also on **who they are, how they relate**, and **what the organization stands for.**

Character, Competence, and the Earned Nature of Trust

In a recent review, **Doty and Fenlason** remind us that **trust is the outcome of both tactical-skill competency and character competency.** Technical mastery alone is insufficient.

Carrying a mission or vision statement in your pocket does not ensure that your daily behavior aligns with its principles. For trust to exist, the organization must first **develop character** — the moral and ethical foundation that ensures actions and decisions reflect the mission and values at every level.

Character and ethics cannot be taught solely in a classroom; they are **forged through consistent actions**. Trust grows each time a leader's words align with their deeds — and erodes the moment they diverge.

As leaders, we also carry the responsibility to **build the character of our followers.** Trust may be earned, but it must also be *given*. Blind, unthinking trust is dangerous, but thoughtful, deliberate trust — grounded in mutual accountability — is empowering.

Trust: Earned, Given, and Guarded

Trust is never static. It must be **earned repeatedly** and **vigilantly maintained.** It can be lost far more quickly than it is built.

Every day, followers evaluate their leaders — consciously or not — deciding whether they can continue to believe in them. That ongoing assessment is based almost entirely on trust.

A leader who is trusted commands not just compliance, but **commitment.** And that difference — between following orders and following willingly — is what separates authority from true leadership.

TRUST IS BUILT BY LEADERS WHO HAVE:

- <u>**Character/Integrity:**</u> Adhere to ethics and moral principles- For people to follow you blindly, you simply must be of sound moral character with honesty, and ethical practice. You can be an authority figure and ensure psychological safety simultaneously.
- <u>**Competency:**</u> Maintain competency- Competency is built by constant training thereby building their experience as a skilled leader as well as leading by example.
- <u>**Quality communication and information sharing skills:**</u> Train in honing communication skills- Your messages must be honest, clear, simple, never cryptic.
- <u>**Responsibility and accountability:**</u> Remain responsible and accountable- Leaders who are responsible and accountable both as a leader and a follower.
- <u>**Personnel Management Human Resource skills:**</u> Train and practice excellent Human Resource Management skills- Skills such as empathy, discipline (boundaries) and conflict management (to name a few) are extremely important.
- <u>**Be Prepared!**</u> Practice and planning as business as usual, rather than putting out fires all the time.
- <u>**Be Prepared!**</u> Prepare for leadership under duress- Decisiveness in the midst of uncertainty. Ability to remain flexible and shift leadership style as the situation dictates.
- <u>**Be Prepared!**</u> Focus on their personal resiliency through personal management- Time management, lifestyle management (burnout awareness and avoidance, and mindfulness & ability to embrace failure).

TRUST IS EVERYTHING

Remember—**trust is more important than anything.**
You can be the kindest, smartest person in the room, but if you are **immoral, incompetent, a poor communicator, irresponsible, unaccountable, unempathetic, short-sighted, or unable to manage stress, your team will turn on you in a heartbeat.**
Trust is the bedrock of leadership. Without it, nothing else matters.

c. TRUST BUILT THROUGH CHARACTER AND INTEGRITY

Trust is built on **character**—the fusion of ethics, integrity, and psychological safety. As **Sweeney et al.** state:

"A healthy organizational climate is one in which members are aware of and committed to a common, clearly articulated set of values. Leaders set the example by demonstrating personal behavior consistent with those values."

Followers depend on their leaders to exhibit honesty, integrity, moral courage, and loyalty. They watch not only what you *say*, but how you *behave*. Leaders who model their values establish **clear moral and ethical boundaries** for their teams.

Honest leaders cultivate transparency and open communication, which are the cornerstones of psychological safety. In contrast, **one-way communication, hidden agendas, arbitrary punishment, or outright deception** breed mistrust. Once trust is eroded, communication collapses—and with it, safety, morale, and performance.

Subordinates must believe their leaders will *do the right thing*. When leaders show moral courage—especially when confronting higher authorities about frontline risks—followers are inspired to act unselfishly for the greater good. Conversely, leaders who waver, dissemble, or compromise principles foster suspicion. And once trust is lost, it is extraordinarily difficult—if not impossible—to regain.

As Sweeney and colleagues remind us, leaders who model integrity build strong, cohesive teams. Those who simply *preach* ethics without embodying them create fragile, skeptical organizations.

Leaders who *coach* integrity and *live* their values are easy to follow. They establish behavioral expectations, enforce fair standards, and invest the time and patience required for authentic character development. By contrast, those who slap a "code of ethics" on the wall and expect compliance without modeling it themselves will quickly lose credibility.

(Sweeney et al.; Doty & Sowden; Doty & Fenlason)

Character Under Pressure
One of the most revealing aspects of character is **how a leader behaves under pressure.** Stress exposes authenticity—it strips away pretense and reveals who we really are.

As **Coach Tony Dungy**, former head coach of the Indianapolis Colts, reflected:

"I try to remember what my dad told me when I would get out of control. He would say, 'Did that help the situation?' When something gets you upset, you have to think about what you can do to improve the situation. Usually, I find that getting angry and venting emotions doesn't really help. In fact, many times it makes things worse. So when I start getting upset, I think about what I can do to help the situation—and that throws me into thinking ahead instead of reacting with anger."
(www.allprodad.com/dungy/o-i-ever-get-angry-yes-and-this-is-what-i-do/)

Too often, leaders allow frustration with "the system" or bureaucracy to morph into anger. But venting rarely helps—and often harms—the team. Constructive leadership requires **self-regulation**: understanding the problem, working within your capacity to improve it, and setting the emotional tone for others.

True integrity under pressure is about composure, not control; about accountability, not accusation. Leaders who can remain thoughtful amid chaos model the very kind of **moral steadiness** their teams will emulate.

The Takeaway

Trust is not a byproduct of personality or title—it is **earned through consistent integrity, authentic communication, and moral courage under pressure.**

Leaders who live their values build trust.

Leaders who only talk about them eventually lose it.

And once trust is gone, **no title, policy, or motivational speech can bring it back.**

"If you are going to be at a place for a long time, you gotta win then also you gotta be who you are or Players read through it, people read through it. So I just want to be real. We are in this business to act as a team so you better get in line early and work it out, figure it out. Everybody's got their strengths and weaknesses and if you are strong in an area and I am weak in an area, cover me up, and I will do the same for you. "

Interview Dec 2016 Andy Reid Coach Kansas City Chiefs

"The truth is sought, General McNair wrote to the army commanders, regardless of whether pleasant or unpleasant, or whether it supports or condemns our present organization and tactics." Greenfield KR, Palmer RR AFG study 1946

Leadership Transparency Regarding Intent to Relay Your Concerns to Your Organizational Leadership: Will your leader tell you that they will relay your concerns to their upper level leadership but not forward that information? If they do not, is that due to lack of comprehension of your concerns due to your inability to convey the concern in a comprehensible manner or is it due to their cognitive overload from other priorities? Is it due to their concerns the organizational leadership will not respond effectively- due to those same reasons? Do they rely on waiting for an opportune moment to assure their leadership is capable and willing to receive this information?

A leader with character will explain either of those to you and explain they cannot promise that they will be capable of relaying your concerns at that moment. You can help them by referring to the techniques described in *WORDS ON "HOW TO WORK EFFECTIVELY WITH YOUR BOSS: HOW TO MANAGE UP!"* page 45 as well as the techniques described in the conflict management and buy in sections in this chapter.

Public humility is not endearing to trust… Always take that person aside.

d.   TRUST IS BUILT THROUGH LEADERSHIP COMPETENCE

(Developed through continuous training, learning, and engagement in the field)

Competence is the second cornerstone of trust. It is built not by authority or title, but by constant engagement, continuous learning, and real-world experience.

In the modern era, experience in the field is more vital than ever. Gone are the days of the "Iron Colonel"—the leader who commands from behind a desk, untested in the environments where their people work. That model survived in the past, often because it was protected by hierarchy and deference. Today, however, teams are far less forgiving. They place their trust in leaders who have "been there before"—those who understand the realities, pressures, and hazards of the front line.

Followers are rightly skeptical of leaders who remain detached from practice. Few are willing to follow someone who does not stay current in the science, techniques, and culture of their field. Modern teams are well-informed and discerning; with instant access to information, they can recognize incompetence or disingenuous claims immediately.

As Sweeney et al. emphasize, *competence may be the most important factor followers use to determine whether to trust their leader.* Competence shapes decision-making, confidence, and credibility. Followers expect their leaders to be:

- Knowledgeable in the technical skills and professional standards required of the team.
- Adept in organizational management and communication.

- Capable of performing under pressure and making sound decisions in crisis.

Competence instills confidence. When leaders demonstrate mastery — through preparation, training, and sound judgment — followers feel secure in both the mission and the person leading it.

Knowing Your Limits

A critical yet often overlooked dimension of competence is self-awareness. Great leaders not only refine their skills but also recognize their limitations — both personal and team-based.

Effective leaders regularly assess their own capabilities, identify weaknesses, and seek opportunities for growth. They also evaluate the team's strengths and vulnerabilities to ensure that responsibilities align with ability.

True competence, therefore, is not perfection — it is continuous improvement. The most respected leaders are those who acknowledge when they don't know something, who seek counsel from experts, and who view learning as a lifelong pursuit rather than a stage completed.

As Sweeney et al. note, competence is not static. It must be renewed through training, reflection, and experience. Without this constant evolution, even the most capable leader risks losing both trust and relevance.

In summary: Character may win hearts, but competence wins confidence.
Together, they form the unshakable foundation of trust.

<table>
<tr><td>

**CREATIVITY IS THE NUMBER ONE QUALITY
TO ASSURE SUCCESS IN THE BUSINESS WORLD!**

When one discusses competency as a necessary character component to become a successful leaders, one must include the need to be innovative - creative. The 2010 IBM study of 1500 CEO's from 33 industries and 60 countries, concluded that "more than rigor, management discipline, integrity or even vision -- successfully navigating an increasing complex world will require creativity." Creative leaders make more business model changes, invite disruptive innovation, change the enterprise, are comfortable with ambiguity, challenge-alter the status quo, and invent! (IBM)

</td></tr>
</table>

"He is not competent because he has no clue what the staff are supposed to be doing around him! He just sits at his computer all day." Comment by staff

e.   TRUST THROUGH PRECISE COMMUNICATION AND INFORMATION SHARING

In the past, leaders often protected themselves by keeping information "close to the vest." The old "need-to-know" communication model insulated the boss from scrutiny and kept subordinates in the dark. Those days are gone.

In the modern era, effective leaders must be skilled communicators. Transparency, collaboration, and clarity are now essential. In healthcare, the consequences of poor communication have been documented extensively over the past two decades. Failures in communication are among the leading causes of medical error, while effective communication and teamwork have been shown to improve patient outcomes and promote psychological safety within teams. *(Sutcliffe KM et al.; Williams RG et al.)*

One of the most overlooked aspects of communication is a leader's ability to clearly convey expectations. Many new leaders assume their subordinates understand their roles, only to discover that assumptions lead to confusion. A simple exercise — meeting with your staff and asking each person to describe their perceived responsibilities — can be enlightening. Comparing those perceptions with the organization's expectations (see Appendix C) often reveals surprising gaps.

Key Principles of Communication for Trustworthy Leadership
While communication strategies are discussed in more detail later in this book, several key reminders are worth emphasizing here:
- Transformational communication: In today's environment, barking orders is counterproductive. Explaining *why* something needs to be done builds understanding, motivation, and buy-in.
- Listen quietly — but not silently: Listening is not the absence of speech; it is the active presence of attention.
- Prioritize information: Communicate the mission broadly enough for understanding, yet precisely enough to avoid ambiguity. Avoid overwhelming your team with irrelevant details. Keep your message clear, concise, and actionable.
- Be consistent and adaptable: Flexibility is essential, but inconsistency destroys trust. Changing tone, message, or standards unpredictably erodes credibility.
- Encourage diverse thinking: Beware of surrounding yourself with "parrots." Agreement feels safe, but innovation requires differing perspectives. Diversity of thought prevents blind spots and groupthink.

Above all, your communication must be simple, honest, and clear. When people know what to expect, they feel secure. When they are left guessing, trust begins to unravel.

f.   Trust Through Responsibility and Accountability

Responsibility and accountability are two of the most misunderstood — and most vital — components of leadership trust.

Responsibility is the duty or obligation to answer for one's actions and decisions within one's sphere of control. Accountability goes a step further — it is the expectation that you will be held answerable for outcomes, even when the circumstances are imperfect.

In leadership, especially in medicine, responsibility is rarely cleanly defined. As systems become more decentralized and interdependent, the temptation grows to say:

"That wasn't my task," or "I wasn't responsible for that decision."

But in truth, delegating authority does not transfer accountability. You may authorize others to act, but you remain responsible for the outcome.

In surgery, for example, a procedure's success or failure may depend on countless variables — timing, personnel, instrumentation, preoperative care, and more. Yet when the outcome falters, the surgeon bears ultimate responsibility. That weight is not unfair — it is the reality of leadership. Patients and teams alike look to the leader for advocacy, ownership, and honesty.

The litigious nature of modern society only amplifies this tension. Acknowledging responsibility for outcomes beyond one's direct control can feel risky, but integrity demands it. Responsibility is not merely about blame; it is about stewardship — accepting ownership of what you can influence and demonstrating accountability for what happens under your command.

Leadership Principles from Doty and Doty
As Joe Doty reminds us, several key principles help reconcile this complex relationship between authority and responsibility:
- A commander can delegate authority, but never responsibility. Authority defines who directs an action; responsibility defines who answers for it.
- A commander is responsible, but not always in control. The absence of total control does not absolve accountability.
- Leaders must ensure subordinates are trained, empowered, and capable of operating independently under the leader's intent.
- Leaders must establish a command climate that encourages ethical action — even when the leader is not present.

Doty and Doty emphasize that the maxim *the commander is responsible for everything the unit does or fails to do*" is philosophical, not literal. Leaders cannot—and should not—micromanage every detail 24 hours a day. But leaders who internalize the principle of being responsible without total control develop habits of thinking, planning, and acting that position their teams for success.
(Doty & Doty)

Practical Lessons from the Field

BUILDING TRUST THROUGH ACCOUNTABILITY MEANS LIVING BY A FEW TIMELESS RULES FROM EFFECTIVE LEADERS:

- Accept responsibility for leading both their subordinates and superiors.
- Tell superiors how they will solve problems, rather than asking how to fix them.
- Lead up and down the chain of command—never complain downward, but advocate upward for your team's legitimate concerns.
- Encourage ownership and autonomy among subordinates without becoming over-controlling.
- Balance discipline with flexibility.
- Publicly take responsibility for team failures, but give full credit for successes to the team. Adapted from Willink and Babin

The Bottom Line

Trust is sustained when leaders communicate clearly, act accountably, and embody ownership.

When people know that their leader is honest, competent, transparent, and responsible—even under pressure—they will follow through uncertainty, adversity, and change.

A leader who takes credit for success loses respect.

A leader who takes ownership of failure earns loyalty.

WORDS ON "HOW TO WORK EFFECTIVELY WITH YOUR BOSS: HOW TO MANAGE UP!"
ACS CLINICAL CONGRESS 2017

1. Know your boss's expectations and personality- Know their views. That likely is the view you need to conform to or sway.
2. Understand your environment/ institutional culture- "you don't need to be a weather man to know which way the wind is blowing".
3. Define your own narrative- establish your brand (team) highlight your team!
4. Build a coalition- Cesar was killed by friends. You cannot hide in this age.
5. You need emotional intelligence-
6. Support your premises with data data data-you must give data! U need support
7. Be patient- Nothing great is build overnight. Great ideas and plans take time. Plod along.
8. Never waste an opportunity- Recognize a good thing when you see it. Use those chance moments that suddenly appear. Look for other opportunities for leverage. Use those chance hallway encounters.
9. It's all about the patient! Outcomes and safety.
10. Getting what you want? Need their attention first- Keep it simple and tailor to your boss's personality- Make your case presentation simple and visual when presenting to nonphysicians -use imagery! It's not that they don't want to listen to you but likely they just don't understand you so YOU need to change your approach.
11. Keep your boss in the loop-Get in the habit of checking in with your boss via email- fill them in on goals, projects and success. Otherwise they either have no clue what you are up to or micromanage you or you could be on a different path altogether.
12. Understand situational leadership- Your role may be different depending on what team you are leading.

Adapted with Permission, David Tom Cooke, MD, FACS, MAMSE, Professor and Founding Chief, Division of General Thoracic Surgery, Vice Chair for Faculty Development & Wellness, Physician-In-Chief, UC Davis Comprehensive Cancer Center, Immediate Past-President, Thoracic Surgery Directors Association

g.   TRUST THROUGH EFFECTIVE PEOPLE MANAGEMENT

(Empathy, Boundaries, and Conflict Resolution)

After decades of enduring the autocratic "boss," the modern workforce no longer tolerates being ruled through fear or hierarchy. People want to be led, not managed; respected, not intimidated.

Healthy leadership therefore requires a constant balance — **firmness without rigidity, empathy without emotional entanglement, and structure without micromanagement.**

A successful leader must understand that **organizational trust** is sustained only when the team feels psychologically safe *and* professionally accountable. To achieve this, leaders must possess — or be trained to develop — strong **human resource management skills**, including empathy, discipline, and conflict resolution.

When the team fails, the leader fails. When the team thrives, the leader has succeeded in creating an environment where both structure and humanity coexist.

Empathy and Care

Many sources cite **empathy** — the ability to understand and share another's emotional perspective — as second only to **competence** in its impact on leadership trust. Leaders who genuinely care about the consequences of their actions on others foster reciprocal care within their teams. When subordinates see their leader sacrifice self-interest for the welfare of the group, loyalty and motivation rise dramatically.

Simple acts — **thanking the team, acknowledging achievements publicly, supporting professional growth, helping to solve local problems, and truly listening** — build immense trust. Yet empathy must be grounded in professionalism. Empathy does **not** mean emotional overinvolvement. Leaders must be close enough to understand their team's emotions but disciplined enough not to be blinded by them. One person, no matter how valuable, can never become more important than the mission. Mutual concern and respect can exist without emotional enmeshment.

(Sweeney et al.; Willink & Babin)

Traits of Empathetic but Effective Leaders

- Consistent yet adaptable — flexible in method but not erratic in principle.
- Humble yet assertive — able to lead with mutual respect, not dominance.
- Open-minded but grounded — welcoming dissenting views rather than surrounding themselves with "parrots."

Discipline, Boundaries, and Feedback

Many leaders fall into the same trap as lenient parents — **avoiding conflict and failing to set boundaries** until a problem erupts. By the time frustration peaks, damage is done: relationships fracture, morale declines, and trust is lost.

A **2016 Harvard Business Review** article challenged the belief that employee engagement alone drives productivity. The authors found that the most significant performance drivers were:

- Effective team performance
- A psychologically safe culture
- Clear goals
- A strong sense of purpose
- The leader's judgment and decision-making ability

Excessive emphasis on engagement, without appropriate boundaries or accountability, can backfire. Unrestricted autonomy leads to inconsistency and fatigue.

Leaders must therefore **define behavioral limits, enforce expectations fairly, and provide consistent feedback.**

Structure does not restrict creativity — it protects it.
(Garrard, HBR, 2016)

Conflict Resolution and Negotiation

Conflict is inevitable wherever humans collaborate. In fact, as **Amy Edmondson** observes, psychological safety does not eliminate conflict — it *enables* it. When people feel safe to speak their minds, disagreement is inevitable. The goal is not to avoid conflict, but to **channel it productively.**

When handled well, conflict sharpens perspective and strengthens teams. When ignored or suppressed, it breeds resentment, silence, and mistrust.

As **an ORNM**, aptly put it: "If we want to reach a solution, we have to stop making everything so personal."

Conflict is uncomfortable because it triggers a **threat response** — the primal fight-or-flight instinct. Yet neither fighting nor fleeing serves a team well. True leadership requires the courage to **pause, listen, and respond rather than react.**

For surgeons and other high-stakes professionals, this can be particularly difficult. Our training rewards decisiveness; hesitation can cost lives. However, in interpersonal conflict, **speed kills.** The best decision often comes only after reflection.

Effective conflict resolution requires:

- Active, nonjudgmental listening.
- Willingness to understand before seeking to be understood.
- Emotional regulation — recognizing and controlling one's instinctive stress responses.
- Focus on the issue, not the individual.

As Edmondson, Weeks, Lee, and Wachs emphasize, leaders who cultivate calm objectivity and patience create environments where disagreement becomes dialogue rather than destruction.

The Bottom Line

Trust is not sustained through authority — it is sustained through **empathy, consistency, and fairness**. Leaders who care but set boundaries, who listen but stay decisive, and who face conflict with courage and composure build teams that are both loyal and resilient.

- Empathy without discipline is weakness.
  Discipline without empathy is tyranny.
- The effective leader strikes the balance — and earns trust through it.

(See also: "Innate Maladaptive Responses to Stress," pp. 81–86.)

STEPS IN A SUCCESSFUL CONFLICT RESOLUTION:

☐ <u>Diffuse defensiveness</u> by assuring the parties that your goal is to establish a win-win resolution thereby assuring that those involved avoid feeling as though they are a victim.

☐ <u>Model good conflict</u> management behaviors through active listening, remaining neutral and avoiding distraction.

☐ <u>Focus the parties away from subjectivity</u> by steering them towards objective findings after collecting factual information.

☐ <u>Create a constructive foundation</u> by avoiding judgmental undertones and other negativity.

☐ <u>Practice effective communication</u> by personally using controlled voice and relaxed body language followed by assuring that the involved parties are aware of these engagement rules as well.

☐ <u>Diffuse the conflict</u> using neutrality and depersonalization of the problem at hand.

☐ <u>Identify and understand the subtle underlying needs of the individuals</u> involved by discovering why the individuals harbor such deep interest in their point of view.

☐ <u>Take pauses to validate</u> your understanding of viewpoints and objective findings.

☐ <u>Engage</u> the involved parties in problem solving to reach an agreement.

☐ <u>Reach consensus</u> via provision of alternatives which steer the parties towards resolution.

☐ <u>You cannot fix everything.</u> Remember that not all conflicts can be resolved, so you may be forced to accept that you could fail to resolve the conflict. There is always a potential that if you appear to be failing to resolve the conflict, you may begin to feel threatened personally (you may fear your potential as a great leader drifting away in the eyes of the involved parties, forcing you to be less objective). In the long run if you lose objectivity this can be more damaging to your efforts than failing to resolve the conflict. Everyone must learn to walk away and agree to reassess the situation later.

Adapted with permission from Stanley R. Wachs, PhD - Wachs Associates

h. BE PREPARED! – PART 1

Trust is built by leaders who treat practice and planning as business as usual, not as crisis response. If your organization spends every day "putting out fires," it's time to reframe your approach. True leadership means preparing your team so that when the unexpected happens, response feels routine. Preparation is not about predicting every event—it's about developing a culture of readiness.

The Art of Planning Without Paralysis

Effective leaders must master the delicate balance between decisive action and deliberate planning. You must be capable of acting amid uncertainty—without becoming paralyzed by indecision—while still recognizing when it's appropriate to pause, gather critical information, and reassess.

- Sometimes waiting for key facts prevents poor choices.
- Other times, hesitation is dangerous, and you must act with the information available.

Leadership often requires making decisions with an incomplete picture. You can't afford to take anything for granted.

Your mission is to maximize success while minimizing risk. That requires preparation, awareness, and disciplined thinking—especially when stress levels are high.

Leading Under Pressure

In moments of overwhelming stress, when priorities conflict and chaos reigns, resist the instinct to react emotionally.

Instead:

1. Step back—create mental space to think clearly.
2. De-emotionalize the situation.
3. Assess the environment and available information.
4. Identify the highest priority.
5. Make a simple plan.

6. Execute that plan.
7. Reassess, adjust as needed, and move to the next priority.

Throughout, maintain situational awareness—monitor what's happening, track the impact of previous actions, and anticipate what's next.

Trust grows when followers see a leader who stays calm, methodical, and forward-looking—even when the world seems to be spinning.

Think About the "What-Ifs"

Preparation is not pessimism—it's foresight.

Leaders must plan for contingencies before the fire starts. As the saying goes, "Have an extinguisher ready before the blaze gets out of control."

That means training your team, rehearsing responses, and identifying potential weak points before they become crises. Planning is not about fear—it's about confidence born of readiness.

Know Your Market

Preparation also means understanding your environment. Every organization—healthcare included—has a market: patients, partners, suppliers, and resource streams.

Even if you don't think of yourself as being in "business," you always have customers and stakeholders. Whether they are patients, referring physicians, administrators, or the community, *value* still drives success. Failure to understand your market—your audience, your partners, and your system's limitations—will lead to poorly designed strategies that fall short of your mission.

Do your research. Know your environment. Anticipate what your "customers" need and expect. That understanding is what transforms plans into successful, sustainable action.

Bottom Line:

Prepared leaders inspire trust because they make readiness routine.

They plan without paralysis, act without panic, and think ahead before the fire ever starts.

THE SCOUT MOTTO IS "BE PREPARED."

It means maintaining a constant state of readiness—**in mind and in body**—to do one's **duty**. **Be prepared in mind** by disciplining yourself to respond appropriately to direction, and by thinking ahead about accidents or unexpected situations that may arise. Through foresight and reflection, you cultivate the ability to recognize what must be done—and the willingness to do it—at the critical moment.

Be prepared in body by developing strength, endurance, and agility, so that when the moment comes, you are physically capable of acting decisively and effectively.

- Baden-Powell, Robert.

---

i.   BE PREPARED! PART 2:

Trust is built by leadership which exemplifies understanding and preparedness for leadership under duress (decisiveness in the midst of uncertainty) as well as adaptability:

(see chapters concerning leadership under duress later in this book for details)

"I tell our residents they need to 'Play like you practice'. We are working diligently to perform pretrauma briefings and debriefings to assure that everyone is clear who has what role and to assure that everyone has an equal voice when it comes to improvement." Joseph Ibrahim, MD, Trauma Surgeon Orlando Regional H.

Leadership competencies effective leaders learn before the crisis occurs:

1. <u>Strong "signal detection and perspective taking"</u>- you must be capable of assessing a situation, make sense of it, then use that information to develop a plan of action. This includes the necessity of requesting more information.
2. <u>Prevention and Preparation</u>- decisiveness after an occurrence begins prior to the event through discussion and resolution of "what if" scenarios.
3. <u>Containment and Damage Control</u>- this requires keen decision making under pressure and precise communication. Inevitably, the on-scene commander needs to take some degree of risk-taking if they want to move forwards.
4. <u>Recovery</u>- resilient teams and commanders understand the need to "bounce back" to pre-disaster characteristics if they want to remain solvent.
5. <u>After action reporting (AAR)</u>- learning and reflecting after the event to discuss what went right and how to improve the response or prevent the incident are key to success. Note that these must be team member LEAD and Not commander LEAD (other than to keep the group on focus).

Adapted from Willink and Babin

AFTER ACTION REPORT (AAR) : DEBRIEFING Adapted from (Sweeney, et al)

(All untoward / adverse events should have group discussion by those involved as quickly as possible to assess for opportunities for improvement)

    A. Case scenario- succinct synopsis, objectivity only

    B. Background- brief history of similar situations- how often, past experiences

    C. Expectations- What did we expect should have happened. What was the intent. Ideally, what should have occurred in chronological order. Objective only.

    D. Situation - What actually occurred-chain of events- steps along the way in chronological order. Subjective comments allowed in this step- but require validation if needed/able. Why was there a deviation/discrepancy?

        1. Was communication clear
        2. Were roles and responsibilities clear
        3. Was situational awareness maintained
        4. Was workload distributed equitably
        5. Errors of omission or commission? Safety net failure?
        6. Resources available or a hindrance
        7. Doctrine / Policy / procedural issues- help or hinder
        8. Sustainment: ***Three ups***- record positive actions and response here- what went right; commendations; heroic efforts.
        9. Improvement: Three downs- ways to be better next time (team, system)

    E. Improvement/ Solutions offered: Items for team. Items for command structure to process. (command relationships, triage and treatment plans, focal points for train)

        1. Specific areas to discuss for the future-
        2. What is being proposed as potentially able to prevent future occurrences
        3. Opportunities for training

Effective leaders understand that all will not remain quiet for long. These leaders are constantly mentally prepared for when "the other shoe drops" and all hell breaks loose. These prepared leaders know when life gets complicated it's easy to become overwhelmed. **It is a known fact that when faced with a significant effect we tend to do one of two things: <u>FIGHT or FLIGHT</u>. It's a natural tendency which we will discuss more at length later on. It's actually easy to either put up our shields and fight or just give in and run or hide but we seldom think of a third option: rationalize and analyze the situation (also to be discussed more at length later on).** The third option takes much more effort and training and few are equipped to deal with threats in that manner. Leaders who are prepared to deal with stress understand that under duress it is best to **simplify, prioritize tasks, execute the highest priority task, set aside time to monitor the effects**, and then **move on to the next priority**. To do that you need…

- Mental strength but endurance for the long haul and knowing your limitations. It's the Chief's job to assure that staff understand that the command must allocate resources based on information they get from the front line.
- Confidence without cockiness / overconfidence- you need to listen. Keep your ego in check.
- Courage / decisiveness without being reckless / stupid- you must be prepared to mitigate risk- understanding that while some decisions can be reversed or altered some cannot be undone. Cannot be reckless - must act on logic not emotions.
- Adaptability, versatility, resilience. You must learn to shift leadership styles as the given situation changes. (More below)
- Composure under pressure without being devoid of emotion- you must remain calm but not robotic- you need to have emotion.
- Understand that if their followers are not fulfilling their duties to expectations then the leader may not have been clear in their expectations.
- Finally, excellent leaders remember to perform an after-action debriefing remembering to assess what went right, what did not go right and how can they improve effectiveness the next time. Adapted from Willink J & Babin L

Adaptability in leadership styles

Most leaders become fixated in one type of leadership for all circumstances. In a conversation in 2015 with Steven Yule and Caprice Greenberg, it was clear that while we tend to think of transactional and transformational as being mutually exclusive, they are in fact part of a spectrum of leadership that leaders must learn to fluctuate between as the situation dictates (see links to conversations below). In his 2000 HBR article regarding leadership, Goleman describes six leadership styles: Coercive, authoritative, affiliative, Democratic, pacesetting, and coaching (definition below). The key to his report is that "leaders who get the best results don't rely on just one leadership style; they use most of the styles in any given week." Understanding the various styles and when to apply them is a key to success. As Patricia Turner, MD (Chair Membership Services, American College of Surgeons) reminded us at the 2016 ACS Clinical Congress **"YOU NEED MORE THAN ONE ARROW IN YOUR QUIVER"**. You simply cannot become fixated on a single leadership style for every situation-environment you work in. It just will not work.

For an interview with Steven Yule and Caprice Greenburg regarding optimal leadership models refer to « LEADERSHIP STYLES IN SURGERY THAT SERVE AS IDEAL MODELS FOR TRAINEES: DO WE EVEN COME CLOSE TO THE PIN? » located in Appendix C at the end of this book

---

GOLEMAN LEADERSHIP STYLES:
- <u>Coercive leaders</u> demand immediate compliance.
- <u>Authoritative leaders</u> mobilize people toward a vision.
- <u>Affiliative leaders</u> create emotional bonds and harmony.
- <u>Democratic leaders</u> build consensus through participation.
- <u>Pacesetting leaders</u> expect excellence and self-direction.
- <u>Coaching leaders</u> develop people for the future.

YOU MUST REMAIN ADAPTABLE AND CAPABLE OF SHIFTING LEADERSHIP STYLES AS THE SITUATION WARRANTS! (Goleman D)

<table>
<tr><td>

LEADER CHARACTERISTICS THAT LEND ONE TO SUCCESS DURING A CRISIS:
. Experience in difficult situations
. Great interpersonal skills
. Strong when needed but let's others work
. Flexible / innovative
. Decisive
Joseph Ibrahim, MD trauma surgeon in action during Orlando Pulse nightclub Mass shooting June 12 2016

</td></tr>
</table>

<table>
<tr><td>

EFFECTIVE LEADERS MISSION PLANNING CHECKLIST-
- ☐ Understanding of global higher mission- that is, what does the commander want? If you don't believe the mission as a leader then you will fail to assert its importance to your team, so if you have doubts then ask questions before you address your team. You are part of something bigger and don't forget it. You need to detach from your immediate tactical mission and understand how your team fits into the main strategic plan. If you have questions it is your job to provide feedback about the ramifications of your concerns. Your team will ask why so you better ask why.
- ☐ Identify resources (personnel, assets) and time available.
- ☐ Empower key personnel within the team ability to critique the plan with possible courses of action. Keep it simple enough so they can REPEAT it back. Remember complex plans create confusion and paralysis.
- ☐ Identify simplest course of action then focus effort on best course of action.
- ☐ Empower key leaders to develop the plan for selected course of action- identify and delegate.
- ☐ Plan for likely contingencies and risk mitigation.
- ☐ Set periods of time to monitor the plan according to information as it emerges.
- ☐ Brief the team participants and supporting elements with emphasis on commander's intent and engage in discussion.
- ☐ Plan for after action debriefing. adapted from: Willink J, Babin L.

</td></tr>
</table>

j. BE PREPARED! PART 3:

<u>Trust is built by leadership which exemplifies personal resiliency through time management, lifestyle management (burnout awareness and avoidance, and mindfulness & ability to embrace failure):</u>
Sustaining Leadership Through Resilience, Time Management, and Emotional Intelligence
The Rhythm of Leadership
Most medical leadership positions are defined by **cyclical highs and lows** — periods of relative calm followed by intense waves of workload, stress, and competing priorities.
Constant exposure to stress has physiological consequences. Chronic pressure suppresses adrenal function, disrupting normal cortisol cycles and leading to fatigue, irritability, and poor decision-making.
If a leader hopes to remain effective over time, they must acknowledge and manage the risk of **burnout**.
Sustained leadership depends not only on skill and intellect, but also on **resilience** — the ability to recover, adapt, and continue forward with purpose.

Resilience: The Foundation of Endurance
As discussed earlier, teams must cultivate resilience to return to pre-crisis function after adversity. The same is true for individuals.
A resilient leader can absorb stress, learn from difficulty, and emerge stronger. Conversely, a leader who neglects personal well-being quickly loses clarity, patience, and credibility.
Failure to build resilience is one of the most common precursors to burnout, and **physician wellness directly impacts healthcare quality and safety.** (Wallace JE; Williams ES)

Sustaining resilience requires intentional investment—through **time management, lifestyle balance, emotional intelligence, and an acceptance of imperfection.**

Time Management: Leadership's Lifeline

No leader has unlimited time to lead their team, fulfill administrative duties, eat, relax, and sleep. Yet in practice, those restorative activities are often the first to go.

Leaders rarely become ineffective by choice—it happens gradually. Common traps include:

- **Tunnel vision:** becoming so focused on the big picture that you miss field-level problems and early warning signs.
- **Micromanagement:** losing trust in subordinates and wasting time on minutiae.
- **Upward interference:** reacting to poor direction from above, constantly diverting your team to manage someone else's "fires."

The mantra "lead a balanced life" sounds noble but is often impractical. **Balance is not about equal time— it's about managed priorities.**

Multitasking only halves efficiency. Dividing attention between personal and professional spheres without clarity leaves both unfulfilled.

The achievable goal is not *balance*, but **deliberate prioritization**—managing what truly matters most in each moment.

Strategies for Effective Time and Priority Management

Distraction and procrastination are the twin enemies of leadership efficiency. Most of us spend too much time on tasks that, in hindsight, were trivial—and underestimate the time needed for truly critical work. The fundamentals remain timeless:

- Get your goals straight.
- Prioritize.
- Plan ahead.
- Delegate what you don't have to do personally.
- Avoid procrastination and distractions.

Even when you manage these well, **outside forces**—supervisors, systems, or crises—will disrupt your progress. That's leadership reality.

There are countless tools for time management (see Brunicardi & Hobson; Covey), but your system must **fit your personality**. A common mistake is spending excessive time *designing* an elaborate time management process instead of doing meaningful work. Over-organization can become a sophisticated form of procrastination.

Find a method that works and keep it simple.

Whether it's a whiteboard, digital calendar, or sticky notes, choose what helps you **focus on priorities without losing time to process management.**

One effective habit: Spend ten minutes at the **start of each day** reviewing priorities, and ten minutes at the **end of the day** reassessing and resetting for tomorrow.

Remember, *no battle plan survives first contact with the enemy*, but having a plan ensures you know where to return when chaos subsides.

And a practical reminder:

If you want to kill your career—don't manage your budget.

Fiscal awareness is time management in action. Neglecting it erodes trust, stability, and leadership credibility.

Emotional Intelligence: The Anchor of Self-Management

Emotional Intelligence (EQ) represents the art of **self-management through self-awareness, self-regulation, and motivation.**

Leaders with high EQ can monitor their emotions, adjust their responses under stress, and remain calm when others lose composure. They also read the emotional climate of their team, using empathy and insight to defuse tension before it escalates.

Without EQ, even technically brilliant leaders fail — because no one will follow someone who cannot manage themselves.

Lifestyle Management: Protecting the Leader

Sustained leadership depends on personal well-being.

Take care of yourself — **do something that makes you happy every day.** *Schedule it, protect it, and do not apologize for it.*

Most importantly, **avoid isolation.**

Isolation is a silent killer of leaders. It breeds mistrust, distorts perception, and amplifies stress. When isolation sets in, leaders become defensive and disconnected, often leading to the very burnout they hoped to avoid.

(See Dr. Wayne Sotile's discussions on resilience and burnout at the Feagin Leadership Conference, Duke University: crisislead.blogspot.com, 2016.)

Learning to Embrace Failure

Failure is not the opposite of success — it is its instructor. Every leader will fail; what matters is how they recover.

Failure simply means the outcome differed from your intent. It may result from process errors, misjudgment, or forces beyond your control. Regardless, failure is an inevitable part of leadership, and acknowledging that truth is liberating.

Key lessons:

- **Failure does not erase trust.** In modern leadership, humility and transparency create connection, not weakness.
- **Failure is an option.** Make decisions, accept outcomes, learn, and move on.
- **Mistakes are inevitable — repetition is not.** Never make the same mistake twice.
- **Learn from others.** You won't live long enough to make them all yourself.
- **Perfection is irrelevant.** Admit your flaws, seek help from the team, and move forward.
- **Check your ego daily.**
- **Own your errors publicly, correct them privately, and move on.**
  (Covey; Brunicardi)

Isolation after failure breeds distrust and accelerates burnout. Connection, humility, and reflection are the antidotes.

Final Thought

Resilient leaders endure not because they avoid stress or failure, but because they **manage both with awareness, structure, and humility.**

Lead deliberately. Rest intentionally.

Fail honestly. Recover fully.

That is the rhythm of sustainable leadership.

> "There are no secrets to success. It is the result of preparation, hard work, and **learning from failure.**" - Colin Powell

C. MORALE AND INFLUENCE:
1. BUILDING MORALE –

At the end of it all, the above topics all relate to building morale. In Sweeney, et al, they discuss that "morale has been motivating, leading to perseverance and presumably success at group tasks, especially under trying circumstances." Time and time again, high performance teams have been shown diminishing performance in the face of diminishing morale. In contrast, previously low performing teams have been shown to perform better and better in the face of high morale. In both cases, morale was directly determined by the team leader. (sweeney) The definition of morale is extremely difficult to explain. However, it appears that understanding the definition may assist one in developing the skills to improve morale in a given situation. In their text, Sweeney, et al explain morale as "a cognitive, emotional and motivational stance towards goals and tasks. It encompasses confidence, optimism, enthusiasm and loyalty." Inevitably it gives a team a common purpose.

The keys to morale are:
- Confidence as noted by past success
- Enthusiasm
- Optimism from positive and caring leadership
- Capability
- Resilience
- Leadership that sets the example
- Mutual trust between leaders and members
- Respect
- Loyalty
- Social cohesion- strong social relationships based on respect and loyalty
- Common purpose
- Devotion and commitment to excellence- avoiding complacency and high intensity training.
- Selfless service- sacrifice for the good of the group.

Morale can be destroyed by:
- Loss of mission clarity and purpose
- Progressive lack of success
- Progressive lack of mutual respect
- Poor leadership.

New leaders facing a unit with low morale must examine the underlying causes. In essence, inconsistency through incongruent assignments or goals, leadership beliefs and values that contradict the mission, and continual assumptions without factual basis tend to drag a group down.

Underlying assumptions are extremely difficult to dissuade. By the point they have become an assumption they are frequently dysfunctional, implicit and guide all unit behavior.

Improving Morale:
As expected morale is affected greatly by:
- Perceived Personal Morale level- How am I with my job?
- Perceived Unit Morale level- unit togetherness and commander relationship

Therefore, to improve morale, a leader must:
- **Build team trust and confidence-** the details of trust are noted above but in general one can improve team and individual and leadership competence, demonstrate integrity (honest and transparent communication), selfless service (share in team hardships), conducting demanding training, providing opportunity for learning and team-building AND maintaining unit member safety (Proper resources, equipment etc.).

- **Maintain discipline**- The Leader must be in control, remain focused. Direction and discipline must be equal and consistent. Must ensure high standards.
- **Establish unit identity**- instill pride in the unit.
- **Instill pride**- Trust and empowerment of unit members along with group decision making. [Sweeney, et al]

2.   INFLUENCE – What is it and how do you "gain" it?

What is "Influence" and why does it matter?

Influence, Buy-In, and Sensemaking: The Core of Modern Leadership

The Evolution from Authority to Influence

Influence is the power to alter another person's behavior without directly forcing them to act. In modern leadership, influence—not authority—is the cornerstone of effectiveness.

In the past, compliance was driven by fear: people obeyed managers to avoid being fired, but their performance rarely approached excellence. Management once meant control—commanding every detail of a unit's operation.

Today, leadership means inspiring commitment, not enforcing obedience. Modern leaders influence through trust, credibility, and shared purpose. Their goal is not to command, but to gain genuine buy-in—to align individual motivation with collective mission.

Sources of Power and Influence

Leaders draw influence from multiple sources, often overlapping:

1. Instrumental Power – Followers comply because the leader controls something instrumental to their success or reward. The influence persists only as long as that control remains.
2. Referent (Admiration-Based) Power – Followers emulate a leader they admire, believing that by mirroring their behavior or values, they too may achieve success.
3. Value Alignment Power – Some followers are drawn to leaders who share their internalized values and beliefs.

As Sweeney et al. note, *transformational leadership* inspires followers to internalize values that prioritize group interests above self-interest. Transformational leaders gain influence by:

- Addressing individual needs
- Providing intellectual stimulation
- Inspiring and motivating through authenticity and vision

Influence can stem from positional authority (formal power) or personal power—derived from expertise, credibility, and relationships.

Among these, expert power—rooted in competence, knowledge, and integrity—remains the most durable. Ultimately, influence is context-dependent. Effective leaders tailor their approach to the motivations and needs of their team. Understanding *why* people follow is just as vital as *how* they follow.

(Sweeney et al.)

Buy-In and Sensemaking: If It Doesn't Make Sense, They Won't Follow

One of the most frequent leadership frustrations sounds familiar:

"Why don't they get it?"

"They're just too stubborn!"

But perhaps the problem isn't comprehension—it's sensemaking.

Karl Weick (1995) introduced the concept of *sensemaking*—the process by which people interpret and structure the unknown. It is the way individuals frame events, assign meaning, and decide how to act. Weick describes it as:

"The placement of items into frameworks, comprehending, redressing surprise, constructing meaning, and the interactive pursuit of mutual understanding and patterning."

Sensemaking is not the same as interpretation. Interpretation seeks deep understanding; sensemaking seeks plausibility — enough understanding to move forward confidently.

In healthcare, especially in modern, fragmented systems, sensemaking is more critical than ever. Once, medical personnel shared common routines and roles. Now, specialization and silos have fragmented those shared understandings. Each professional frames the same situation through a different lens.

If a new directive, policy, or safety initiative doesn't make sense within someone's existing framework, it will be dismissed as irrelevant — or worse, threatening.

Therefore, if you want people to follow you, you must ensure that your message makes sense in their frame of reference.

You don't need them to grasp every nuance — you need them to find meaning and plausibility in what you are asking them to do. Marc g, Daved van Stralen, Karl Weick

Practical Application: The Need for Framing and Context

Dr. Richard Karl, MD, FACS, pilot and former Chair of Surgery at the University of South Florida, shared an analogy that captures this perfectly:

"Medicine is far more complicated than aviation, but many of the safety tools from aviation could reduce medical errors — if implemented properly.

But you can't just slide a checklist under the operating room door and expect it to work."

The takeaway is simple: change requires context.

If it doesn't make sense, it won't stick.

People must internalize why a change matters and how it aligns with their work. Only then will true buy-in occur.

Cultural Change and the Power of Habit

Changing a culture begins with understanding *why* people do things the way they do. Charles Duhigg, in *The Power of Habit*, explains that behavior is built on a cycle of cue → response → reward. Over time, these cycles become automatic — forming habits that define culture.

Leaders often try to change systems with mandates, punishments, or "sledgehammer" reforms, overlooking the underlying cues and rewards that shape behavior.

Duhigg's framework suggests that sustainable change requires:

1. Observation – Watch the daily routines. Understand existing cues and rewards.
2. Diagnosis – Identify which cues trigger unhelpful responses.
3. Replacement – Substitute new cues or rewards that better align with organizational goals.

You can't destroy a habit — you can only reshape it.

And you can't reshape what you don't understand.

Thus, effective leaders start by observing before imposing. They question before mandating. They analyze habits before punishing behavior.

"It's not dynamite we need — it's insight."

(Weick; Duhigg)

The Bottom Line: Influence Requires Understanding

True influence arises from empathy, credibility, and clarity — not from authority or volume.

People will follow when:

- The message makes sense in their context.
- The leader embodies the values they promote.
- The process respects existing human habits while guiding them toward better ones.

You can't order people to believe.

But you can help them make sense — and once they do, they will follow you willingly.

Experienced surgeon, on dealing with conflict in leadership-
"We had a conflict today with the new intern and another staff member. The staff person stated that they were not going to let an Intern be their leader. The intern was very excited about their new role until this conflict arose. I explained to the intern that there are two ways to deal with someone who absolutely refuses to follow your lead. You can demand that they follow you in which case they may outright refuse or give in but disrespect you OR you back down and belittle yourself enough by asking their opinion on how they would like to handle that situation or give them some options. "

3. HOW DOES ONE KNOW IF THEY HAVE REACHED THE POINT THAT THEY ARE A SUCCESSFUL LEADER?

Most leaders, when asked, "How do you know if you're an effective leader?" respond honestly: *You never really know for sure.* Unless you have objective data showing improvement in productivity, safety, and satisfaction, leadership effectiveness is often only recognized in retrospect.

Sometimes it's not until you leave that colleagues tell you, "Your leadership was exactly what this organization needed"—or conversely, that things improved after you were gone. Leadership impact is often felt before it's measured, and its lessons are clearest in hindsight.

Over the years, I've posed this question to many leaders. Here are some of their most common—and insightful—answers:

- *They may not love you; they may not even like you – but they trust you.*
- *When your team trusts you, they take initiative and share candid information that prevents you from being blindsided.* (Sweeney)
- *Good leaders build teams that function well even when they're not around.* If operations run smoother without you, you may be managing, not leading.
- *When a team member falls short, they tell you immediately – and then they fix it.*
- *If you want to gauge a leader's intelligence, look at the people they hire.*

Trust, empowerment, and team performance in your absence are far more telling than titles or accolades.

Where Does a New Leader Start? — Putting It All Together
What if you're a new leader—either stepping into your first formal leadership role or taking on a new position and wanting to start fresh? Where do you begin?
Leadership development programs, books, and mentors are invaluable starting points. But one of the greatest misconceptions about leadership is that you must be a "Swiss Army knife"—great at everything. Experience teaches otherwise.

The most effective leaders understand their **strengths and limitations**, build around them, and recruit complementary talents. True success comes from **assembling teams whose strengths compensate for your weaknesses**. No one excels in every domain, and pretending otherwise leads to frustration and mediocrity. As Rath and Conchie remind us in *Strengths-Based Leadership*- It's a misperception that all of us should be well rounded leaders. If you spend your life trying to be good at everything, you will never be great at anything. Although our society encourages us to be well-rounded, this inadvertently breeds mediocrity. They found no leader with world-class strength in every area. The paradox is that **leaders who strive to be competent at everything often become the least effective.** The best leaders excel in a few areas and empower others to lead in the rest.

The Complexity of Healthcare Leadership

Leadership in healthcare is uniquely complex. We constantly balance **quality and safety** (for patients and staff), **service expectations** (access, communication, compassion), and **organizational imperatives** (costs, productivity, and outcomes).

It's easy to get lost in these competing demands and forget the basics. In her 2017 Association for Surgical Education Presidential Address, **Dr. Mary Klingensmith** reminded us of the foundational behaviors leaders must uphold daily—simple, human, and essential.

Top Ten Things I Must Do as a Leader *(Klingensmith, 2017)*

1. Run a better meeting.
2. Communicate clearly.
3. Deliver on what I promise.
4. Be careful not to overpromise.
5. Remember what it was like not to be the leader.
6. Don't desire leadership just for power's sake.
7. Don't micromanage—delegate clearly and let people execute.
8. Remember your followers are people—thank them and ask about their lives.
9. Even your most successful team members still need mentorship.
10. Listen more than you talk.

These may sound simple, but they are the essence of sustainable leadership.

Avoiding Common Pitfalls

One frequent leadership pitfall is assuming that staff already understand their **roles and responsibilities** as leaders and followers. More often than not, they don't—and they've received little guidance or training in these areas.

When stepping into a new role, take time to ask:

- "What do you believe you're responsible for?"
- "What training have you received to fulfill that responsibility?"

Their answers may surprise both you and them.

Often, simply clarifying expectations creates more progress than restructuring an entire system.

Frameworks for Leadership Development

For those who want to go deeper, many excellent frameworks exist. One I particularly value is the **FourCe-PITO Leadership Framework**, described by **Drs. Callahan and Grunberg** in *Military Medical Leadership*. This model defines **four domains of leadership**—

- **Character** – *Who the leader is*
- **Competence** – *What the leader knows and does*
- **Context** – *When and where leadership occurs*
- **Communication** – *How the leader interacts*

These domains operate across **four levels of interaction**—

- **Personal**

- **Interpersonal**
- **Team**
- **Organizational**

In a personal conversation Dr. Grunberg explain to me that their model highlighted below which he covered during their **Uniformed Services University Bushmaster Combat Training Course (2016)**. It remains one of the most complete frameworks for understanding and teaching leadership, especially in complex environments like healthcare.

Grunberg

Final Reflection: The Measure of Leadership

Leadership success is rarely measured by titles, metrics, or recognition. It's found in quieter indicators:

- The trust of your team.
- The initiative they take when you're absent.
- Their willingness to tell you the truth, even when it's hard.
- The strength of the organization after you've moved on.

Ultimately, the goal is not to be **admired**, but to be **trusted**- not to be **indispensable**, but to have built a team that thrives without you.

When you reach that point, you may not need to ask whether you are a successful leader—your team will already be living the answer.

UNIFORMED SERVICES UNIVERSITY FOURCe-PITO Framework LEAD MODEL		
PERSONAL LEADERSHIP identify core values, develop self-awareness, understand service cultures, communicate effectively	CHARACTER- Demographics, personality, attributes, values	INTERPERSONAL LEADERSHIP- share core values, Enhance emotional intelligence, work in dyads. communicate difficult information,
COMPETENCE- KSA-skills, knowledge, role-SPECIFIC, transcendent.	LEADERSHIP LEVELS personal interpersonal team organizational	CONTEXT- physical, psychosocial, cultural, situational.
TEAM LEADERSHIP- build team values, understand group dynamics, work in small groups, communicate under stress.	COMMUNICATION- verbal-non-verbal, sending-receiving.	ORGANIZATIONAL LEADERSHIP- inspire core values, learn strategic vision, understand various cultures, communicate to large groups

Leader-Follower Framework (LF-2) with the same elements for follower as well as leader development Formerly the -PITO Framework LEAD MODEL Courtesy of Dr. Neil Grunberg, USUHS; (Callahan-Grunberg)

TEAM LEADERSHIP SKILLS: GOOD OR BAD 'MAYOR'?

In his book, 'Logic of Failure: recognizing and avoiding error in complex situations' Dörner describes an experiment where they asked experimental participants to be "mayor of Greenville" a complex system of interlocking, ecological and political components. Two distinct personalities came out of the experiment: The successful/ good Mayor and the unsuccessful / Bad Mayor. Understanding these characteristics is key for any potential leader to lead any team successfully in any disaster. (Dorner)

SUCCESSFUL / GOOD "Mayor"	UNSUCCESFUL / BAD "Mayor"
Innovative and stable.	Unstable.
Made more good decisions than bad.	Focused on less important but more easily solved issues.
Made more possibilities for influencing the fate of Greenvale.	Took events at face value and regarded them as unconnected.
Considered not just the primary goal but also its potential effects on other sectors of the system.	Changed the subject under discussion far more, when they encountered a difficult situation.
Acted more complexly: decisions took different aspects of the entire system into account, not just one.	Exhibited ad-hocism; they are too ready to be distracted.
Asked more why questions, about causal links behind events.	Aimless switching of fields of focus at one point and single mindedness; preoccupation with a project to the exclusion of all else.
Able to reach a decision that is totally different than a prior decision.	Decisions always resemble prior decisions.
Find ways to focus on the right fields of endeavor and continue to focus on those fields over time.	Merely recapitulate their behavior.
Reflected on own behavior, made efforts to modify behavior.	Walks away from difficult problems or solves them by delegation.
Capacity to tolerate uncertainty	Incapacity to tolerate uncertainty

-"Most leaders do not want to accept metrics that make them look bad". Col Mary Edwards, MD, FACS Army Surgical Consultant

-Never underestimate the value of fortuitous "golden opportunities", but never forget that not all "golden opportunities" turn out to be opportunities. So when asked to volunteer or participate ALWAYS take these seriously-don't be flippant- don't over promise! If you agree, then give it your attention and retire from that duty in good faith.

- I often think the only thing I have perfected is getting the right information or right people at the right place at the right timing in a controlled manner because clearly the folks I work with are a lot smarter than me. A lot can be said for packaging! No leader wants to read reams of information- they just want to know what the problem is, what is the consequence of ignoring it, what solution you are offering and risks and benefits of that proposal.

CHAPTER II BASIC LEADERSHIP SKILLS REFERENCES

- The Arbinger Institute. The Outward mindset: how to change lives and transform organizations. Berrett-Koehler publishers. 2019
- Harvard Business Review: On Leadership (Vol 2). Harvard Business School Publishing Cooperation, 2020
- Higgins RSD, Mathews JB, Rosengart TK, Wong SL. Surgical Chairs Playbook. ACS. 2023.
- Rowland PA, Lang NP. Communication & Professionalism Competencies: a guide for Surgeons. Cine Med 2007.
- Scoggins CR, Pollock RE, Pawlik TM. Surgical Mentorship and leadership: Building for success in Academic Surgery. Springer.2018.
- ACGME and ABS. The General Surgery Milestone Project A Joint Initiative of The Accreditation Council for Graduate Medical Education and The American Board of Surgery July 2015. http://www.acgme.org/Portals/0/PDFs/Milestones/SurgeryMilestones.pdf assessed 110616
- ACGME Holmboe ES, Edgar L, Hamstra S. The Milestones Guidebook Version 2016. http://www.acgme.org/Portals/0/MilestonesGuidebook.pdf assessed 110616

- ACGME. The Six ACGME competencies: what the RC's expect from programs. New program directors Pre-course. 2008.
- Ackoff RL. The Future of Operational Research is Past The Journal of the Operational Research Society Vol. 30, No. 2 (Feb., 1979), pp. 93-104
- American College of Surgeons. Non-technical skills matter too: Nation's doctors, payers and surgical stakeholders recommend teamwork, communication training and standardized processes to improve safety-
NEWS FROM THE AMERICAN COLLEGE OF SURGEONS AND THE AMERICAN ACADEMY OF ORTHOPAEDIC SURGEONS | FOR IMMEDIATE RELEASE. American College of Surgery Press release. Aug 5 2016. https://www.facs.org/media/press-releases/2016/skills-080516
- *Barnard, Chester I. (1938). The Functions of the Executive. Cambridge, MA: Harvard University Press. OCLC 555075.*
- Brunicardi FC, Hobson FL. Time management: a review for physicians. J Natl Med Assoc. 1996 Sep;88(9):581-7.
- Callahan CW, Grunberg NE. Military Medical Leadership in Fundamentals of Military Medical Practice. Schoomaker EB, Smith DC eds, Washington DC Borden Institute. 2017.
- Covey SR. the Seven Habits of Highly Effective People: restoring the Character Ethic. New York NY. Free Press; 2004.
- Dörner D. *The Logic of Failure: Recognizing and Avoiding Error in Complex Situations*. Reading, MA: Perseus Books; 1996.
- Doty J, Doty C. Command Responsibility and Accountability. MILITARY REVIEW 2012 Jan-Feb:35-38.
- Doty J, Fenlason J. Its not about trust; its about thinking and judgment. Military Review 2015 Mar-Apr 149-154.
- Doty J, Sowden W. Competency vs Character? It must be both! Military review. 2009 Nov-Dec 69-76.
- Duhigg C. The power of habit: why we do what we do in life and business. NYNY random house. 2014.
- Edmondson AC. *Teaming: How Organizations Learn, Innovate, and Compete in the Knowledge Economy. John Wiley & Sons 2012.*
- Garrard L, Chamorro-premuzic, T. The dark side of high employee engagement. HBR Aug 16 2016, Accessed Aug 16 2016) https://hbr.org/2016/08/the-dark-side-of-high-employee-engagement)
- Ginter PM, Swayne LM, Duncan WJ Strategic management of Healthcare organizations. Blackwell business. Malden MA. 1999.
- Greenfield KR, Palmer RR (ed) Army Ground Forces Study No 1. Ch II Administration of training under GHQ –p23 in **The Army Ground Forces - ORIGINS OF THE ARMY GROUND FORCES: GENERAL HEADQUARTERS U.S. ARMY, 1940-1942 Study No. 1 Historical Section   •   Army Ground Forces. 1946**
- *Grunberg, N. E., Barry, E. S., Callahan, C. W., Kleber, H. G., McManigle, J. E., & Schoomaker, E. B. (2019). A conceptual framework for leader and leadership education and development. International Journal of Leadership in Education, 22(5), 644-650. https://doi.org/10.1080/13603124.2018.1492026*
- Goleman D. Leadership that gets results. Harvard Business Review. 2000;78:78-93
- Hughes, Daniel J. (ed.) *Moltke on the Art of War: selected writings*. (1993). Presidio Press: New York, New York. p. 45, 92.
- IBM. IBM 2010 Global CEO Study: Creativity Selected as Most Crucial Factor for Future Success-Fewer than half of CEOs Successfully Handling Growing Complexity; Diverging priorities in Asia, North America, and Europe. IBM Newsroom. May 18 2010   https://www-03.ibm.com/press/us/en/pressrelease/31670.wss
- Klingensmith ME. Presidential Address: Leadership and followership in surgical education. Am Journal of Surgery. 2017.213(2):207-213.
- Kolditz TA. *In Extremis Leadership: Leading As If Your Life Depended On It.* San Francisco, CA: Jossey-Bass; 2007.
- Lancaster LC, Stillman D: When Generations Collide: Who They Are. Why They Clash. How to Solve the Generational Puzzle at Work. New York, NY, HarperCollins Publishers, 2003
- Lee L, Berger DH, Awad SS, Brandt ML, Martinez G, Brunicardi FC. Conflict resolution: practical principles for surgeons. World J Surgery.2008;32(11):2331-2335.
- Lobas JG. leadership in academic medicine: capabilities and conditions for organizational success. Am J Med. 2006;119(7):617-621.
- Northouse PG. Leadership: Theory and practice. 6th ed. Los Angeles. Sage. 2013.
- Pearce CL, Hoch JE, Jeppesen HJ, Wegge J. New forms of management. J Personnel Psychol 2010;9:151-3.
- Pearce CL, Sims HP. Vertical versus shared leadership as predictors of the effectiveness of change management teams: an examination of aversive, directive, transactional, transformational, and empowering leader behaviours. Group Dyn: Theory Res Pract 2002;6:172-97.
- Pollack H. Doctors, military officers, firefighters and scientists seen as among America's most prestigious occupations: Yet engineering is what the highest percentage of adults would encourage a child to pursue *The Harris Poll*September 10, 2014. http://www.theharrispoll.com/politics/Doctors__Military_Officers__Firefighters__and_Scientists_Seen_as_Among_America_s_Most_Prestigious_Occupations.html accessed 110516
- Shipper ES, Hardaway JC. Garvey EM, Logghe H. Talking through time: trends in communication and the evolving patient-physician relationship. Bulletin ACS. 2016;101(8):19-23.
- Sweeney PJ, Matthews MD, Lester PB. *Leadership in Dangerous Situations*. Annapolis, MD: Naval Institute Press; 2011.
- Simone JV. Leadership lessons from Machiavelli that are not "Machiavellian". Simone's OncOpinion. Oncology Times Oct 25 2015
- Sutcliffe KM, Lewton E, Rosenthal MM. Communication failures: an insidious contributor to medical mishaps. Acad Med. 2004 Feb;79(2):186-94
- Ten Cate O. Entrustment as assessment: recognizing the ability, the right and the duty to act. Journal of graduate medical education. 2016;8(2):261-262.
- Wachs SR. Put Conflict Resolution Skills to Work. J Oncol Pract. 2008; 4(1): 37–40. http://europepmc.org/articles/PMC2793934
- Weick KE, Sutcliffe KM, *Managing the Unexpected: Resilient Performance in an Age of Uncertainty*. San Francisco, CA: John Wiley; 2007.
- Williams RG[1], Silverman R, Schwind C, Fortune JB, Sutyak J, Horvath KD, Van Eaton EG, Azzie G, Potts JR 3rd, Boehler M, Dunnington GL. Surgeon information transfer and communication: factors affecting quality and efficiency of inpatient care. Ann Surg. 2007 Feb;245(2):159-69.
- Weeks D: The Eight Essential Steps to Conflict Resolution: Preserving Relationships at Work, at Home, and in the Community. New York, NY, Tarcher/Putnam, 1994
- Wallace JE, Lemaire JB, Ghali WA. Physician wellness: a missing quality indicator. Lancet. 2009 Nov 14;374(9702):1714-21.
- Williams ES, Manwell LB, Konrad TR, Linzer M. The relationship of organizational culture, stress, satisfaction, and burnout with physician-reported error and suboptimal patient care: results from the MEMO study. Health Care Manage Rev. 2007 Jul-Sep;32(3):203-12.
- Willink J, Babin Leif. Extreme Ownership: how U.S. Navy SEALs Lead and Win. St. Martin's Press. NY NY 2015.

For interviews with experts in these areas please refer to these blog posts at the end of the book. www.Crisislead.blogspot.com

III.   HUMAN ERROR: WHY DO WE MISS WHAT'S RIGHT IN FRONT OF US?   (WHAT GORILLA?)

Questions to ask prior to reading this chapter:
- **How does human error relate to crisis management?**
- **Effects of hindsight bias after accident occurrence.**
- **What gorilla? introduction to heuristics.**
- **Influences that increase our susceptibility to heuristic tendencies: complacency, distraction, fatigue, etc.**

OBJECTIVES: UNDERSTANDING ADVERSE EVENTS: INSTIGATING FACTORS AND PREVENTIVE MEASURES: Getting down to the basics

A. <u>HUMAN ERROR</u>

1. <u>INTRODUCTION</u>:
   Discuss Adverse events, instigating factors and preventive measures: WHY DO WE CARE?
2. <u>HUMAN ERROR</u>: Discuss the Causes and Effects of *Human Error* in instigation or propagation of patient care problems.
3. <u>CONFIRMATION BIAS- Discuss reasons</u> why I thought that made sense?
4. <u>COMPLACENCY</u>- Discuss whether I was just lazy or caught off guard?
5. <u>OR DISTRACTIONS</u>- Discuss the importance of avoiding distractions
6. <u>TRAINING TO REDUCE ERROR-</u> is that even possible?

B. MALADAPTIVE BEHAVIOR DURING A CRISIS- Briefly discuss maladaptive behavior leading into Crisis management as a result of stress secondary to a threat response.

C. SYSTEMS ISSUES AND TEAMWORK: Briefly discuss the need to understand the importance of teamwork in this error prone environment

HOW DOES HUMAN ERROR RELATE TO CRISIS MANAGEMENT?

When disaster strikes, human error may be a primary, secondary or combined component during the event. We typically think of human error as the direct cause of any negative event (such as I just transected the common bile duct or ordered the wrong medication, or dose) but error can play a secondary role when the team misses the opportunity to mitigate a disaster created by external events or a mistake. In some cases, a single event can be propagated by a multitude of sequential errors.

As reviewed in detail in ***CRISIS MANAGEMENT LEADERSHIP IN THE OPERATING ROOM: prepare your team to survive any crisis***, adverse events in health care were a bit of an unknown until the publication of the 1999 Institute of Medicine report. Since that report became public, multiple studies and malpractice reviews have linked the initiation or perpetuation of adverse events and crises to human error and communication breakdown. Failure to manage these events can quickly transform them into a DISASTER! Similarly, the same human factor mistakes implicated in adverse events, cause loss of situational awareness (or blindness) to the problem directly in front of us, resulting in delayed or complete failure to respond to the crisis that is unfolding before our eyes- we just ignore the obvious. Clearly, any organization interested in prevention of adverse events or rapid response to a critical situation MUST understand and pass along this knowledge of human factor errors.

Human Error: The Hidden Core of Adverse Events

Human error remains one of the most significant contributors to organizational crises and adverse outcomes. As **Dr. James Diehl,** author of *Does Cockpit Management Training Reduce Pilot Error?*, explained to me in a personal conversation, studies in both **aviation** and the **United States Coast Guard** have demonstrated that the majority of aircraft and cutter failures stem from human error. Importantly, they also showed that **team training** can either prevent such failures altogether or equip teams to respond appropriately and avert disaster.

In our conversation, Dr. Diehl recalled that aviators and the Federal Aviation Administration were **initially resistant** — even in the 1980s — to acknowledging the role of human error. It was far more comfortable to attribute failures to mechanical issues or external forces than to internal human factors. Diehl

James Reason, in *Managing the Risks of Organizational Accidents*, defines human error as *"the failure of planned actions to achieve their desired goals — without the intervention of some unforeseeable event."* In other words, most human errors arise not from negligence or malice, but from normal cognitive limitations within imperfect systems. Reason

In the aftermath of any disaster, however, it remains easier — and emotionally satisfying — to **blame individuals** than to dissect the complex organizational, cultural, and cognitive conditions that enabled the failure. This tendency to condemn rather than analyze explains why **error reporting and analysis** remain inconsistent, incomplete, and often underutilized in healthcare.

Evidence from Healthcare: The Fabri Study

A 2008 study by **Dr. Peter Fabri** and colleagues provides a striking illustration. Reviewing **9,830 surgical procedures**, they found that **78.3%** of all complications were associated with a **medical error**. In **three-quarters** of those cases, the error contributed to more than half of the adverse outcome. Most alarmingly, in **25%** of cases the patient either **died or sustained permanent injury.**

Unlike many studies that emphasize system or communication failures, Fabri's data showed those accounted for only **4%** of complications. Instead, the majority reflected **human performance issues**:

- **Errors of technique** – 63.5%
- **Mistakes (doing the wrong thing)** – 20%
- **Slips (doing the right thing incorrectly)** – 58%
- **Errors in judgment** – 29.6%
- **Inattention to detail** – 29.3%
- **Incomplete understanding of the problem** – 22.7%

When I discussed these findings with Dr. Fabri, he emphasized that during the entire study period, **no sentinel events** were reported — yet countless errors still occurred. "For every sentinel event that makes the headlines," he estimated, "a thousand other errors take place quietly, unnoticed, and unreported." Fabri

The Broader Lesson

These findings underscore an uncomfortable truth: **our most frequent failures are not mechanical or systemic — they are human.**
And yet, because most do not culminate in tragedy, they remain hidden.

Like aviation in the 1980s, medicine continues to grapple with resistance to acknowledging human error as a natural part of complex performance. Until we shift from blame to understanding, from condemnation to **learning**, our systems will remain vulnerable to repeating the same preventable patterns.

INEVITABLY, OUR FAILURE (OR DELAY) TO RECOGNIZE A THREATENING CHANGE IN OUR ENVIRONMENT IS DIRECTLY ATTRIBUTED TO THESE FACTORS!

IS THERE ANY VALUE IN LEARNING ABOUT HUMAN ERROR AND IT'S RELATIONSHIP TO NEGATIVE CONSEQUENCES IN PATIENT CARE?

Before we start this section, I might address this question from the outset. ONE, previously Dr. Carol-Ann Moulton warned me that attempting to force trainees to second guess their actions can potentially paralyze them. As we will discuss, our brain rapidly fills in the gaps for us so we can move quickly but keep in mind that heuristics is built for speed, not accuracy. TWO, training to recognize and avoid error before it occurs is difficult, but as Pat Croskerry discussed with me (see below) it is not impossible. With this knowledge I have become more aware, but let's face it, I am still at risk due to the conditions to be discussed in a moment.

If these caveats are true then why bother with this education?

Personally, I have found understanding the origination of error helps me understand my limitations and from that I understand:

1. **TEAMWORK PAYS OFF**: I have learned to heed words of warning from others (it does not hurt to stop and consider what they are saying) and I monitor others for potential errors in crucial steps in a process.
2. **STOP GAPS**: I utilize a brief mental pause before I start a crucial part of a procedure, especially a point of no return, that all is well. Some pauses deserve a team reminder.
3. **TEAM MONITORING**: Trauma teams have learned that by having a Trauma lead standing at the foot of the bed, who is not occupied in any specific activities, situational awareness can be maintained and it is less likely to miss something.

http://crisislead.blogspot.com/2016/10/interview-with-carol-anne-moulton.html

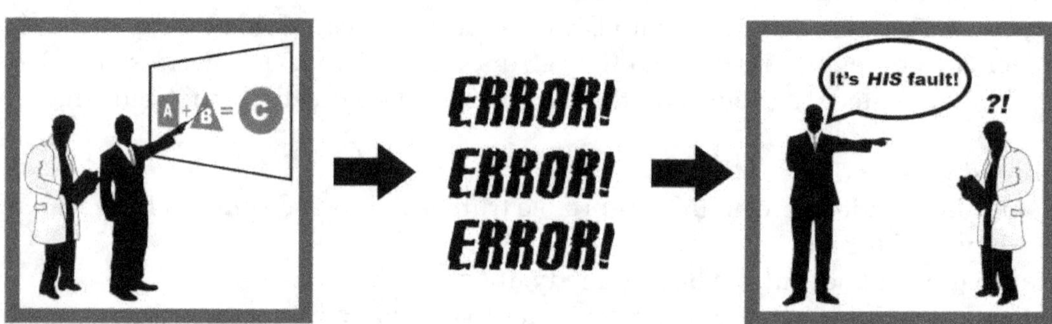

Regardless of pre-emptive planning, a non-contemplative / reactive investigational review may assume guilt and assign blame rather that a root cause analysis as it is quicker to condemn individuals or teams rather than understand the progression of events. Vincent

EFFECTS OF HINDSIGHT BIAS AFTER ACCIDENT OCCURRENCE:

After any untoward event, it is not uncommon for people to automatically assume that the person most closely associated with that event did something wrong. In spite of all the planning to prevent misadventures from occurring and the resemblance of a supporting organization, after most events associated with a poor outcome, a reactive investigational review assumes that an individual or team is totally responsible for the negative outcome. It is easier to condemn individuals or a team than to understand the underlying issues responsible for a bad outcome. Assuming that error was the sole cause of the event is typically easier for individuals or entire systems to accept rather than accept that there were multiple causes to the event. Vincent

"ERRORS UPSTREAM AND DOWNSTREAM TO THE U.P. ASSOCIATED WITH WRONG SURGERY EVENTS IN THE VHA."

"The Universal Protocol has been associated with prevention of wrong surgery procedures; however, such events still occur." Of 308 Root Cause Analysis (RCA) reports of wrong surgery events, 48 (16%) would have occurred despite adherence to the universal Protocol and a well-performed time out. "Future prevention of wrong surgery events will require diligence upstream and downstream from the UP, the participation and communication between multiple stakeholders, and application of new technologies and procedures". Paull DE, et al Am Jnl Surgery July 2015

The natural assumption has been that when a wrong site spine surgery (WSSS) occurs it is due to the surgeon violating standard protocol of the universal protocol and level marking with a fixed device. After meeting with several spine surgeons to discuss the persistence of WSSS it was clear that this was not always the case and that other solutions should be sought as follows:

A. Education is necessary to all staff to assure everyone is aware that in spite of following protocols, mistakes are still possible due to:
1. Distraction, Fatigue
2. Routineness of procedure: Complacency
3. Communication problems including handoff
4. Equipment or Staff problems during localization.
5. Patient characteristics: body habitus, spinal deformities, vertebral morphological variant.
6. Confirmation Bias: accepting of inadequate views due to positioning in lieu of alternate / additional imaging or secondary confirmation with additional expert

B. Repeat localization images if the incision is changed, the patient is moved or the retractors are moved.
C. Assure preoperative and intraoperative images are visible to ALL team members.
D. Routine use of second surgeon / Radiologist who assesses the validity of the level in difficult cases as noted above at a minimum and if possible in all cases (need change in technology so that the radiologist can see the image and see what the surgeon sees).
E. Establish sterile cockpit and absolute concentration w/ no distractions during crucial stages. Lipshy Am J Surg 2016

WHAT GORILLA?

Perception, Cognition, and the Missed "Gorilla"

Shortly after the introduction of **laparoscopic cholecystectomy** in the early 1990s, it became apparent that **laparoscopic common bile duct injuries (LCBDIs)** were occurring at nearly **twice the rate** seen with traditional open procedures. The early assumption was clear and damning: such injuries represented **care below the standard**, and only **inexperienced surgeons** made these mistakes.

That assumption did not hold up under scrutiny.

In 2003, **Dr. Way, Dr. Hunter, and colleagues** reviewed **252 videos** of LCBDI cases. What they discovered challenged the prevailing narrative. In **97% of cases**, the surgeons were **unaware** that an injury had occurred during the operation. These were not reckless or poorly trained operators. Rather, the injuries occurred because of a **visual perception illusion**.

The researchers concluded that the surgeons had become **subconsciously committed** to a mental model that everything was normal. Despite objective evidence to the contrary—clearly visible in retrospect—their **perceptual and cognitive frames** prevented them from recognizing the abnormal anatomy unfolding in real time. They were, quite literally, **blind to the error as it happened.**

This finding underscores a profound truth: even skilled and experienced surgeons are vulnerable to **cognitive bias** and **situational blindness.** When feedback contradicting one's expectation is subtle or arrives under stress, the mind may dismiss it. **Corrective feedback loops** that should trigger a reevaluation often fail to engage.

Subsequent studies have confirmed that **laparoscopy demands higher cognitive load, sustained concentration, and greater mental stress** than open surgery. These stressors amplify the risk of **perceptual and judgment errors**, reinforcing the need for **formal training in intraoperative stress management and cognitive resilience.**

To address these challenges, we must confront a difficult question—one that extends far beyond the operating room:

How can we miss the "gorilla" standing directly in front of us?

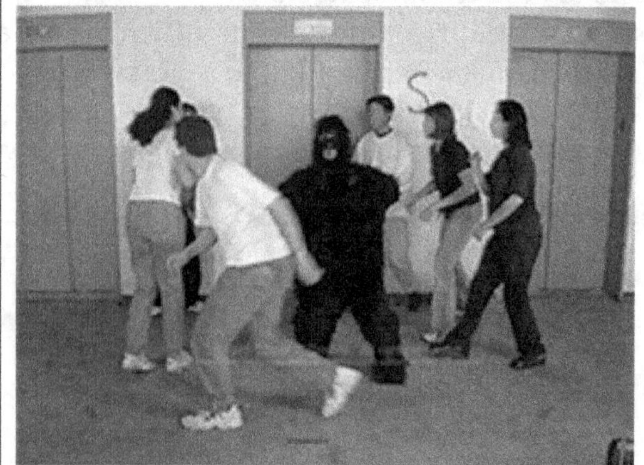

THE HARVARD 'INVISIBLE GORILLA'

- 2004 Harvard Group Nobel Prize in Psychology.
- 50% of participants totally *missed the gorilla.* It was as though the gorilla was invisible.
- We are missing a lot of what goes on around us.
- We have no idea that we are missing so much.

Figure provided by Daniel Simons. @ Simons, D. J., & Chabris, C. F. (1999).

Gorillas in our midst: Sustained inattentional blindness for dynamic events.

Perception, 28, 1059-1074. www.dansimons.com; www.theinvisiblegorilla.com

In 1999 Harvard Simons and Chabris designed an experiment where observers were asked to count how many times a basketball was passed around the room. At the end of the experiment, 50% of observers missed that a "Gorilla" passed through the middle of the room and stood in the middle of the players for several seconds before moving off to the side. It was as if the Gorilla was totally invisible. [Simons]

Daniel Kahneman (author of *Thinking, Fast and Slow*) summarized this to me as:

a. "We can be blind to the obvious."

b. "We are also blind to our blindness." [Kahneman]

Humans' innate habit of missing the "gorilla" in the room can be costly in terms of dollars and potentially lives lost.

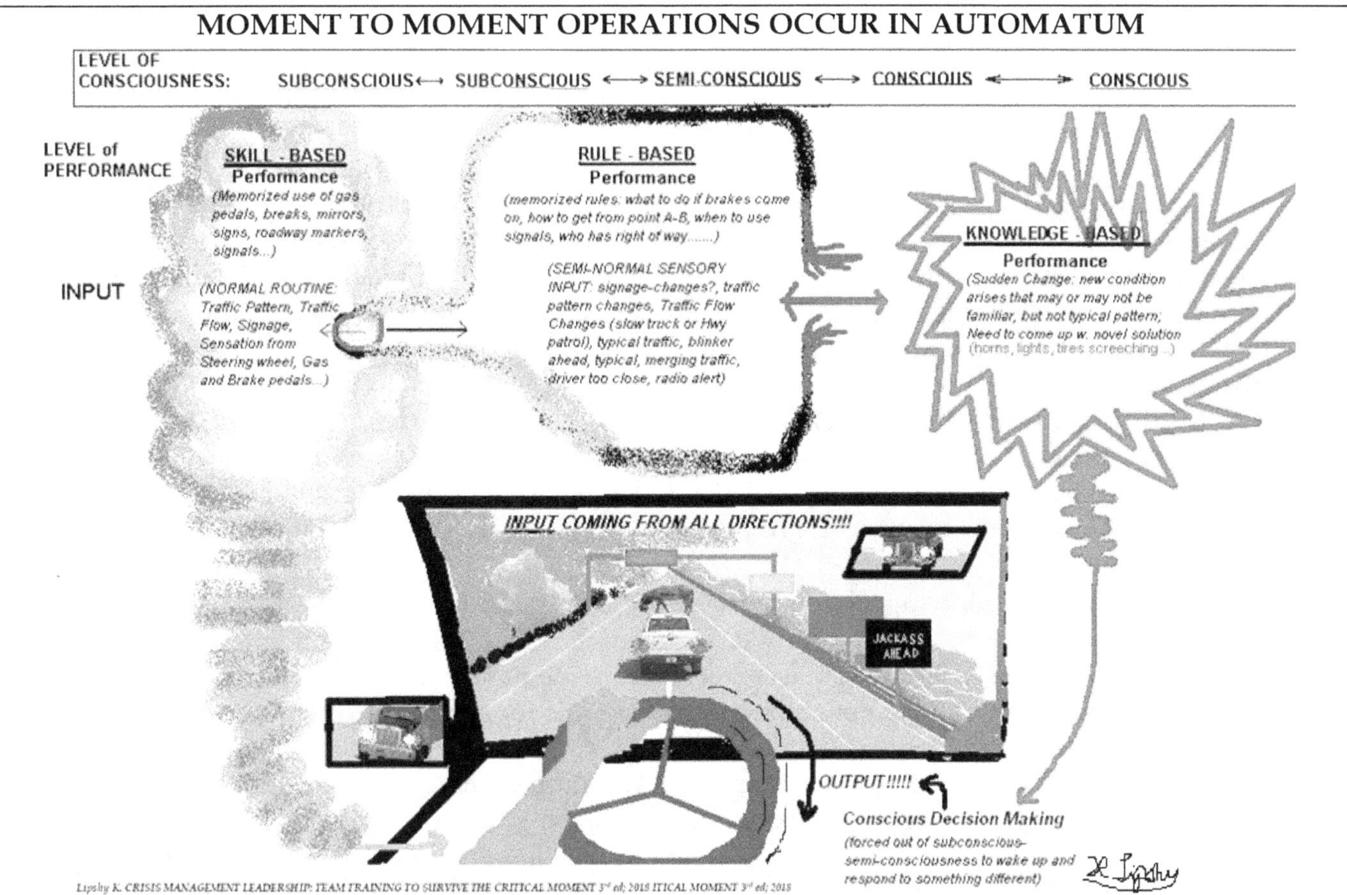

Lipshy K. CRISIS MANAGEMENT LEADERSHIP: TEAM TRAINING TO SURVIVE THE CRITICAL MOMENT 3rd ed; 2018 ITICAL MOMENT 3rd ed; 2018

The majority of the time we function under the *Skill-Based level of performance*. This performance level consists predominately at the automatic level. We have subconscious input that is processed using memorized sets of actions. Our brain takes in this subconscious sensory input, analyzes it into the most probable construct based on past experience and produces a subconscious action (Heuristics). We see the normal traffic pattern on our typical way to work. We start the car, pull out of the drive, use the gas, brakes, turn signals, steering wheel with very little thought. This process is fast and reasonably accurate (but not completely).

When a new variable opens up for us, we move into the *Rule-Based Level of performance*. This forces us temporarily out of the "ozone" and into reality (semi-consciousness) for brief periods of time. Someone pulls in front of us, traffic slows down, a traffic alert overhead, etc., causing us to wake up and adjust into a semiconscious area. We still use prior rules and behavior learned previously but we are not required to stay there for long. We go back to listening to the radio, pushing the gas pedal, occasionally looking in the mirror, etc.

Sudden changes, especially when these are unexpected or in our distant memory, force us into alertness (consciousness). We may attempt to solve these using skill-based or rule-based behaviors, but this is unsuccessful so we need to process and perform using *Knowledge-based* skill sets.
Someone slams on their brakes ahead or some obstacle appears and traffic comes to a halt. We need to wake up and determine what to do next (sit and wait, look for an alternate route, get out of the way of emergency vehicles, etc.). The real problems come in if we mentally do not accept that the situation has changed and remain in lower levels of function This may or may not be effective depending on the level of change, the level of threat, the need to rapidly make alternate decisions. We probably will end up with erroneous analysis of the situation leading to an erroneous action. The skill-based and rule-based performance levels are typically very fast but do not provide what we need when something is unexpected and new to us. Unfortunately, knowledge-based behavior is slow and typically cannot keep

up with these scenarios. Solutions? Yes, we train for these types of scenarios using knowledge-based behavior until they become skill-based.

The Rasmussen SRK model described error in judgement based upon these skill-based, rule-based, and knowledge-based cognitive functions as follows:

Skill-based are slips/lapses in routine tasks (e.g., putting keys in the fridge); **Rule-based**are applying the *wrong* rule (e.g., using an old pump's settings for a new one); and **Knowledge-based** are errors in novel situations due to insufficient understanding (e.g., trial-and-error when a new machine breaks). These help move beyond blaming workers to understanding *why* errors happen for better system fixes, with skill-based being most reliable and knowledge-based least reliable.

Types of Errors
- **Skill-Based Errors (Slips & Lapses):**
    - **When:** Performing familiar, routine tasks (e.g., driving, typing).
    - **Why:** Lack of attention, distraction, fatigue, or switching tasks.
    - **Example:** Forgetting to put the car in park before getting out.
- **Rule-Based Errors (Mistakes):**
    - **When:** Following a known procedure but applying it incorrectly or using an outdated rule.
    - **Why:** Misapplication of a correct rule, inadequate plan, or flawed assumptions.
    - **Example:** Using a general maintenance rule for a specific, different piece of equipment.
- **Knowledge-Based Errors (Mistakes):**
    - **When:** Facing a new or unexpected situation with no pre-set rules.
    - **Why:** Insufficient knowledge, poor problem-solving, or cognitive overload.
    - **Example:** Trying to diagnose a complex, unique machine failure without enough information.

Adapted from *Rasmussen, Jens* (May–June 1983). "Skills, rules, and knowledge; signals, signs, and symbols, and other distinctions in human performance models". IEEE Transactions on Systems, Man, and Cybernetics.* SMC-131983 *(3): 257–266.* doi:*10.1109/TSMC.1983.6313160.* S2CID *1525146 – via IEEE Xplore.*
Cook R, Rasmussen J. 'Going solid': a model of system dynamics and consequences for patient safety. Qual SAF health care. 2005;14:130-13
Deceased 2018

Heuristics: The Brain's "Best Guess" Mechanism

We frequently hear the term heuristics used to describe the brain's ability to process large amounts of information and generate a rapid, experience-based "best guess" about what is happening. Daniel Kahneman defined heuristics as *"a simple procedure that helps find adequate, though often imperfect, answers to difficult questions."*

Heuristics allow us to function efficiently in complex environments. Most of the time, our actions occur at what is known as the skill-based level of performance — the automatic level. Here, subconscious sensory input is continuously processed against stored experience to produce familiar, almost reflexive responses. This level of function is what allows us, for instance, to drive to work along a familiar route while thinking about something entirely different. It is fast, efficient, and generally accurate — until the environment changes.

When something unexpected happens — a car cuts in front of us, traffic slows abruptly, or a warning light flashes — we shift temporarily into the rule-based level of performance. At this stage, we are partially pulled from our automatic "cruise control" mode into a semi-conscious state of awareness. We rely on previously learned rules ("when this happens, do that") to respond and then often slip back into automatic behavior once the situation stabilizes.

However, when a sudden or novel event occurs—something outside our memory or pattern recognition—we are forced into full consciousness. Our subconscious shortcuts and previously learned rules are no longer adequate. We must engage in deliberate, analytical problem-solving—what cognitive scientists refer to as the knowledge-based level of performance.

At this level, we must pause, observe, interpret, and decide using conscious reasoning rather than habit or intuition. It is a slower process but one that is essential when facing unfamiliar or high-stakes situations. As James Reason noted, many critical errors arise when individuals attempt to solve new problems using skill- or rule-based responses instead of engaging the conscious, knowledge-based system.

ERROR INCREASED BY 2 COMMON FACTORS:

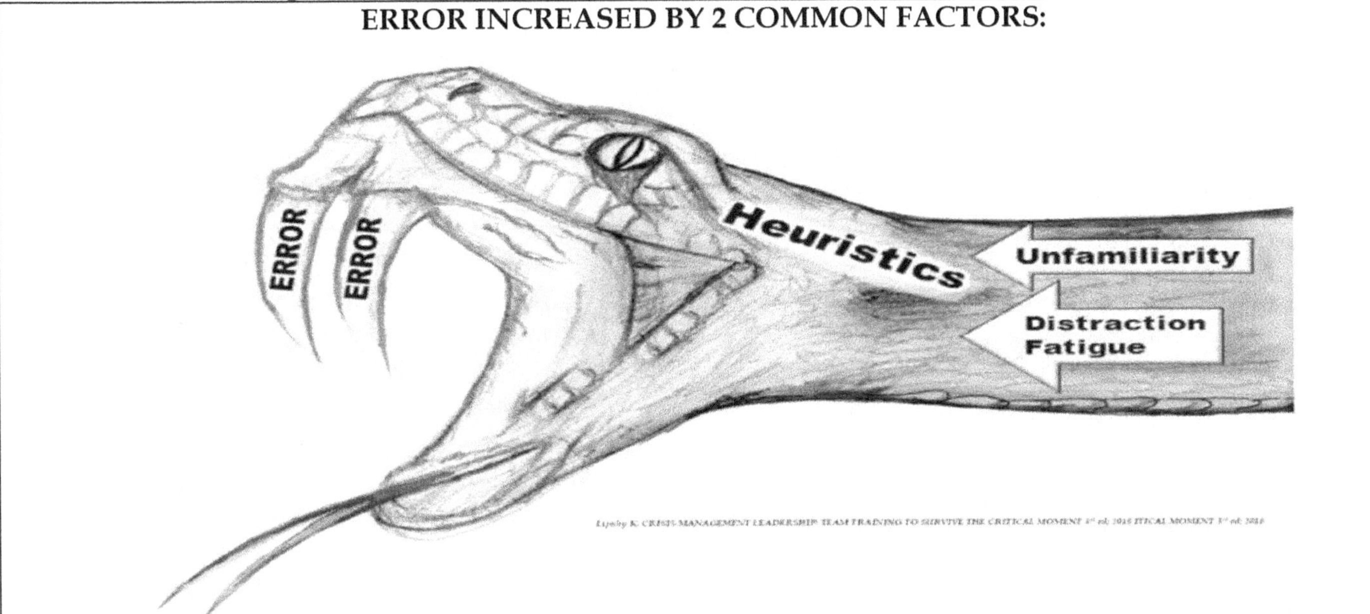

The risk for error increases by the incremental degrees of unfamiliarity of the circumstances and distraction/fatigue. Our innate behavior is to analyze the information put before us as rapidly as possible to develop a solution that is familiar to what is stored in our memory.

Gonzales, Gonzales, Weigman, Sharps, Siddle, Weick, Drawing by Bradley Lipshy

INFLUENCES THAT INCREASE OUR SUSCEPTIBILITY TO HEURISTIC TENDENCIES:
In addition to our **state of arousal**, our tendency to fall prey to prior modeling to sensory input is drastically augmented if we are **unfamiliar** with that stimulus or we are victim to **lapses of consciousness** (**STRESS, ANXIETY, FATIGUE OR DISTRACTION**). Gonzales, Gonzales, Weigman, Sharps, Siddle, Weick
(known in the Anesthesia and Emergency Medicine world as the HALTS: Hungry, Angry, Late or Lazy, Tired, or Sick)

WHY DON'T WE RECOGNIZE THESE ERRORS? CONFIRMATION BIAS!

- Based on past experience, our mind creates an image where such an image does not really exist.
- It is as though once we commit to a judgment, any contradictory evidence is discounted in favor of any confirmatory evidence

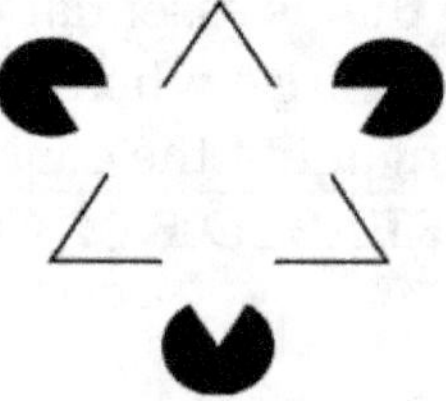

Gaetano Kanizsa triangle

Kanizsa, G. Margini quasi-percettivi in campi con stimolazione omogenea. *Rivista di Psicologia.* 1955;49(1):7–30.

While a *positive attribute* may be that this process works quickly and relatively effectively, on the *negative side*, it potentially can provide faulty solutions. That is, defects in the output can arise as a result of errors at any point in the sequence of input interpretation. Way, Reason, Hastie. Hogarth, Hoffman Reason clearly summarized the potential pitfalls in this processing, as *"the price we pay for this automatic processing of information is that perceptions, memories, thoughts, and actions have a tendency to err in the direction of the familiar and expected."* Reason

Optical illusions are classic examples of how this process can work quickly but can also be deceiving. One early example of how our mind simply fills in the blanks in its attempt to be fast and efficient is the 'Kanizsa' triangle. When we look at the three figures we automatically visualize a white triangle. This triangle itself does not exist, but we persistently see a white triangle that is brighter than the surrounding white area.

Once we commit to a judgment (there must be a triangle there), any contradictory evidence is discounted in favor of any confirmatory evidence (now the triangle will not go away). *Once our mind has made up its mind it is not going to change its mind!* This is known as **CONFIRMATION BIAS**. This is not a character flaw, since cognitive biases seem to be a normal feature in the way Humans reason.Fisher, peterson

Cognitive Bias in Action: When the Mind Sees What It Wants to See
One of the most compelling demonstrations of **confirmation bias and perceptual illusion** is **Edward Adelson's 1995 Checker Shadow experiment**. In this visual illusion, two checkerboard squares—one seemingly in shadow and one in light—appear to be drastically different shades of gray. In reality, they are **exactly the same color**.
The mind, however, interprets the surrounding context and **constructs a "reality"** consistent with what it expects to see. The brain automatically adjusts for lighting, contrast, and shadow, generating a perception that feels undeniably correct yet is entirely false.
(*Adelson E. Checkershadow Experiment, 1995. Massachusetts Institute of Technology. "These checkershadow images may be reproduced and distributed freely."*) See also P292, Lipshy 2013
http://web.mit.edu/persci/people/adelson/checkershadow_downloads.html
This illusion perfectly mirrors what occurs in the operating room, the ICU, and every other high-stakes environment where our perception is filtered through expectation and bias.

Hill-Climbing Heuristics: The Reluctance to Change Course
In our original textbook (page 294), we discussed **Dr. Evie Fioratou's work** exploring why anesthesia teams sometimes fail to perform a surgical airway when endotracheal intubation attempts have repeatedly failed. Her team found that providers often fall victim to a **"hill-climbing heuristic."**

In this model, the brain seeks the most direct route toward a desired goal—in this case, successful intubation—and resists any action that seems to move *away* from that goal. The very act of considering a surgical airway feels like failure, a step "uphill" from the intended path.

One emergency physician I spoke with found a simple, powerful solution:

"Before every intubation, I mark the cricothyroid notch with a marker, place a Betadine-soaked gauze and scalpel on a tray next to the bed, and ask the residents what they'll do if they get into trouble."

By **preparing the cricothyrotomy tray in advance**, he reframes the surgical airway as just another tool—not a defeat. This small ritual reduces psychological resistance and transforms an avoided option into a viable, rehearsed contingency.

Confirmation Bias: Seeing What We Expect to See

Confirmation bias occurs when individuals interpret information in a way that confirms their existing beliefs, ignoring evidence that contradicts them. In medicine, this bias can be deadly. The following real-world cases—shared by experienced clinicians—illustrate its impact with painful clarity.

Case 1: The Intubation That Was "Fine"

"We had a patient who vomited right as the anesthesia provider was intubating. The patient deteriorated quickly. I asked the provider several times if he was sure the tube was in place, and he insisted it was fine. When I suggested we reintubate, he became angry—offended that I implied an error. Ten minutes later, another provider removed the tube, reintubated under direct vision, and the patient's hemodynamics improved immediately."

Even highly skilled providers can become **anchored to an assumption**—in this case, that the tube was secure—and interpret all evidence through that lens.

Case 2: The Missing Clamp

"I remember a case where a bulldog clamp was missing. We searched everywhere and took plain films, convinced someone had made a mistake. We even assumed it was thrown away. Finally, someone ordered a lateral chest X-ray—and there it was. We had simply assumed it couldn't possibly still be inside."

Here, **assumption overruled logic.** The team's collective confidence in their own process prevented them from questioning the obvious.

Case 3: The Misplaced Incision

"When I drain an abscess, I always start with a needle to identify the collection. A patient came in two days after the ED drained and packed an abscess. The ED provider said they pulled out *dry* packing—something that should have alerted me. I reopened the same incision, nothing came out. Frustrated, I numbed again, explored deeper—still nothing. Finally, I stepped back, re-evaluated, extended the incision in the opposite direction, and pus poured out like a geyser. I was convinced the first incision had to be correct. Big mistake. I ignored my own pattern of practice."

Even seasoned surgeons are vulnerable to **self-confirmation bias**—the tendency to overvalue prior assumptions, especially when they align with one's own prior experience or ego.

The Broader Lesson

These examples—whether visual illusions, failed airways, or surgical missteps—remind us that **our brains are pattern-making machines**. Under stress, time pressure, or fatigue, we default to the familiar and subconsciously filter out contradictions.

The antidote is not perfection, but **awareness**.

By acknowledging our susceptibility to these biases—and creating deliberate strategies to counter them—we become safer, more reflective leaders and clinicians.

In crisis or calm, humility and vigilance are the true safeguards against the mind's most persuasive illusion: the belief that "I can't be wrong."

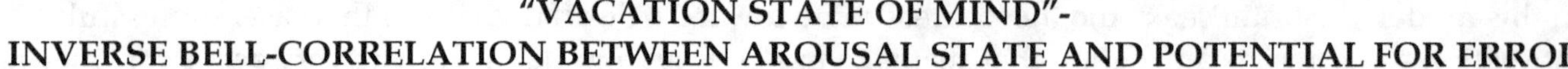

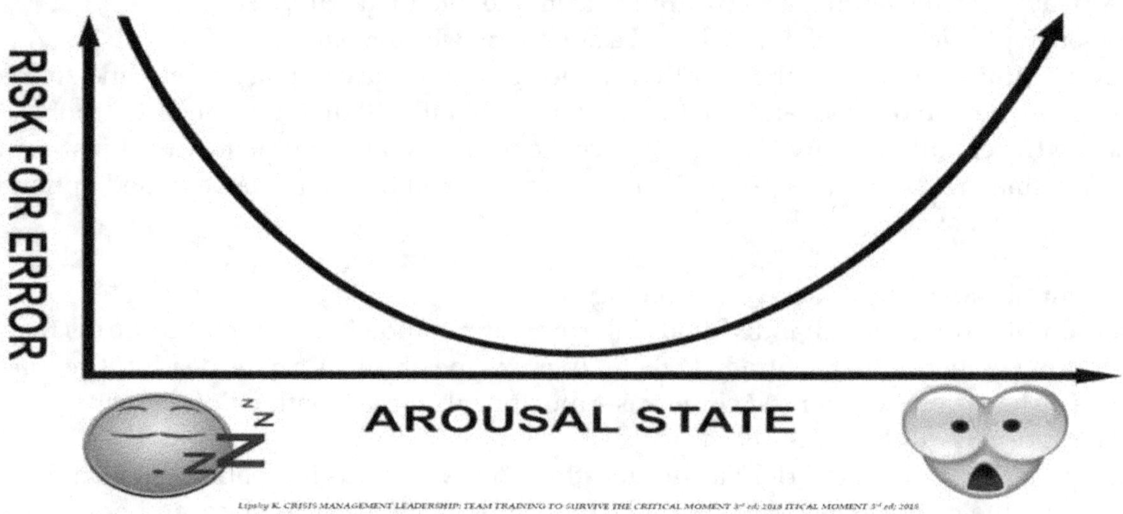

Vacation State of Mind: Risk for error based on arousal state. According to Daniel Kahneman, your risk for making an error is heightened when you are overly relaxed (lazy) and overly stressed or panicked. When you are highly aroused, you tend to be more focused and suspicious.
Adapted with permission from: Kahneman D. *Thinking Fast and Slow*. New York, NY: Farrar, Straus and Giroux; 2011. 62

The Comfort Trap: How Familiarity Breeds Vulnerability

It is human nature to enter a **deep state of skill-based performance** when executing familiar, routine tasks. In this state, actions become automatic, requiring minimal conscious effort. While efficient, this mode of operation can also render us vulnerable when the unexpected occurs.

The **wilderness rescue literature** is replete with cautionary tales of what has been termed the *"vacation state of mind."* This mindset is characterized by:

a) poor preparation,

b) lack of alertness, and

c) loss of situational awareness once one enters a realm of perceived familiarity. Kahneman

In essence, familiarity breeds complacency. When people believe an activity will unfold predictably, they subconsciously down-regulate vigilance. Most of us go through daily life assuming events will proceed normally, with little expectation of surprise. This same pattern—complacency born of routine—appears repeatedly in analyses of **wilderness accidents, aviation errors, and medical crises**. Victims are often not unskilled or careless; they are simply **unprepared for a sudden deviation from the expected.**

As **Nakhleh and Spath** observed, *"Humans do poorly at routine, repetitive tasks. They are susceptible to boredom and distraction."*

Mood and Cognitive Vigilance

Psychologist **Daniel Kahneman**, in *Thinking, Fast and Slow*, describes how mood shapes our cognitive engagement.

- When we are in a **happy or relaxed state**, we tend to let our guard down. We may be more creative and intuitive but also **less vigilant and more prone to error.**
- When we are **sad, tense, or under pressure**, we become more **analytical, suspicious, and deliberate.**

In a personal conversation, Kahneman refered to this as a shift between *cognitive ease* and *cognitive strain*. When the mind is at ease, it prefers shortcuts—relying on intuition and assumption rather than analysis. When under strain, it slows down, double-checks, and seeks control.

It seems counterintuitive, but our greatest cognitive lapses often occur **not in crisis**, but in **comfort**. When we feel safe and relaxed, we are **least likely to question our assumptions or verify our conclusions.**

The Peril of Jumping to Conclusions

The same principle applies to our tendency to **"jump to conclusions."**

In familiar, low-threat environments, this heuristic serves us well—it saves time and mental energy. But in **unfamiliar or high-stakes situations**, premature conclusions can be catastrophic. Acting on incomplete information without pausing for reflection transforms efficiency into error.

In short, **the brain's efficiency under familiarity becomes its liability under surprise.** Personal conversation with Daniel Kahneman

The Takeaway

Whether hiking a familiar trail, flying a routine route, or performing a standard procedure, leaders must guard against the **comfort trap**. Vigilance is not only required in crisis—it must be cultivated in calm. The challenge for every professional is to remain **alert within familiarity** and **analytical within ease**.

The moments that feel safest are often when we are most at risk of missing what matters most.

COMPLACENCY:

"There is no such thing as a low threat day. It is the leader's job to keep the team on the edge and ready to react if needed. We get too complacent and act as if nothing could go wrong. " Lt Dave Grossman 'On Combat' PERSONAL COMMUNICATION

Half the surgeons report having witnessed intraoperative complications directly related to surgeon stress. Most surgeons believed that stress management training would be beneficial in surgery. Anton, Stefanidis et al

Distraction and Performance: Lessons from Aviation to the Operating Room

Over the past several decades, extensive research across high-risk industries has demonstrated the **negative impact of distractions on human performance**. Nowhere has this been studied more rigorously than in aviation, where early recognition of distraction-related accidents led to the development of **"distraction-reducing" protocols** such as **load-shedding** and the **sterile cockpit rule**. These measures—pioneered by Dismukes, Latorella, and others—have since become foundational in aviation safety training and human factors research.

In recent years, medicine has begun to follow suit. Researchers have increasingly turned their attention to the **operating room (OR)** and other procedural settings to better understand how distractions affect team performance and patient safety.

The Wheelock Study: Dissecting Distractions in the Operating Room

In a landmark paper published in the *Annals of Surgery* (June 2015), and in a personal conversation, **Dr. Angela Wheelock** explained they meticulously analyzed the nature and frequency of intraoperative distractions. Their findings were both eye-opening and deeply unsettling:

- On average, they observed **seven distractions per case**—roughly **one every ten minutes**.
- The **most frequent** distraction came from **external personnel entering the OR**, 81% of which were **unnecessary**.
- The second most common was **case-irrelevant conversation** within the surgical team—often initiated by other surgeons—especially during "non-stressful" periods. These off-topic discussions correlated with **poorer team performance**.

Among all sources of disruption, **equipment-related issues** were found to generate the **highest stress levels**, particularly among nursing staff. Although these technical disruptions occurred less frequently—about once every 90 minutes—they produced disproportionate psychological strain.

Acoustic distractions such as **phone calls and pages** also ranked high, causing **increased workload for anesthesia teams** and **heightened stress among surgeons**. One of the study's more surprising findings was that **resident teaching** itself contributed to communication breakdowns; when attendings engaged with residents, **nursing communication to the attending team decreased**, potentially delaying responses to intraoperative needs.

Ultimately, Wheelock's team concluded that even **minor distractions — such as misplaced cautery pedals — can significantly elevate stress and impair performance**.

(*Wheelock A, et al., 2015; Arora S, 2010; Healey AN, et al., 2006–2007; Savoldelli GL, 2010; Sexton JB, 2000; Sevdalis N, 2007–2008; Wiegmann DA, 2007; Zheng B, 2008.*)

The Broader Evidence: How Distraction Impairs Surgical Performance

Subsequent studies have reinforced and expanded on these findings.

- **Sami et al. (2012)** reported that the **primary stressors** experienced by surgeons were **technical difficulties, equipment malfunctions, and team-related factors** — all of which heightened perceived workload and reduced performance.
- **Feuerbacher et al. (2012)** demonstrated that **younger, less experienced surgeons** were particularly vulnerable to distraction. In simulated laparoscopic cholecystectomies, distractions such as phone calls, clanging trays, or unrelated conversations led to **major technical errors**, with **interrupting questions** being the most detrimental.
- **Moorthy et al. (2003)** further confirmed that stressors — such as **verbal mathematical tasks, background noise (80–85 dB)**, and **time pressure** — caused significant increases in errors and reductions in dexterity.
- At the **Mayo Clinic**, a study in **cardiothoracic surgery** revealed that **surgical errors correlated directly with increases in "flow disruptions."** These included **communication failures, equipment problems, extraneous interruptions**, and **training-related distractions**, with **team communication breakdowns** being the strongest predictor of error.

(*Sami et al., 2012; Feuerbacher RL, 2012; Moorthy K, 2003; Mayo Clinic Study, 2015.*)

The Unseen Burden: Fatigue, Burnout, and Environmental Stress

While the aviation industry has spent decades studying environmental stressors, **healthcare has been slower to recognize distraction and fatigue as systemic threats to safety.** Despite the growing body of literature, research into **environmental stress, cognitive load, and distraction within surgical teams** remains sparse.

Yet the implications are undeniable: **fatigue, burnout, and environmental overload** silently erode performance and situational awareness. They create fertile ground for cognitive biases, lapses in vigilance, and teamwork breakdowns.

As in aviation, the solution is not merely to eliminate distractions — an impossible task — but to **train for them**, to **build resilient teams** capable of maintaining composure and focus under dynamic, high-stress conditions.

In the cockpit or the operating room, the threat is rarely the distraction itself — it is the team's failure to recognize, recover, and refocus after it occurs.

ROUTINE DISTRACTIONS INCREASE MISTAKES!

- During a simulated laparoscopic cholecystectomy surgeons (aged 27-37) were distracted by **NOISES***, **QUESTIONS****, **CONVERSATION*****, and **COMMOTION.**
- Younger, less-experienced surgeons are more prone to distraction in the OR - and to make surgical errors as a result.*
- Participants did much worse in the afternoons, although conventional fatigue didn't appear to be an issue.
- 44% of 2nd, 3rd, & research year surgical residents made **serious errors**, particularly when they were being tested in the afternoon.
- By comparison, only 1 surgeon made a mistake when there were no distractions.
- Interrupting questions caused the most major errors (such as damage to internal organs, ducts and arteries), followed by sidebar conversations.
    - *   A cell phone would ring, followed later by a metal tray clanging to the floor.
    - **   Questions posed about problems developing with a previous surgical patient -necessary conversation
    - *** Off to the side talking about politics, a not-so-necessary but fairly realistic distraction

Feuerbacher RL, Funk K, Spight D, Diggs B, Hunter J. Realistic distractions and interruptions that impair simulated surgical performance

---

IN THE O.R., BACKGROUND NOISE
IMPEDES CRITICAL INFORMATION SHARING!

- *Fifteen surgeons with 1-30 years OR experience were tested with the following noise levels:*
    - **Conversational noise levels**: 70 dB vs. Music 74.2 dB
    - **Drills / powered instruments:** 131 to 140 dB
- Average noise levels found in the OR decrease communication effectiveness.
- Even predictable sentences can be distorted by background noise.
- Communication was much WORSE when sound levels are higher.
- **Performance was poorer when the sentences were low in predictability**- While in general, it is much more difficult to communicate when it is noisy, a poor outcome is even more likely when communication involves conversations that carry critical information that is unpredictable in the midst of excessive background noise.

Personnel should be aware that the combination of noise, music, and engagement in a task can lead to substantial breakdowns in communication! Moorthy

---

Minor disturbances during a laparoscopic procedure, such as wrong scissors, can increase patient morbidity and mortality by 40%. way

---

For an interview with the FAA, Dr. Pellegrini and Dr. Baxter in Toronto on Fatigue and Performance, myths and truths, see Appendix C at the end of this book.

SITUATIONAL AWARENESS- Heuristics, distraction, fatigue, and unfamiliarity can lead to loss of situational awareness. Leadership roles in maintaining situational awareness are discussed in sections that follow.

MALADAPTIVE BEHAVIORS SEEN IN RESPONSE TO STRESS / ANXIETY:

One should take a moment to consider that these error prone potentials in our normal human function are seen even when we are not stressed or threatened. As is discussed later in this guide, humans under stress have a heightened risk for maladaptive behavior. Several responses are seen by an observer when a person becomes stressed and anxious and enters a fight or flight mode. There are nine basic categories of maladaptive behavior seen:

- **Sound Anomalies**
- **Inability to speak**
- **Intrusive Thoughts**
- **Automatic Pilot**
- **Memory loss**
- **Sense of time deceleration**
- **Denial**
- **Tunnel Vision**
- **Panic**
- **Over-steering**
- **Dissociation / Paralysis**

(For further discussion on maladaptive response to a threat go to section IV.F. CRITICAL PAUSE - ANXIETY / MALADAPTIVE RESPONSE CONTROL AT THE START OF THE CRITICAL MOMENT MALADAPTIVE BEHAVIORS SEEN IN RESPONSE TO STRESS / ANXIETY)

CAN WE TRAIN OUR BRAIN TO AVOID MAKING ERRORS?

COGNITIVE FORCING STRATEGIES:
TRAIN: Acquire knowledge of error theory and develop a sense of self-awareness for risk for error. Learn pattern recognition approaches.
RECOGNITION: Understand most likely types of error that would be encountered and develop plan to recognize and to address these.
CRITICAL CHECKPOINT PAUSES: Train to take a step back and assess those situations more carefully when these are encountered (Denial, Exclusion, or one goal errors).
PROTOCOLS: Train for and Develop specific protocols for the most predictable and most dangerous errors (Universal Protocol).

Recognizing and Preventing Error: Training the Mind to See What It Misses

Failure to recognize that we are *about to* commit — or have *already* committed — an error is alarmingly common. As discussed previously, this failure lies at the heart of most human and organizational breakdowns. The question, then, is not whether we make errors, but **how we prevent them when they are most likely to occur.**

Cognitive Forcing Strategies: A Mental Guardrail Against Bias

Pat Croskerry, MD, one of the foremost authorities on cognitive error in medicine, described to me in a personal conversation the use of **"cognitive forcing strategies"** — mental techniques designed to *abort latent errors before they manifest.*

According to Croskerry, the foundation for minimizing bias involves principles most of us already practice:

- Providing specific, deliberate **training**, particularly through **simulation.**
- **Decreasing reliance on memory** and simplifying task complexity.
- **Reducing time pressure** whenever possible.
- **Improving feedback loops** and accountability structures.
- And critically, **minimizing distractions** during key decision or procedural moments.

Yet, as Croskerry emphasizes, none of these measures fully address **the moment when an error is imminent** — that instant when intuition collides with uncertainty and our brain doubles down on an incorrect assumption.

So how do we train ourselves to recognize error *as it unfolds*?

Step 1: Develop Insight and Situational Self-Awareness

The first step is to cultivate **self-awareness of our vulnerability to error.**
Experts are not immune to mistakes; they are simply **more aware of when they are at risk.** Experienced professionals recognize when their performance is degrading, when their focus is slipping, or when fatigue and emotion cloud judgment.
This form of **metacognition — thinking about one's own thinking —** enables leaders to self-monitor and self-correct before errors solidify. As Croskerry and others have shown, awareness itself is a protective factor.

Step 2: Train to Step Back and Reflect
The second step is to practice **mental detachment at critical junctures.**
Croskerry advocates for the routine use of what he calls **"reflective pauses."** This involves deliberately stepping back from the immediate situation, even for a second or two, to reassess assumptions and consider alternative explanations.
"You must train yourself to step back from the noise and ask — 'What else could this be?'"
This process, while seemingly simple, builds the habit of **interrupting heuristic thinking —** the fast, automatic mental shortcuts that often lead to bias.

Pattern Recognition: A Double-Edged Sword
Pattern recognition is one of our most powerful cognitive tools — and one of our greatest liabilities. It allows humans (and machines) to process vast amounts of data quickly and recognize familiar configurations, "seeing the forest through the trees." However, as **Jim Holbrook, EdD**, an expert in High Reliability Organization (HRO) principles, reminded me:
"Pattern recognition is a primordial process built for speed, not accuracy."
It is designed to provide rapid answers, not perfect ones. While instinctive or trained responses may often be correct, they are not infallible. Professionals constantly walk a fine line between **missing subtle cues that suggest the wrong course** and **becoming paralyzed by overanalysis.**
The goal of deliberate training is to **tune your filters —** to learn which cues are irrelevant noise and which demand attention. Through repetition, feedback, and simulation, leaders and clinicians can improve their ability to detect meaningful anomalies without succumbing to distraction or hesitation.

As described by **Willink and Babin (*Extreme Ownership*)** and **Rorke Denver (*Damn Few*)**, elite military operators cultivate this skill through scenario repetition. They learn to sense subtle environmental changes — a door slightly ajar, a pattern of silence, a flicker of movement — and act decisively. Sometimes these instincts avert disaster; other times, they lead to false alarms. What matters is the ability to recognize potential anomalies **without losing composure or halting progress.**
In high-risk professions, there is a razor-thin margin between **paralyzing paranoia and justified vigilance.**

Step 3: Anticipate Common Bias Traps
The most common cognitive errors fall into a few predictable categories:
- **One goal–one solution bias:** "There has to be only one problem."
- **Exclusion error:** "It must be anything but this."
- **Denial:** "Everything is fine."

By acknowledging these tendencies, leaders can preemptively build mental checkpoints. At critical moments — after a distraction, when events deviate from plan, or when intuition conflicts with data — pause briefly and ask:
"What am I assuming? What might I be missing?"
This simple act of reflection — taking just seconds — can break the chain of error before it hardens.

Step 4: Establish Standardized Protocols for High-Risk Scenarios
For situations that are inherently error-prone, **written or mental protocols** serve as anchors for decision-making.

The **Universal Protocol** in surgery is a classic example.
Verifying the patient, marking the correct site and laterality, and confirming consent may seem rudimentary, yet these cognitive forcing steps prevent catastrophic outcomes such as wrong-site surgery. Unfortunately, most clinicians develop such forcing strategies only **after** they or a colleague make a mistake. Over time, these experiences accumulate into a personal "library of lessons learned," shaping future vigilance. The goal is to **formalize that wisdom early** — to make it teachable, transferable, and habitual before error occurs.

"Teaching people about bias helps them avoid it," Croskerry told me, "but teaching them to *recognize* it while it's happening — that's the real challenge."
Through awareness, deliberate reflection, and disciplined training, leaders and clinicians can rewire their cognitive instincts — not to eliminate error, but to catch it before it catches them.
(Croskerry P., "Cognitive Forcing Strategies in Clinical Decision-Making and Diagnostic Failure.")

<table>
<tr><td>

FAILURE TO RECOGNIZE A PATTERN CAN SPELL DISASTER:

"We learned the hard way that failure to recognize a pattern can be disastrous. After canoeing all day, we camped above a waterfall at the confluence of two rivers. Thunderstorms pushed through during the night. When we awoke in the am, we were surprised to see that the water level was up about 2 feet. If that was not enough, we marveled at the rapid flow of the large trees floating downstream and commented that we would reach our destination much sooner than we had planned. It was not until we heard the locomotive roar of the falls that we realized our stupidity in failing to put all this together."

</td></tr>
<tr><td>

TRAIN TO LOOK FOR AND RESPOND TO DISCREPANCIES (THE CHANGES YOU DID NOT EXPECT "It just does not look right").

One should identify potential circumstances in their profession that could result in a catastrophe and rehearse these under controlled circumstances to gain the mental and muscle memory needed to respond appropriately in an emergency. Example-practice engine failure in controlled circumstances. Remember that a discrepancy to an novice may be entirely different to an experienced person. To a novice a scenario may be novel and problematic while that same scenario may not be of any concern to the experienced person because they have seen or heard of this and know what to do. The more experienced person will note the way an inexperienced person will react to a crisis in their verbal and physical reaction. In some cases, it may be obvious that the novice has not picked up on the changes/discrepancy in total but their subconscious knows something is not right. An experienced person can use this to realize when an inexperienced person may need more training.

The question should then come to mind of how do you recognize that what you are experiencing is a new experience vs a known experience and do you know you are using the correct scenario solution? You cannot train for everything but if you train well, when a deteriorating situation occurs, you apply what you know (pattern recognition) and pay attention looking for the expected response. If that does not occur, then begin the process of looking for another known experience. The real problem is when you become misdirected and don't realize it. Your perspective (experience, personality, prejudices) can often lead you to miss the discrepancy; it can be very difficult to step back and understand why you are failing to realize the problem in front of you- recognition and training should help.

</td></tr>
<tr><td>

RECOGNIZING A MISTAKE BEFORE IT OCCURS:

"I had not heard anything about a patient's labs yet and I needed to reorder the PPN for another provider who was on leave. I checked the labs and the Glucose was 890! My knee jerk reaction was that this person was just placed on PPN and he must not have tolerated it and needed some insulin in the bag. It struck me as odd though so just paused for a moment and then I checked his past sugars and they were all fine. It hit me that lab result must be wrong so asked the nurses if they checked a finger stick yet and they had not, so they did. It was 143."

</td></tr>
</table>

ERRORS OF OMMISSION OR COMMISSION

In our discussion about the book *Crew Resource Management for the Fire Service*, Represntative Lubnau mentioned that under duress 60% of **FIRE FIGHTER** errors are those of COMMISSION -where we carry out a task incorrectly and the rest are errors of OMMISSION - where we neglected to carry out a task element.

Dr. Carla Pugh (University of Wisconsin) presented their assessment of residents' success or failure to recognize an operative error occurred (typically errors of commission or omission) and their comprehension of the steps necessary to adapt to the new uncertain situation- i.e. reverse/salvage the error. (D'Angelo AL, Pugh CM et al) Their study highlighted two major questions:

1. Do we rehearse the case in advance to identify the most likely critical points where a mistake is going to occur allowing us to pause and assure the mistakes are avoided? Dr. Pat Croskerry advised me that this is an opportunity in critical thinking we often avoid but need to address. Dr's Zenati and Tarola in West Roxbury discussed with me their use of the HUB system to introduce alerts during cardiac bypass and valve procedures. These alerts notify the team at critical steps where the team needs to focus on and avoid errors of omission.

2. Do we have the capability to understand when an error occurs what mechanics are needed to salvage / reverse the error?

TEAMWORK:

Hopefully by now it is readily apparent that as an individual we are susceptible to mistakes. One thing I have learned from the past is that if you continually ignore or refute your teammates and their suggestions you will miss an error sooner or later. Secton IV.I. FOLLOWERSHIP, TEAMS and TEAMWORK! Covers the essentials of teamwork. Healthcare is extremely complicated and success in avoiding error and increasing the safety of our patients and staff is NOT a one person venture. Our world is far more complex than the other High Reliability Organizations and we simply have to help one another and assist in preventing the perpetuation of an errro.

Chapter III Human Error References

- Adelson E Checkershadow Experiment *http://web.mit.edu/persci/people/adelson/checkershadow_downloads.html accessed October 30 2012; ©1995.*
- Arora S, Sevdalis N, Nestel D, Tierney T, Woloshynowych M, Kneebone R. Managing intraoperative stress: what do surgeons want from a crisis training program. *Am J Surg.* 2009;197(4):537-543.
- Arora S, Hull L, Sevdalis N, et al. Factors compromising safety in surgery: stressful events in the operating room. *Am J Surg.* 2010;199:60–65.
- Arora S, Sevdalis N, Nestel D, et al. The impact of stress on surgical performance: a systematic review of the literature. *Surgery.* 2010;147:318–330.
- Arora S, Tierney T, Sevdalis N, et al. The Imperial Stress Assessment Tool (ISAT): a feasible, reliable and valid approach to measuring stress in the operating room. *World J Surg.* 2010;34:1756–1763.
- Callison, D; Key Words, Concepts and Methods for Information Age Instruction: A Guide to Teaching Information Inquiry.
- Croskerry P. Cognitive Forcing Strategies in Clinical Decision-making. Ann Emerg Med 2003; 41(1):110-120.
- Croskerry P. Diagnostic Failure: A cognitive and Affective approach. *In Advances in Patient Safety: From research to Implementation (Vol 2:Concepts and Methodology.*, Henriksen K, Battles JB, Marks ES, Lewin DI. Rockville MD. Agency for Healthcare Research and Quality; 2005.
- D'Angelo AL, Law K, Cohen E, Ray R, Shaffer DW, Pugh C. Error management: Do residents Identify Operative Errors as Reversible? Annual Meeting of the Association for Surgical Education Conference Dates: 12-16 April 2016 Location: Boston, Massachusetts.
- Denver R. Damn Few: making the modern SEAL warrior. New York, NY: Hyperion; 2013.
- Diehl, A. *"Does cockpit management training reduce aircrew error?"* Proceedings of the Twenty-Second International Seminar of the International Society Of Air Safety Investigators. Canberra, Australia. November 4-7, 1991. *ISASI Forum.*1991;24(4):46.
- Dismukes K, Young G, Sumwait R. Cockpit interruptions and distractions: effective management requires a careful balancing act. *Aviat Safety Rep Syst Directline.* 1998;10:4–9.
- Fabri PJ, Zayas-Castro JL. Human error, not communication and systems, underlies surgical complications. Surgery. 2008;144(4):557-565.
- Feuerbacher RL, Funk K, Spight D, Diggs B, Hunter J. Realistic distractions and interruptions that impair simulated surgical performance by novice surgeons. *Arch Surg.* 2012;147(11):1026-1030.
- Fioratou E, Flin R. No simple fix for fixation errors: cognitive processes and their clinical applications. *Anaesthesia.* January 2010;65(1):61-69.
- Fischer J. Editorial opinion: is damage to the common bile duct during laparoscopic cholecystectomy an inherent risk of the operation. *Am J Surg* 2009;197:829-832.
- Gonzales L. *Deep Survival: Who Lives, Who Dies and Why.* New York, NY: WW Norton; 2003.
- Gonzales L. *Everyday Survival: Why Smart People Make Dumb Mistakes.* New York, NY: WW Norton; 2008.
- Hassan I, Weyers P, Maschuw K, et al. Negative stress-coping strategies among novices in surgery correlate with poor virtual laparoscopic performance. *Br J Surg.* 2006;93(12):1554-1559.

- Hastie R, Dawes RM. *Rational Choice in an Uncertain World, the Psychology of Judgment and Decision Making*. Thousand Oaks, CA: Sage Publications; 2001.
- Healey AN[1], Primus CP, Koutantji M. Quantifying distraction and interruption in urological surgery. Qual Saf Health Care. 2007 Apr;16(2):135-9.
- Healey AN, Sevdalis N, Vincent CA. Measuring intra-operative interference from distraction and interruption observed in the operating theatre. *Ergonomics*.2006;49:589–604.
- Hoffman DD. *Visual Intelligence: How We Create What We See*. New York, NY: WW Norton and Co.; 1998.
- Hogarth RM. *Educating Intuition*. Chicago, IL: University Chicago Press; 2001.
- Institute of Medicine, Committee on Quality Health Care in America. Crossing the Quality Chasm: A new health system for the 21st century. Committee on quality of health care in America. Washington, D.C.: National Academies Press; 2001.
- Kahneman D. *Thinking Fast and Slow*. New York, NY: Farrar, Straus and Giroux; 2011.
- Lipshy KA. Invited response to Paull et al, errors upstream and downstream to the universal protocol associated with wrong surgery events. Am J Surg. 2016 Apr;211(4):827-9. doi: 10.1016/j.amjsurg.2015.07.035. Epub 2016 Feb 23.
- Moorthy K, Munz Y, Dosis A, Bann S, Darzi A. The effect of stress-inducing conditions on the performance of a laparoscopic task. *Surg Endosc*. 2003;17(9):1481–1484.
- Nakhleh RE. Error reduction in surgical pathology. Arch Pathol Lab Med. 2006;130(5):630-632
- Paul DE, Mazzia LM, Neily J, Mills PD, Turner JR, Gunnar W, Hemphill R. Errors upstream and downstream to the universal protocol associated with wrong surgery events in the Veterans Health Administration. Am Jnl Surg 2015;210(1):6-13.
- Reason J. *Human error*. New York, NY: Cambridge University Press; 1990.
- Reason J. Understanding adverse events: human factors. *Qual Health Care*. June 1995;4(2):80-89.
- Reason J. *Managing the Risks of Organizational Accidents*. Burlington, VT: Ashgate; 1997.
- Sami A, Waseem H, Nourah A, Areej A, Afnan A, Ghadeer A,[1] Abdulaziz A, and Arthur A.Real time observations of stressful events in the operating room. Saudi J Anaesth. 2012; 6(2):136–139.
- Savoldelli GL, Thieblemont J, Clergue F, et al. Incidence and impact of distracting events during induction of general anaesthesia for urgent surgical cases. *Eur J Anaesthesiol*. 2010;27:683–689.
- Sevdalis N, Davis R, Koutantji M, et al. Reliability of a revised NOTECHS scale for use in surgical teams. *Am J Surg*. 2008;196:184-190.
- Sevdalis N, Undre S, McDermott J, Giddie J, Diner L, Smith G. Impact of Intraoperative Distractions on Patient Safety: A Prospective Descriptive Study Using Validated Instruments. World J Surg (2014) 38:751–758.
- Sevdalis N[1], Forrest D, Undre S, Darzi A, Vincent C. Annoyances, disruptions, and interruptions in surgery: the Disruptions in Surgery Index (DiSI). World J Surg. 2008 Aug;32(8):1643-50.
- Sevdalis N, Healey AN, Vincent CA. Distracting communications in the operating theatre. *J Eval Clin Pract*. 2007;13:390–394.
- Sexton JB, Thomas EJ, Helmreich RL. Error, stress, and teamwork in medicine and aviation: cross sectional surveys. *BMJ*. March 2000;320(7237): 745–749.
- Sharps MJ. *Processing Under Pressure: Stress, Memory and Decision-Making in Law Enforcement*. Flushing, NY: Looseleaf Law Publications; 2010
- Siddle B. *Sharpening the Warriors Edge: The Psychology and Science of Training*. 10th ed. Belleville, IL: PPCT Research publications; 2008.
- Simons D, Chabris C. Gorillas in our midst: sustained inattentional blindness for dynamic events. *Perception*. 1999;28(9):1059-1074.
- Vincent C. *Patient safety*. Chichester, UK: Wiley-Blackwell; 2010
- Vincent C, Moorthy K, Sarker SK, Chang A, Darzi AW. Systems approach to surgical quality and safety. *Ann Surg*. 2004;239(4):475-482.
- Way LW, Stewart L, Gantert W, et al. Causes and prevention of laparoscopic bile duct injuries: analysis of 252 cases from a human factors and cognitive psychological approach. *Ann Surg*. 2003;237(4):460-469.
- Weick KE, Sutcliffe KM, *Managing the Unexpected: Resilient Performance in an Age of Uncertainty*. San Francisco, CA: John Wiley; 2007.
- Wheelock A, Suliman A, Wharton R, Babu E, Hull L, Vincent C, Sevdalis N, Arora S. The Impact of Operating Room Distractions on Stress, Workload, and Teamwork. Ann Surg 2015; 261(6):1079–1084.
- Wiegmann DA, El Bardissi AW, Dearani JA, Daly RC, Sundt TM Disruptions in surgical flow and their relationship to surgical errors: an exploratory investigation. *Surgery*. 2007;142(5):658-665.
- Willink J, Babin Leif. Extreme Ownership: how U.S. Navy SEALs Lead and Win. St. Martin's Press. NY NY 2015.
- Zheng B, Martinez DV, Cassera MA, et al. A quantitative study of disruption in the operating room during laparoscopic antireflux surgery. *Surg Endosc*.2008;22:2171.
- http:// crisislead.blogspot.com/2016/10/interview-with-carol-anne-moulton.html

IV. CRISIS MANAGEMENT LEADERSHIP DURING THE *CRITICAL MOMENT*: MANAGING ANXIETY, MALADAPTIVE BEHAVIOR, LEADERSHIP, FOLLOWERSHIP, COMMUNICATION, RAPID PROCESS DECISION MAKING UNDER DURESS- HOW TO SURVIVE THE CRITICAL MOMENT

- Introduction to time critical decision making.
- Bringing order to chaos: the critical pause during the critical moment.
- Problem recognition-problem solving pathways.
- The first step in solving a problem is to recognize there is a problem!
- Situational awareness vs load shedding.
- Anxiety and maladaptive behavior.
- Leadership under duress.
- SA-Situational Awareness.
- Followership.
- Communication.
- Time critical decision making.
- Words of advice from experienced chiefs.
- Debriefing.

IV.A. INTRODUCTION TO LEADERSHIP UNDER DURESS: RESILIENCE - THE ABILITY TO RETURN TO A NORMAL STATE FOLLOWING AN ADVERSITY.

THE CRITICAL MOMENT- the **decisive moment** when all hell has broken loose and **the team relies on their leader to establish a sense of control and order to the confusion**. The faster a team returns to a **stable state** the higher the likelihood of surviving. The sooner the team has a sense of normalcy, the sooner they become functional again. There is potential for a successful pathway to the return to normalcy during a crisis, but that all depends on the ability of the team leader and team to

1. Rapidly recognize the situation as being abnormal. SIZE UP THE SITUATION.
2. Control self and team membership behavior.
3. Perform damage control and risk assessment.
4. Develop a plan.
5. Then act (and reassess).

As will be explained, teams that work through this process in sequence can rapidly restore order. Those that panic and attempt to rectify the situation without establishing order, typically worsen the situation. Resiliency depends entirely on optimism, coping mechanisms, and team trust, ALL of which can be trained for in advance. Team leaders must instill optimistic thinking during adversity, as optimistic teams control their own destiny. ^{Sweeney PJ, Matthews MD, Lester PB}

The Myth of Immediate Reaction in Medicine

Clinicians often resist the idea that medicine requires an **organized, methodical process**, believing instead that **immediate action** is always necessary. While this instinct stems from a desire to help—and while there are indeed situations that demand rapid engagement — it is a misconception that *every* medical scenario requires instantaneous reaction.

In some high-risk fields, such as **combat or aviation**, immediate instinctive responses are sometimes the only path to survival. However, medicine rarely mirrors the chaos of an ambush on the battlefield. Only a handful of situations — such as a **sudden airway obstruction** or **massive external hemorrhage** — demand unthinking reflexes and immediate intervention.

In contrast, **most clinical crises** can be managed through a structured, **rational, and analytic process** that, when executed by a well-trained team, can unfold within **two to three minutes** — a span that feels long in panic but short in practice.

Far too often, however, I observe the opposite: **rapid conclusions, raised voices, and diminished listening.** Haste replaces judgment; noise replaces communication. The assumption that speed equals effectiveness can lead teams astray and amplify error.

The key is **discernment** — knowing **when to engage reflexively** and when to **pause, assess, and organize.** Effective teams develop both instincts: the ability to act immediately when the situation demands it, and the discipline to apply deliberate structure when it does not.

IV.B. BRINGING ORDER TO CHAOS: IT ALL STARTS WITH THE CRITICAL PAUSE DURING THE CRITICAL MOMENT

STOP!!! It all seems pretty simple: *restore order, perform damage control, perform a risk assessment, contain further damage, make a plan, execute the plan and then reassess.* Unfortunately, in the midst of a crisis, these steps are frequently averted and short cuts to resolution sought, usually leading to **discord and disaster!**

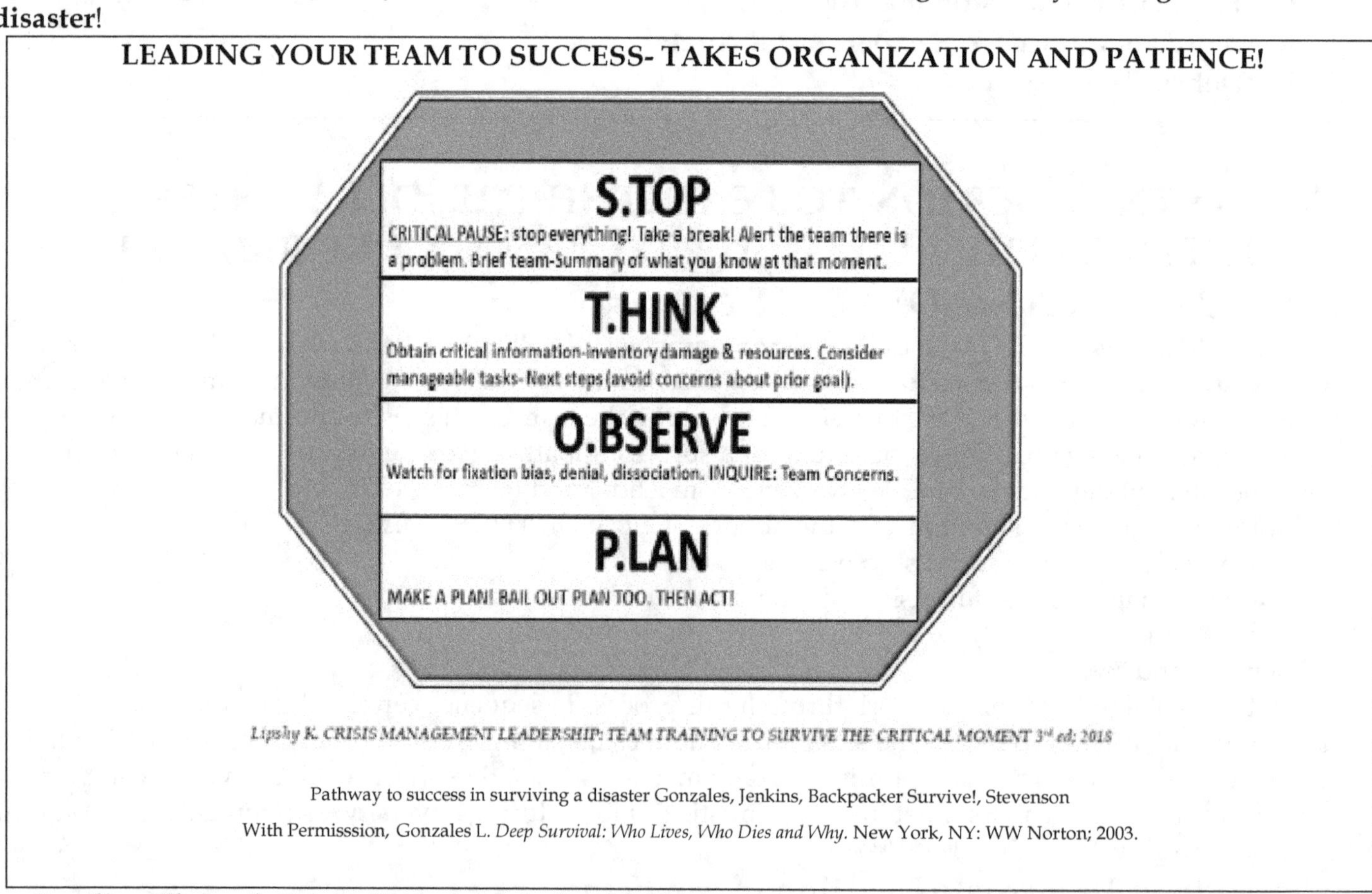

Lipshy K. CRISIS MANAGEMENT LEADERSHIP: TEAM TRAINING TO SURVIVE THE CRITICAL MOMENT 3rd ed; 2018

Pathway to success in surviving a disaster Gonzales, Jenkins, Backpacker Survive!, Stevenson

With Permisssion, Gonzales L. *Deep Survival: Who Lives, Who Dies and Why.* New York, NY: WW Norton; 2003.

Leading Through Crisis: Organized Action in Chaos

Leading a team through a crisis demands **organization**. The wrong steps taken at the wrong time can compound confusion and turn a manageable event into disaster. High-risk industries have developed complex crisis protocols for such situations, but for those who do not operate in these environments daily, it helps to rely on a **simple, memorable framework**.

Under stress, when cognitive load peaks and panic threatens to take over, **simplicity saves lives**. Laurence Gonzales, in *Deep Survival*, describes one of the most effective algorithms for regaining control: **S.T.O.P. — Stop, Think, Observe, Plan.**

S.T.O.P. — A Mnemonic for Crisis Organization

1. **STOP! SIT!**
   Halt all activity. Acknowledge the problem out loud and brief your team immediately. Stopping allows everyone to control anxiety, fear, and dissociation. Clear your mind, steady your breathing, and establish a shared awareness: *"We have a problem. Here's what we know so far."*

2. **THINK.**
   Take inventory. Identify resources, assess damage, and assign manageable tasks. Focus not on the end goal but on the **next immediate step.** Forget all competing obligations and concentrate on the task at hand.

3. **OBSERVE.**
   Gather information. Ask questions. Inquire actively. Situational awareness comes from collective observation — ensure everyone's input is heard.

4. **PLAN.**
   Develop a strategy based on available information. Be bold but cautious. Then **act.**
   According to both aviation and military experts, one of the most frequent failures during crisis is not poor planning — it is **failure to execute.** Under duress, people freeze, doubt themselves, or forget to move forward.

This simple sequence may seem basic, but under acute stress it can be the **mental lifeline** that separates chaos from control. Once you've reestablished focus using S.T.O.P., the more advanced principles of crisis management can follow naturally.

Simplifying Crisis Management Leadership

Any threatening situation can be managed successfully — if you have either **experienced it before** or have **trained through failure**. But what happens when the event is unfamiliar, or when confusion dominates? The natural human response is often **panic**, especially in leaders who feel the weight of responsibility.

In these moments, remember: **organization, not urgency, restores control.**

Even the most complex crisis can be managed by following **a few rehearsed, simplified steps.** When leaders consciously calm themselves and their team, resolution typically follows within a minute. Conversely, when leaders act in haste or panic, recovery often takes much longer — delayed by backtracking from avoidable mistakes.

And above all, remember one of the most important leadership lessons:

"When you're lost, seek help."

In crisis leadership, humility and teamwork are not signs of weakness — they are the foundations of survival and recovery.

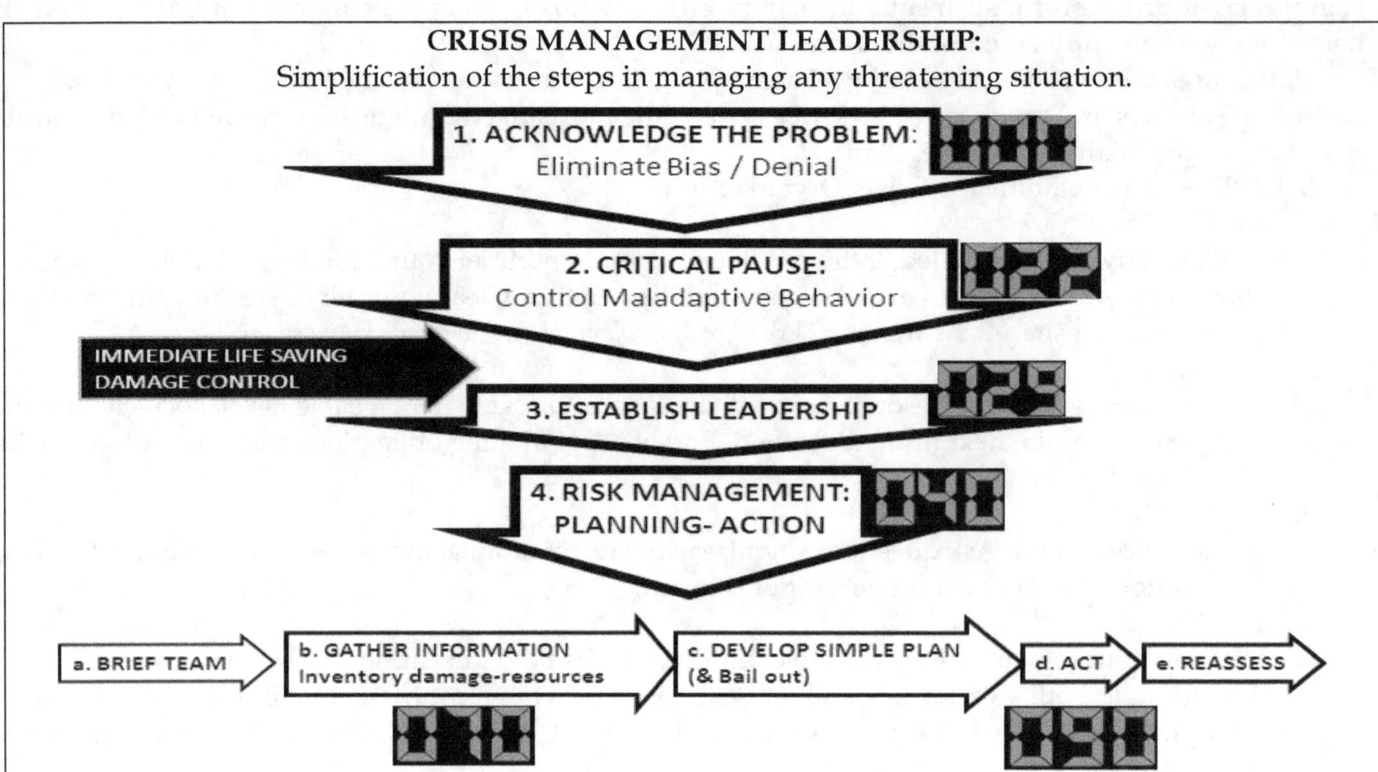

(Time frames indicated in seconds are based on personal experience in what it typically takes to reach these steps. It always feels much longer in real time. Even the time from when the geese took out the engines on US Airways Flight 1549 and the plane subsequently landed in the Hudson River was only a couple of minutes).

VI.C. CRISIS MANAGEMENT - TIME CRITICAL/ RAPID PROCESS- DECISION MAKING IN THE MIDST OF THE CRITICAL MOMENT

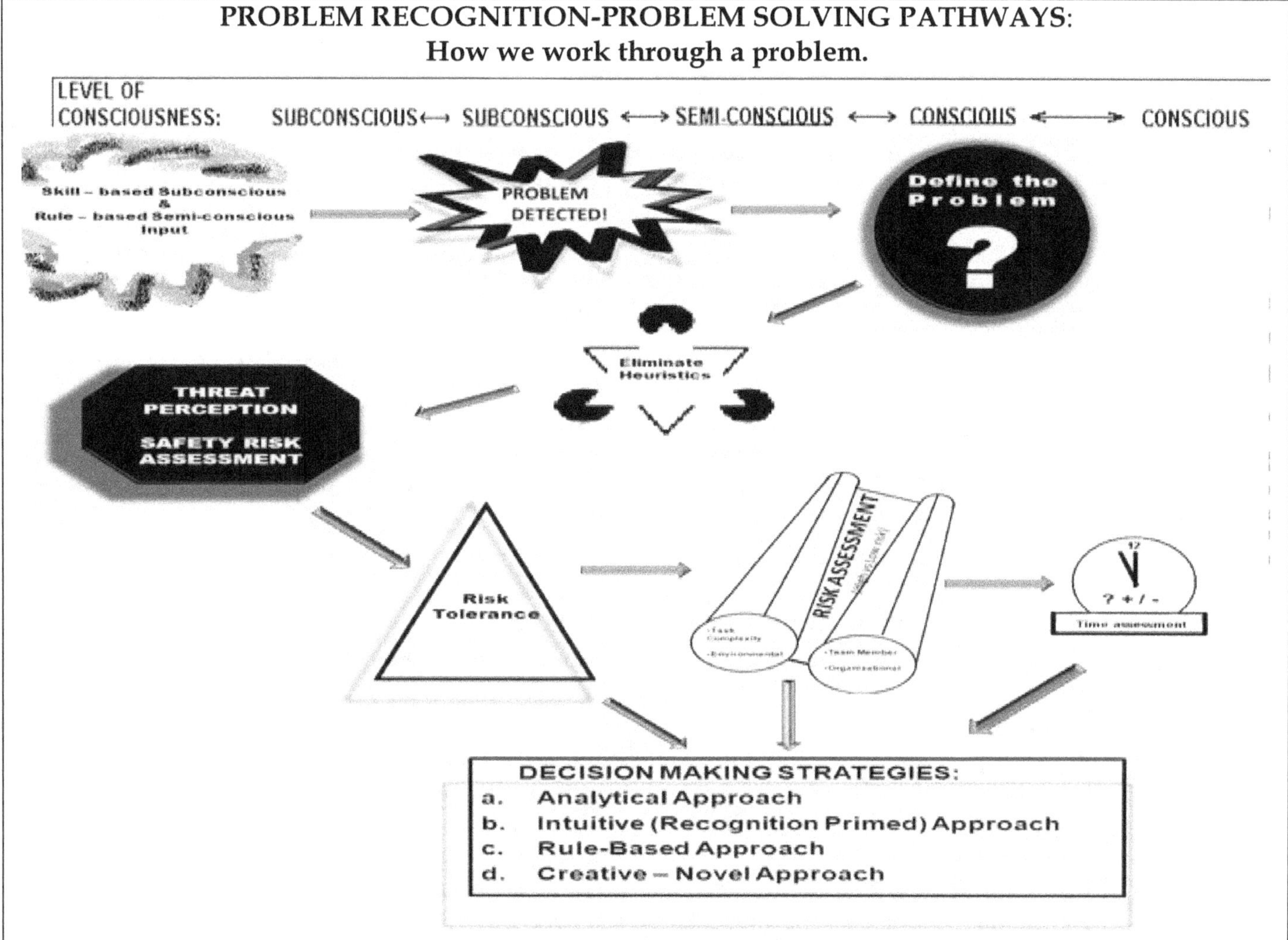

Lipsky K. CRISIS MANAGEMENT LEADERSHIP: TEAM TRAINING TO SURVIVE THE CRITICAL MOMENT 3rd ed; 2015 ITICAL MOMENT 3rd ed; 2015

Problem Recognition-Problem Solving Pathways—How we work through a problem: Initially one breaks out of their typical Skill-based subconscious pathway to discover an unexpected problem. Once the problem is detected, the observer must determine what the problem is. If they are successful in eliminating biases and other heuristic errors they must then determine what threat/safety risk the problem poses to their environment. Three processes then must occur: a) determination how much risk the team can tolerate, b) what is the risk to their current objective and team based on what is going on around them, and c) how much time they have. Once that occurs the observer can determine what strategy to use based on one of four common type of problem solving approaches.

Adapted with permission from: Pauley K, FlinR, Yule S, Youngson G. Surgeons intraoperative decision making and risk management. *Am J Surg*. 2011;202:375-381.131

Cohen I. Improving time-critical decision making in life-threatening situations: observations and insights. *Decision Analysis*. 2008;5:100–110.132 Pauley, Cohen

Problem Recognition and Decision-Making Under Duress

As discussed previously (*Human Error: Why Do We Miss What's Right in Front of Us? – "What Gorilla?"*), our daily thought processes are largely **automated**. Every moment, our senses collect vast amounts of **visual, auditory, olfactory, and proprioceptive** information. Yet, we are only consciously aware of a fraction of it. The question, then, is: *how do we recognize when something is wrong?*

When confronted with a problem, the human mind conducts a tremendous amount of **unconscious problem-solving**—a complex, behind-the-scenes process that runs almost continuously. To truly understand how we solve problems under duress, we must first appreciate how our brain processes information under normal circumstances.

Normal Cognitive Processing

During routine activities, input is gathered and processed primarily at the **subconscious or semi-conscious** level. Most habitual tasks—whether driving to work or performing a familiar procedure—occur automatically, guided by **heuristics** and pattern recognition.

Only when a situation deviates from expectation does our brain "wake up," shifting from **automatic** (skill-based or rule-based) processing to **knowledge-based**, fully conscious reasoning. Unfortunately, even in these moments, our natural heuristic tendencies can introduce **confirmation bias** or **fixation**, keeping us functioning at a lower cognitive level than the situation demands.

Simplified Model of the Problem Recognition–Solving Process

Drawing from Gary Klein's work (and my conversation with Lt General Van Riper) on decision-making, the process can be viewed as a series of deliberate steps:

A. Problem Detection

The first step is simply realizing that something is wrong. This detection may occur consciously or subconsciously, but recognition is essential for any further analysis.

B. Problem Definition

Next, we define the problem—ideally using **pattern recognition** to match current cues with previous experiences or known patterns. Accurate framing of the problem determines whether subsequent actions will succeed or fail.

C. Situational Assessment

Experienced individuals often claim they can "size up the situation in a second or two." This rapid cognitive scan involves four overlapping phases:

1. **Threat Perception:** Identify elements that pose risk—patient comorbidities, anatomy, BMI, adhesions, unexpected findings. Ask: *Have I seen this before? Is it serious? Do I have time? Can I overcome it?*
2. **Risk Tolerance:** Assess how much risk you (and your team or organization) are willing to accept in this context.
3. **Risk Assessment:** Evaluate risk level by category:
   - **Task complexity** (e.g., equipment malfunction, unexpected blood loss, inaccurate results)
   - **Environmental factors** (e.g., lighting, positioning, temperature, equipment failure)
   - **Team dynamics** (e.g., poor communication, inexperience, bravado, failure to recognize problems)
   - **Organizational pressures** (e.g., productivity targets, open conversion rates, inadequate staffing or supplies)
4. **Time Analysis:** Estimate how much time is available for decision-making—whether seconds, minutes, or longer—and adjust your strategy accordingly.

5.
D. Time-Critical Decision-Making

When time is limited, decisions rely heavily on **rapid pattern matching** and **rule-based reasoning**. Information is integrated with prior experience — our **mental and procedural memory "library."** We detect patterns that resemble familiar scenarios and apply the most fitting response.

Responses typically fall into three categories:

1. **Rule-Based:** Applying a known protocol or standard practice (most common).
2. **Adaptive/Improvised:** Creating a new solution on the spot when precedent is lacking (rare but necessary in novel crises).
3. **Consultative:** Seeking input or assistance when the situation exceeds one's immediate knowledge or capability (common and often prudent).

Ultimately, the capacity to recognize, define, and respond to problems under stress depends on **deliberate training and disciplined awareness.** The clinician who has practiced pausing to think — even for seconds — before acting is far more likely to choose correctly when the unexpected occurs.

Recently I received a call from the ED just one hour after I walked into my house. They stated a female patient was seen elsewhere the night prior and told they had appendicitis and the CT scan said there was swelling and inflammation of the appendix. Since the patient was tachycardic and febrile, I called in the team. Upon arrival to the ED the scenario was not that clear. The further I delve into this the more I was convinced this was a Tuboovarian abscess so I did not cancel the CT they had already ordered. CT was delayed waiting on the pregnancy test and team was on the way in. After an exam confirmed my suspicion about PID, I called our Gynecologist.

Patient went to the room and as I was about to scrub, the housekeeper said there was call from the lab in the holding area so I went to see what that was about, then realized my access card was in the OR and now I was locked out. Without going into details, further distracting events proceeded as we pushed thru the case. I identified a normal appendix but could not figure out why I was so lost. Finally, I admitted to the Gynecologist I was lost and could not understand why. He pointed out that the beefy red engorged object in front of me was the uterus and the inflamed object to the left was the infected tube. Well now everything was completely obvious. Why did I not see that? Could it be that this was the 20th hour that I had been awake? Aggravated and distracted by the other events? It definitely served as a reminder how easy it is to get lost when you least expect it and always ask for help.

"The ultimate measure of a man is not where he stands in moments of comfort and convenience, but where he stands at times of challenge and controversy". Martin Luther King Jr.

IV.D. PHASE ONE: RECOGNITION THAT THERE IS A PROBLEM

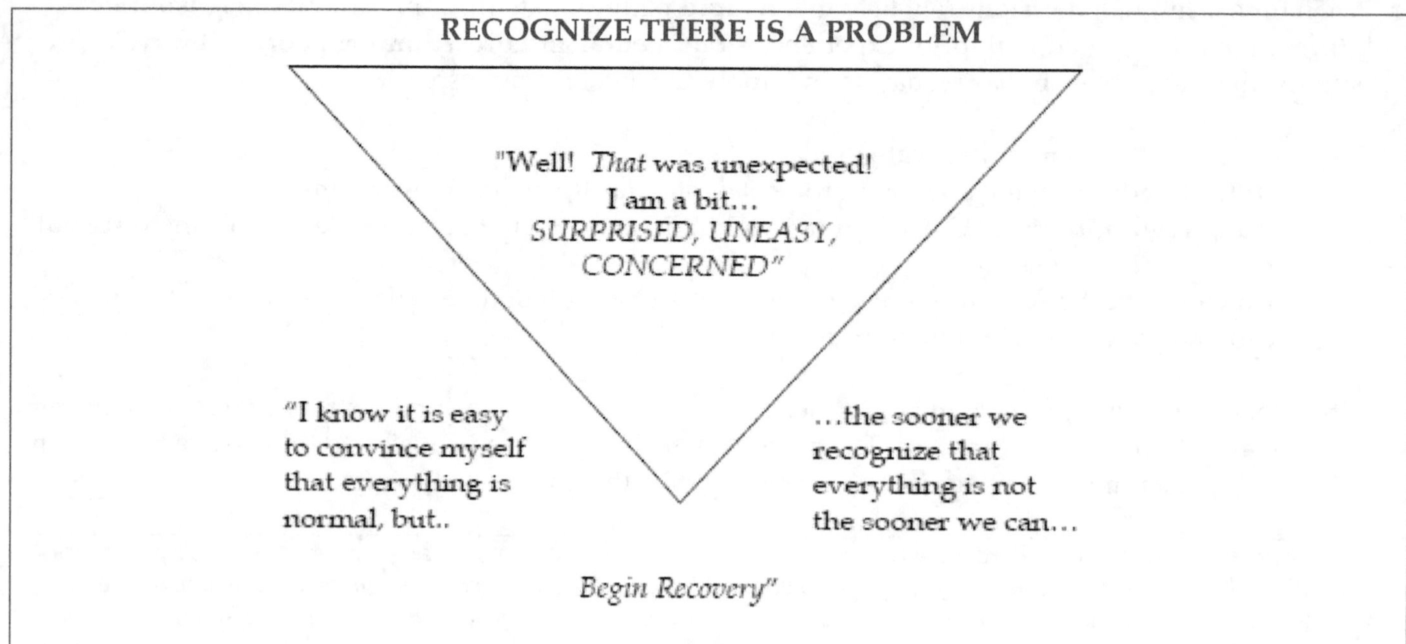

When one first recognizes that something unexpected arises they need to have trained themselves to *trust their instincts* rather than rely upon protective responses that try to lead them to believe all is normal. Avoid Heuristic Confirmation / Normalcy bias, convincing you all is okay.
Adapted from: Weick KE, Sutcliffe KM. *Managing the Unexpected: Resilient Performance in an Age of Uncertainty*. San Francisco, CA: John Wiley; 2007. 88

HOUSTON- WE HAVE A PROBLEM!

Jack Swigert, Apollo 13, stated calmly without hesitancy

"THE FIRST STEP IN SOLVING A PROBLEM, IS RECOGNIZING THAT THERE IS A PROBLEM":
Michael Lechman, MD

As noted previously in our discussion regarding normalcy-bias, having expectations about an event can create a *blind spot*. The blind spot occurs as one disconfirms evidence to the contrary of what they believed to be true. As in, "everything is just fine, it's all good." The same can be said for when the unexpected occurs: you usually know when something *unexpected* has happened because that is the moment you feel *anxious, concerned, surprised, leery…* yet instead of seizing the opportunity, we ignore our subconscious warning system. In his book '*BLINK*', Malcolm Gladwell points out that experts typically do not fully comprehend the processes whereby they are able to discern that a specific situation has occurred, they simply know based on their experience that something happened and that based on past experience they were successful when they utilized a specific measure to handle that situation (whatever it was). In fact, if one analyzes the event, more often than not, what the expert thought they were using to overcome that situation, likely was not really what they were doing (it was just instinctual so it was subconscious).

It is easy at this moment for you to convince your-self that everything is normal, and indulge in your confirmation bias that everything is okay. As will be explained below, the sooner one recognizes the unexpected has occurred and all is *not* normal, the sooner recovery can happen.

IS THERE A PROBLEM HERE TO DETECT?	Hum?
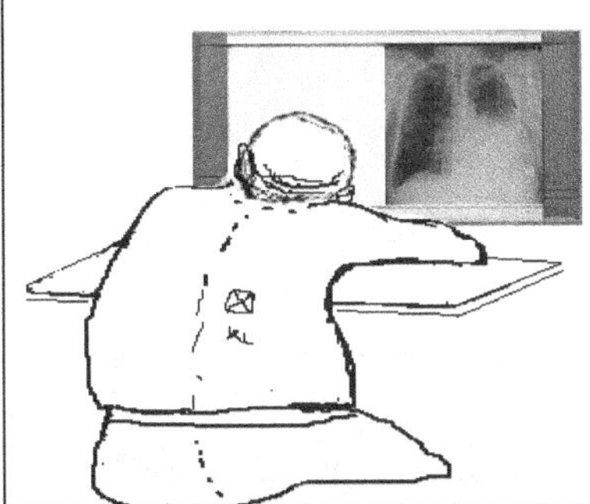	Something just does not feel right. *True Story!* *My first week as a brand new intern, sent to the ward to do a paracentesis. Had my spiral medical procedures manual with with everything ready to go, but something did not feel right until the patient spoke up.*

To survive a threatening event, one has to do five essential processes:

1. **Detect that there is a problem.**
2. **Identify what that problem is.**
3. **Analyze the problem.**
4. **Perform a threat analysis (i.e. SIZE UP THE SITUATION).**
5. **Determine one's options and make a plan.**

Successful leaders are able to determine there is a problem, identify what the problem is, analyze it with use of intuition and some additional information, perform a threat assessment and begin the planning process in a few seconds.

PROBLEM DETECTION AND PROBLEM ANALYSIS:
Two of the least understood processes necessary when performing under pressure are:
a. PROBLEM DETECTION: how do we detect that something has gone wrong?

b. PROBLEM ANALYSIS: when we have acknowledged that there is a problem that needs to be addressed, how do we analyze the situation so we understand what the problem is?

Before I try to summarize this process in a manner that I could understand, you must understand the difficult nature that Human Factors Psychologists face in assessing these situations. If you have ever interviewed an expert in a high-pressure field, then you can understand the immense challenge faced in interviewing a surgeon to tease out their thinking processes. In my experience, it can sometimes be a bit frustrating to ask experts in high pressure fields how they synthesize information during a period of challenge. I recently asked Colt McCoy (past University of Texas Quarterback) how he has learned to focus on the receiver but not loose contact with the locations of the defenders. He explained that this took years of practice, but that for a deeper discussion, I should speak with his Father, Coach Brad McCoy. Fortunately, his father provided me with a very interesting explantation. (Go to http://crisislead.blogspot.com/ for my conversation with Coach Brad McCoy on training quarterbacks and leadership)

I also had a similar conversation with Rorke Denver (Navy SEAL commander) when I asked him the same question. He promptly explained that they tried to escape whenever their psychologists came to ask them that same question and that they succeed thru vigorous training. I asked Tom Kolditz, Patrick Sweeney, Mike Mathews, Dave Grossman and a slew of others, what military experts have learned regarding an expert's response to pressure in the field. They all say the same thing - it's tough to tease information from these experts, because they always attempt to walk away. Frankly, until I began to research this area, I did not realize that in the majority of circumstances, experts really have no idea how they solve problems under pressure. For this reason, I interviewed experts in the field to tease out the components of this process so we can all understand it better.

ITS ALL ABOUT TIME!

Time frames are relevant! For the trained team the time frame from event detection to definitive action is fast! Consider the following events:

NFL Football huddle: 30 seconds

NFL Hike to touchdown pass: 2-4 seconds.

NFL Punt or kickoff return of 100 yards: < 10 seconds

NBA Fastbreak for two-point slam dunk, 3-5 seconds.

MLB double play from crack of the bat to out at first, 4-5 seconds.

The only way these players react and respond so rapidly is thru continued training till they get it right every time.

Learning the rules for problem detection, identification, analysis, assessment and action only helps if you incorporate this into your training. YOU MUST Rehearse so these actions occur in your team as rapidly as possible. If all you do is ignore the team around you, you just wasted valuable time and opportunity to intervene.

1. Problem Detection

In Section II (*Human Error: Why Do We Miss What's Right in Front of Us?*), we discussed the **Rasmussen Decision-Making Model**, which describes how humans operate at three cognitive levels—**skill-based, rule-based, and knowledge-based** processing. Most of the time, we hover within the **subconscious, skill-based zone**, allowing learned behaviors and patterns to guide our daily decision-making.

What we did not explore in detail is how an **expert transitions into knowledge-based processing**—how they realize that something has changed or gone wrong. Most of what we know about this comes from **Gary Klein's research on problem detection** and naturalistic decision-making (as put into action during live combat and Marine troop training by Lt Gen Van Riper).

In his 2005 paper *Problem Detection*, Klein emphasizes that **before any corrective action can occur, a person must first recognize that a problem exists.** This may sound self-evident, yet it is one of the most common failure points in crisis management. The sooner one detects that an event is taking an **unexpected and undesirable course**, the more time there is to analyze, plan, and act—potentially preventing disaster. Unfortunately, as discussed earlier, our perception is often **selective and biased**, and we may fail to recognize even the most obvious cues (the proverbial "gorilla in the room").

Recognizing the Cue

Problem detection depends on the presence of a **cue**—a signal that the current situation is diverging from expectation. This cue alerts us that a **routine or recovering process** has shifted into a **deteriorating one**. Cues can vary widely in form and timing:

- **Immediate and obvious:** A sudden change in wind direction during a wildfire, instantly placing a crew in danger; or a surgeon's subconscious awareness that *"something doesn't look right"*—for example, a missing ureter.
- **Delayed or subtle:** Small deviations that accumulate over time, producing no clear alarm until the situation has already become critical.
- **Negative cues:** The *absence* of an expected event, such as a pulse oximeter ceasing to display a normal pattern, can also serve as a trigger for detection.

The Role of Pattern Recognition

At all times, our subconscious mind is scanning for patterns—attempting to **make sense of incoming sensory data** from multiple channels. When something does not fit our expected pattern, we experience an internal jolt of uncertainty that may or may not reach conscious awareness.

Experts differ from novices not because they avoid error, but because they **actively test their assumptions**, seeking to distinguish between **true anomalies** and **inconsequential aberrations.** They are constantly comparing what they *expect* to see with what is *actually happening.*

How Problems Are Detected

Problem detection often occurs through one or more of the following mechanisms:

a. **Direct contradiction:** What we expected to happen is replaced by something obviously different.

b. **Cumulative discrepancies:** Several small deviations accumulate over time until a threshold of concern is reached.

c. **Micro-cues:** Subtle indicators recognized only by those with deep experience or "hyperawareness"—the skilled sailor sensing a shift in wind or the surgeon intuitively detecting abnormal tissue tension.

Constructing the Mental Model

Once awareness emerges, the expert begins to construct a **mental model**—a dynamic "story," "map," or "picture" that integrates sensory data into a coherent framework. This allows them to hypothesize what might be occurring and decide whether the situation represents a **real deviation** or a **false alarm.** However, this same mechanism can also be **deceptive.** The brain tends to fit new information into **familiar patterns**—a process that expedites decision-making but can lead to dangerous misclassification if the **wrong pattern** is applied. When this happens, every subsequent solution may be aimed at the wrong problem.

In summary:

Effective problem detection is not a passive process—it requires **awareness, curiosity, and disciplined doubt.** Experts develop this capability not merely through experience but through deliberate practice in recognizing subtle cues, questioning assumptions, and validating or revising their mental models in real time.

ERRORS OF OMMISSION OR COMMISSION (CONT):

One of the real issues faced by surgeons is when we commit an error of omission or commission and the problem is not recognizable because the symptom has not yet occurred. By definition there is a discrepancy between what was supposed to occur and what did. The problem exists, but may not be symptomatic until it may be too late or we have to undo what we just did. For example, I just did an anastomosis with a circular stapler but failed to assess the completeness of the rings or I did a choledochojejunostomy but did not put in the back wall of sutures, etc. (for details about errors of omission and commission refer above to the section on error creation). Maybe someone in my family forgot to turn off the gas on the stove. The actual problem that needs to be recognized is that the gas is flowing freely but at the instant I omit that step, it is traditionally not a problem just yet (but will be in a minute when the symptom of gas smell is evident or I have a panic attack wondering if I remembered to turn off the gas).

2. Problem Analysis and Decision-Making

When asked what they do after recognizing a problem, most experts—especially those without formal training in psychology or human factors—respond simply:

"Well, I size up the situation."

That description is accurate but not particularly useful when teaching novices how to think and act under pressure. So, what does "sizing up" really mean?

From Recognition to Diagnosis and Action

According to Gary Klein, once a problem is detected, the next step is to identify and define it—to diagnose what's wrong—and then to plan a course of action to resolve or mitigate the situation. His *Recognition-Primed Decision (RPD) Model* describes how experts use prior experiences, pattern recognition, and mental simulation to make rapid, effective decisions in complex environments.

Experienced individuals first search for familiar cues and attempt to match the current situation to a stored pattern—a mental model built through training, prior exposure, or education. Once a pattern is recognized, they mentally simulate a likely course of action to see whether it fits the current scenario. If it "feels right," they proceed. If the mental simulation produces warning signs or contradictions, they abandon that idea and rapidly construct an alternative.

Key insight: In high-stakes environments, *a workable solution is often better than the perfect one that comes too late.*

As Klein noted in his studies of fire commanders, effective leaders integrate intuition and analysis. They rely on intuition to recognize patterns quickly but verify through mental simulation before acting. A purely intuitive approach risks catastrophic error if the wrong pattern is matched; a purely analytical approach, meanwhile, is often too slow for rapidly evolving crises.

Decision-Making in Surgery: The Calgary Model

Building on Klein's framework, Cristancho and colleagues at the University of Calgary examined how surgeons make intraoperative decisions under stress. Their 2013 study distinguished between decision-making during routine versus non-routine moments. In non-routine situations, surgeons follow a recurring three-stage process:

a. Situational Assessment: Gathering initial information and identifying cues that something is wrong.

b. Reconciliation: Collecting and analyzing data to confirm what has changed and why.

c. Planning and Implementation: Developing and executing a course of action based on that analysis.

This framework aligns closely with your crisis leadership model—where successful leaders draw from experience, pre-implementation planning, pattern recognition, and bias awareness to pause, brief the team, gather information, project outcomes, plan, act, and then reassess.

Poor leaders often short-circuit this process—acting too quickly out of anxiety or freezing midway through analysis—leading to delayed or inappropriate responses.

In a 2016 follow-up study, Cristancho's team discovered that expert surgeons often perform dual-track cognition during crises:

- They execute damage control measures immediately, while simultaneously gathering and interpreting information about the evolving situation.
- They actively seek missing information, even when uncertain whether it is absent, a process the authors called "transforming information."

This transformation differs between novices and experts.

- Novices focus narrowly on immediate facts and short-term outcomes.
- Experts look for broader patterns, interpreting how new information alters both immediate and long-term consequences.

The ability to oscillate between immediate response and analytical reflection is what distinguishes a competent operator from an adaptive expert. [Cristancho]

Training to Avoid Missing the Obvious

Many trainees ask, *"If denial is such a natural response, how do I know when I'm denying reality?"*

A simple analogy helps: imagine using a GPS navigation system that suggests a route, but as you follow it, something feels wrong—you notice landmarks that don't match expectations. You consciously interrupt your automatic behavior, reassess, and reorient yourself. That moment—when you choose to question your "peripheral brain"—is the essence of cognitive forcing, a concept emphasized by Pat Croskerry and the Critical Thinking Institute (see prior section on error management).

You cannot consciously analyze every step; overthinking leads to paralysis by analysis. Instead, you must learn to recognize warning signals that indicate when automatic behavior may be unsafe. Like driving, effective decision-making involves three phases:

1. Develop foundational skills and pattern familiarity.
2. Recognize early warning cues that signal deviation.
3. Interrupt automation, reassess, and decide whether to continue or change course.

With practice, leaders and clinicians learn to integrate experience, situational cues, and team feedback into fluid mental models that balance intuition with deliberation. This ability—to pause, process, and proceed deliberately—is the essence of expert-level decision-making under duress.

IV.E. SITUATIONAL AWARENESS: TUNNEL VISION vs LOAD SHEDDING. WHY DO WE MISS WHAT IS IN FRONT OF US?

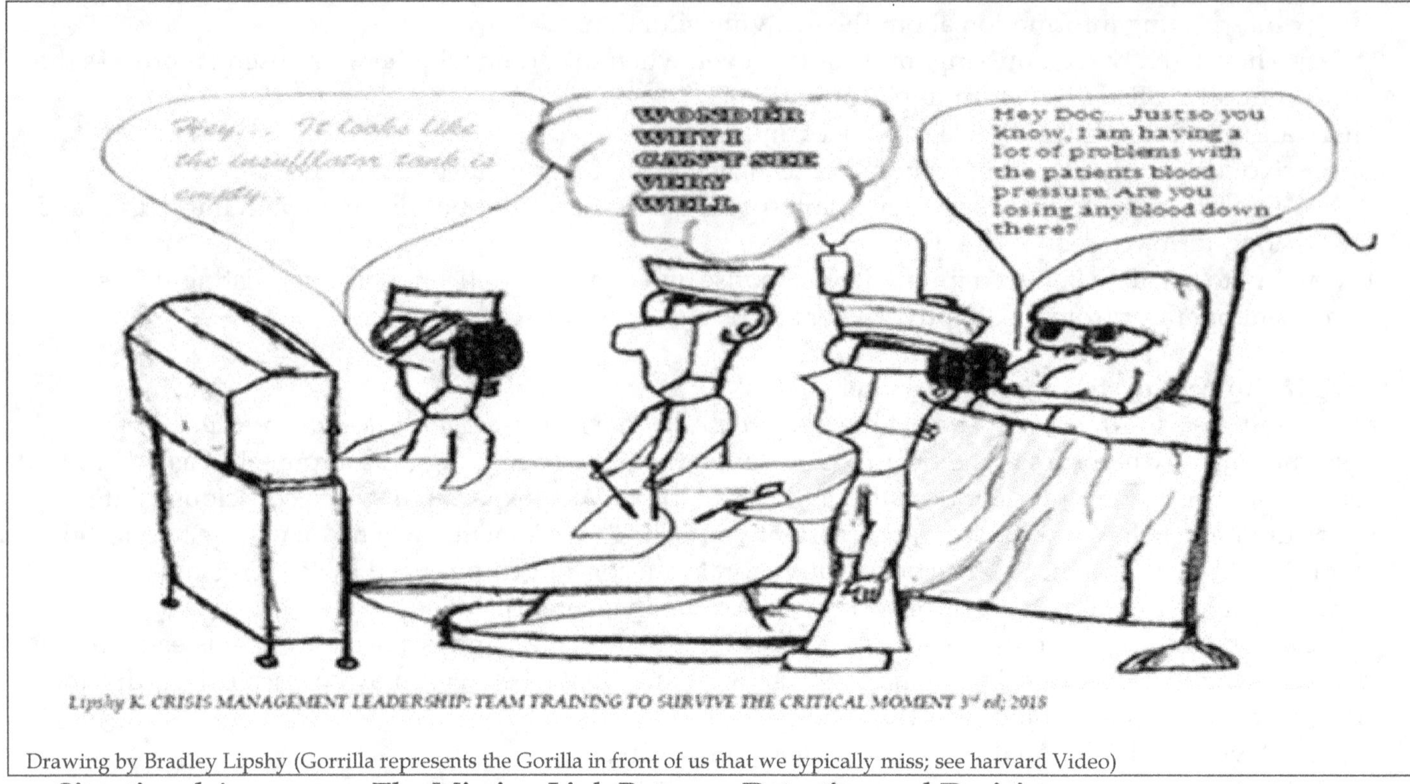

Drawing by Bradley Lipshy (Gorrilla represents the Gorilla in front of us that we typically miss; see harvard Video)

Situational Awareness: The Missing Link Between Detection and Decision

We will explore **Situational Awareness (SA)** in greater depth later in this book, but it is important to connect its principles here—particularly as they relate to **problem detection and analysis.**

As healthcare professionals, we often work in **environments of intense focus**, where our attention narrows to the immediate task at hand. This hyper-focus, while necessary for precision, frequently leads to **attentional tunneling**—a form of cognitive blindness in which we lose awareness of the larger environment. We may filter incoming sensory information to reduce distractions, but in doing so, we risk missing critical cues from our surroundings.

Over time, experienced clinicians learn to **filter and prioritize** incoming data, distinguishing between relevant and irrelevant stimuli. Yet even with experience, much of the information reaching us is subtle—signals or cues that do not directly command attention. Unless our **teams are trained in structured communication and shared situational awareness techniques**, we remain vulnerable to **missing the earliest signs of deterioration**—even when those signs are as obvious as "the gorilla standing right in front of us."

Lessons from Aviation: Managing Cognitive Load

Pilots, like surgeons, must constantly balance two competing dangers:

1. **Information overload**, where too much sensory input overwhelms decision capacity, and
2. **Information omission**, where vital cues are ignored or unseen.

To manage this balance, pilots are trained to practice **"load shedding"**—a deliberate process of eliminating or deprioritizing extraneous tasks or stimuli in order to focus on what appears most critical. When properly executed, load shedding enables efficient decision-making under pressure, allowing pilots to concentrate on the essentials of flying the aircraft.

However, this same skill can become dangerous when **the wrong information is filtered out.** History has shown that numerous aviation accidents resulted from pilots focusing narrowly on one malfunctioning indicator while missing the true root cause — often displayed elsewhere on the instrument panel.

As **Samuel Elfassy**, Senior Director of Corporate Safety, Environment, and Quality at Air Canada, explained to me, *"People who work in high-risk industries must continuously rehearse maintaining balance — avoiding distraction from irrelevant inputs while not becoming trapped in tunnel vision."*

Stress further compounds the problem. Under duress, **breathing patterns become erratic**, and hypoventilation can directly impair both **attention** and **night vision** in pilots. In medicine, similar physiological effects of stress — tachycardia, shallow breathing, narrowed vision — can degrade clinical performance and situational awareness at the precise moment when clarity is most needed.

Bridging Awareness and Action

Maintaining situational awareness requires a deliberate and practiced effort to manage cognitive bandwidth — **to perceive, comprehend, and project** the environment in real time (Endsley, 1995). The expert clinician must continually toggle between **focused attention on the immediate task** and **peripheral awareness of the broader system** — the patient, the team, and the environment.

In crisis situations, success depends not just on what the leader sees, but on what the **team collectively perceives and communicates.** Structured briefings, closed-loop communication, and cross-monitoring — concepts borrowed from aviation crew resource management — are essential to overcoming the limitations of individual attention and preventing errors that stem from lost situational awareness.

In summary:

While problem detection and analysis begin the cognitive process of crisis management, **situational awareness sustains it.** The ability to maintain a wide perceptual field — balancing focus with peripheral sensitivity — is what distinguishes high-performing teams in aviation, surgery, and every other high-risk profession.

IV.F. ANXIETY/MALADAPTIVE RESPONSE CONTROL AT THE START OF THE CRITICAL MOMENT – THE VALUE OF THE CRITICAL PAUSE -

SURVIVAL ARC

RECKONING

DELIBERATION

DECISIVE MOMENT

Lipsky K. CRISIS MANAGEMENT LEADERSHIP: TEAM TRAINING TO SURVIVE THE CRITICAL MOMENT 3rd ed; 2018

Adapted with permission from: Ripley A. *The Unthinkable: Who Survives When Disaster Strikes and Why.* New York, NY: Three Rivers Press; 2009. 133

Pathway to Survival! How to overcome the odds in virtually any anxiety provoking situation!

A. **SURVIVAL ARC / COMBAT SURVIVAL TRAINING**: Immediate personal (team) hazard response via adaptive vs maladaptive behavior. Within the first few seconds, individuals must progress through the "survival arc" and either avoid maladaptive behavior or fail. This truly takes Combat Survival Training.

B. **ESTABLISHMENT OF ORDER VIA EFFECTIVE TEAM LEADERSHIP & COMMUNICATION**: Shortly thereafter, the team needs to organize by declaring a leader. Followers must understand who is in charge, their roles and effective communication techniques.

C. **DELIBERATE POSITIVE ACTION PHASE**: Once order has been restored, damage control followed by risk assessment, containment, planning, execution and reassessment are needed. [Ripley with approval]

Controlling Oneself in Crisis: The Leader's Critical Pause

Effective team leaders must possess the ability to **control themselves under pressure**, employing adaptive behaviors that steady both their own performance and that of the team. In the midst of crisis, **you must stop everything—if only for a moment—to control anxiety.** This brief, deliberate pause serves as the anchor for all subsequent decision-making.

Team members instinctively look to their leader for composure and direction. They expect not merely competence, but *calm authority*—a steady presence amid chaos. The leader's demeanor becomes the emotional thermostat for the group; if the leader projects panic, the team will amplify it. If the leader projects steadiness, the team can begin to recover its rhythm.

In **military and first responder** environments, this ability is often described through two intertwined attributes:

- **Mental toughness**—the capacity to maintain focus and clarity despite internal turmoil.

- **Hardiness** — the sense of control over external events, even when circumstances appear overwhelming.

As Sweeney, Matthews, and Lester emphasize, **team resilience** in such fields depends heavily on the selection and training of leaders who embody these qualities. In most other high-risk professions — particularly in medicine — these attributes are not innate; they must be **taught, modeled, and practiced** through deliberate training and education.

The First Seconds Define the Outcome

The **first few seconds** following a critical event often determine the ultimate outcome. Leaders who can rapidly recognize the situation, contain their emotions, and implement structured reasoning are more likely to guide their teams toward recovery rather than collapse. Understanding how humans **think under stress** enables leaders to foster **advantageous, compensatory, and adaptive responses** — and to recognize and intercept **disadvantageous, decompensatory, maladaptive behaviors** before they cascade into dysfunction. These processes are universal across all hazardous environments — from the cockpit to the battlefield to the operating room.

The Survival Arc: Reckoning, Deliberation, and the Decisive Moment

When faced with crisis, individuals pass through what **Amanda Ripley**, author of *The Unthinkable: Who Survives When Disaster Strikes — and Why*, describes as the **Survival Arc**. This arc unfolds in three stages:

1. **Reckoning** – The moment of realization that something catastrophic has occurred.
2. **Deliberation** – The mental process of orienting oneself, evaluating options, and formulating an initial plan.
3. **The Decisive Moment** – The point at which one acts — decisively, adaptively, and with resolve.

Each stage requires successful navigation before moving to the next. Failure to progress through any stage — remaining in denial, panic, or indecision — can stall or derail both individual and team performance. Leaders who understand this progression can help their teams traverse these stages more efficiently, turning confusion into coordination.

The Critical Pause

Admiral **William H. McRaven**, in his 2014 University of Texas commencement address, captured this principle succinctly:

"Every SEAL knows that under the keel, at the darkest moment of the mission, is the time when you must be calm and composed — when all your tactical skills, your physical power, and all your inner strength must be brought to bear. If you want to change the world, you must be your very best in the darkest moment."

This concept — the **Critical Pause** — is at the heart of crisis leadership. It is the brief but deliberate moment when the leader resists the instinct to react impulsively, instead taking control of their physiology, emotions, and cognition. It is during this pause that clarity emerges, allowing the leader to transform fear into focused action.

In summary:

The effective crisis leader is defined not by speed or bravado, but by **composure and adaptive**

control. When everything seems to unravel, it is the leader's calm, deliberate presence — the critical pause — that steadies the team and reclaims order from chaos.

Lipsky K. CRISIS MANAGEMENT LEADERSHIP: TEAM TRAINING TO SURVIVE THE CRITICAL MOMENT 3rd ed; 2018

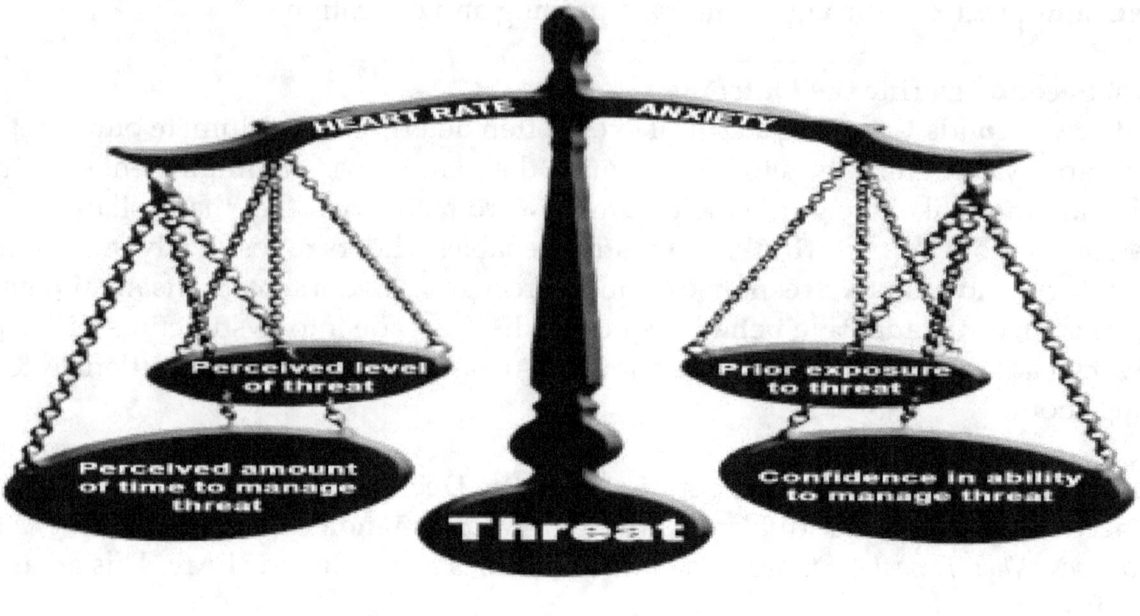

Anxiety is all a matter of balance. Anxiety is all a matter of how you perceive the threat: a) how much of a threat is it to you, b) have you been exposed to this threat before, c) how much time you have to deal with the threat, and d) how much confidence you have in managing the threat. By decreasing anxiety you can decrease your heart rate, gaining control of fine and complex motor function. If any one of these becomes out of balance the threat is perceived as overwhelming, anxiety picks up and the heart rate increases further debilitating the victim.

Adapted with Permission from: Siddle B. *Sharpening the Warriors Edge: The Psychology and Science of Training.* 10th ed. Belleville, IL: PPCT Research publications; 2008. 87 Siddle

Anxiety, Maladaptive Behavior, and the Critical Pause

The cognitive pitfalls discussed earlier — confirmation bias, fixation, and heuristic shortcuts — occur even in calm, routine settings. When **stress and anxiety** are added to this already fragile cognitive system, the likelihood of **maladaptive behavior** increases dramatically.

Under perceived threat, the human body defaults to a primitive survival mechanism — the **"fight or flight" response.** While evolutionarily adaptive for escaping predators, this reaction is decidedly counterproductive in surgery, medicine, or any high-risk team environment where composure and precision are required.

The Critical Pause: The First Step in Any Crisis

The **first step in managing any crisis** is to **stop everything** — to create a deliberate, conscious **pause** before acting. This momentary interruption of automatic behavior allows leaders to control their **physiological arousal** and **prevent emotional hijacking**.

The **critical pause** is not inaction — it is intentional control.

It is the leader's conscious override of instinct.

Only after this pause can the leader think clearly, assess accurately, and direct others effectively. Without it, the mind is ruled by adrenaline, perception narrows, and judgment deteriorates.

Understanding Anxiety and Its Origins

Anxiety represents the body's **biochemical response** to perceived threat—primarily driven by the **release of epinephrine (adrenaline)** and its effects on heart rate, breathing, and alertness. While this surge can heighten performance in brief, controlled doses, it becomes destructive when unregulated.

In healthcare, anxiety often arises not from external danger but from **internal cognitive and moral conflict**. Whether novice or expert, providers share remarkably similar thoughts in moments of crisis:

- *Am I doing the right thing for this patient?*
- *Am I doing enough?*
- *Did I cause this problem — or make it worse?*
- *Should I act now or wait for more data?*
- *Should I call for help — or will that make me look incompetent?*
- *If this goes badly, will I be blamed? Will my reputation suffer?*

These are the inner monologues of uncertainty—**the noise of self-doubt** that accompanies crisis. They mirror the universal human fear of loss: loss of control, competence, credibility, or even life itself.

Yet, when properly reframed, these thoughts can be **harnessed** into productive vigilance. Awareness of one's anxiety is the first step toward mastering it.

Perception Determines Threat

Anxiety is not determined solely by circumstance but by **perception**—how the threat is interpreted. Four primary factors influence whether an event triggers adaptive focus or paralyzing panic:

1. **Magnitude of Threat:** How serious does this situation feel to you or your team?
2. **Familiarity:** Have you encountered this type of problem before?
3. **Time Pressure:** How much time do you believe you have to respond?
4. **Confidence:** How competent and prepared do you feel to manage it?

Tipping even one of these variables in your favor—through **training, rehearsal, or self-regulation**—can dramatically improve performance. As confidence and familiarity rise, perceived threat decreases, and anxiety becomes manageable.

From Anxiety to Panic: When Control is Lost

Anxiety becomes **panic** when the situation is perceived as **inescapable or dismal**—when cognitive control collapses and instinct dominates. Panic is the ultimate **maladaptive response**: reasoning disintegrates, communication fails, and coordinated action ceases.

Preventing panic requires **early recognition** of escalating anxiety and the immediate use of **countermeasures**—controlled breathing, brief timeouts, grounding techniques, and team-based reassurance. In essence, the leader's calm must become the team's anchor.

In summary:

The human body's first instinct in crisis is survival, not clarity. To be effective under pressure, leaders must retrain instinct—**replace reflex with reflection.** The **critical pause** is the bridge between primitive reaction and purposeful action, transforming fear into focus and chaos into control.

EMOTIONAL CONTROL VS PANIC AND CHAOS

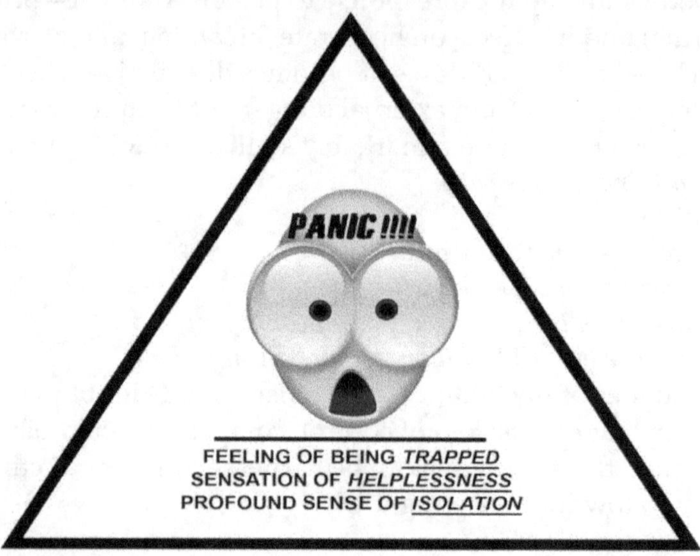

Three Conditions are required to cause panic and chaos. These three conditions compounded with dread, typically result in panic. Learning to control these will limit or eliminate panic from a team. Dread is a result of uncontrollability, unfamiliarity, impossibility, suffering, unfairness and compounded by the degree of destruction. 23

Adapted with permission from: Dörner D; The Logic of Failure: Recognizing and avoiding error in complex situations. Reading MA Perseus Books, 1996. Dorner

The psychology of panic is very complex, but survival experts have simplified this response by breaking the origination of panic into three components:

    a. A feeling of being *trapped*

    b. A sensation of *helplessness*

    c. A profound sense of *isolation*

This response to a situation can be amplified by a sense of **dread**. Dread is a result of uncontrollability, unfamiliarity, impossibility, suffering, unfairness, and it is compounded by the degree of destruction.

ANXIETY RESPONSE CONTROL TO CURTAIL MALADAPTIVE BEHAVIOR

What use is it to understand the origination of our anxiety response? In a personal conversation, Thomas Kolditz (author of *In Extremis Leadership*) summarizes this process best when he explained that it is safer to control your fear, stay relaxed and remain outwardly focused than to become inwardly focused on your personal injuries. Unfortunately, most of us focus on those things we fear as described above and forget the "*mission*". By understanding this natural response, we can reduce its negative effects. By decreasing your response to anxiety, you can decrease your heart rate, gaining control of fine and complex motor function. If any one of these becomes out of balance then the threat will steadily be perceived as overwhelming. As the other issues come into play anxiety picks up and the heart rate increases further debilitating the victim.[87] What can be done about this? It takes training and practice but it can be done and has proven successful in many very high-risk environments.

CONTROLLING YOUR ANXIETY! *PRACTICE TO CONTROL YOUR FEAR!*

HOW MILITARY AND FIRST RESPONDERS COMBAT ANXIETY IN THE MIDST OF OVERWHELMING STRESS AND ANXIETY

    a. **COMBAT-TACTICAL BREATHING**

    b. **VISUALIZATION (rehearsal)**

    c. **CONFIDENCE IN ABILITY TO BEAT THE ODDS**

Combat (Tactical) Breathing: Regaining Control of the Body

Of all the body's automatic responses to fear and its resulting surge of adrenaline, respiration is the most controllable. Controlled breathing runs counter to instinct; it requires conscious focus and outward attention at a moment when the body urges panic.

The method is simple but powerful:

- Inhale slowly for four seconds.
- Hold the breath for four seconds.
- Exhale slowly for four seconds.

This technique, widely taught to military and civilian combatants, increases lung volume, maintains oxygenation, and prevents the hyperventilation that leads to excess carbon dioxide loss and impaired cerebral function.

Equally important, controlled breathing diverts focus away from distressing sensory input. After combat, warriors are often given purposeful tasks to redirect their attention from the stress of recent battle; tactical breathing serves the same purpose. It shifts attention to a simple, benign process—breathing—thereby reducing emotional overload.

Practice this technique during moderate stress—while driving in traffic, standing in line, managing conflict at work, or addressing an irate colleague. By training under low-stakes conditions, you condition the response for when it truly counts.

(Grossman, On Combat; Kolditz, In Extremis Leadership)

Visualization: Mental Rehearsal for Success

Just as elite athletes mentally rehearse success, trained combatants visualize themselves overcoming the threat they face. This primes both mind and body to respond appropriately when the real challenge arises, increasing the likelihood of survival and success.

Rao et al. describe this as mental training or mental imagery—the process of constructing a motor or cognitive response to a stimulus before it occurs. Visualization effectively pre-programs the behavioral and neural pathways necessary for decisive action.

(Rao et al.)

Confidence: The Warrior Mindset

Confidence is the belief in one's ability to overcome adversity. It is not bravado or denial—it is disciplined optimism grounded in preparation.

When stress rises, avoid catastrophic thinking and instead reframe: *There is always a solution. There is always a way forward.* Repetition of calm, directive self-talk reinforces emotional regulation ("Be calm. Be silent. Breathe.").

This mindset is core to combat survival: warriors may face impossible odds, yet their focus remains fixed on the mission, not their mortality. Success, not fear, dominates their attention. They rely on their tools, their training, and their discipline to maintain composure and concentration.

(Grossman; Rao et al.)

Getting in the Zone: Outward Focus vs. Inward Focus

Leadership under pressure demands outward focus—a conscious awareness of the environment, the team, and the unfolding situation. As Tom Kolditz, author of *In Extremis*

Leadership, explained in a personal conversation, great leaders maintain an outward perspective even in chaos.

Experienced leaders often describe "flattened emotions" during crisis—a calm detachment that allows clear assessment and decisive action. This occurs when attention turns outward toward the mission and the environment, rather than inward toward fear or self-doubt.

> **STRESS INOCULATION**
> Inoculate against the stress to reduce the fears. The best method to control anxiety under duress is to train to control anxiety under duress. Grossman D. *On Combat.*

By contrast, inward focus—obsessing over one's emotions, worries, or injuries—narrows perception and paralyzes performance.

Leaders must also prevent their team members from becoming inwardly focused. In high-risk environments, individuals under stress can fixate on personal concerns or fear of failure. The effective leader intervenes—assigning purposeful tasks, redirecting energy, and restoring outward attention. When eyes and minds turn outward, performance stabilizes and control returns.

(Kolditz, In Extremis Leadership, Department of Behavioral Sciences and Leadership, U.S. Military Academy, West Point)

Applied Lessons in Leadership Resilience

For a real-world example of these principles in action, see "Resiliency—Lessons on Leadership through the Eyes of Daniel Linskey, Boston Police Chief and Incident Commander during the 2013 Boston Marathon Bombing" (Appendix C). Chief Linskey's experience exemplifies tactical calm, adaptive focus, and decisive leadership under extreme duress.

> *"I remember one particular canoe trip that went wrong really fast. In the middle of the night a wicked storm came through. When we got up, the water was four feet higher and large trees were moving down the river. That should have tipped us off to the bad scene that was about to unfold. Prior groups went thru the falls we were about to go over and they told us they were typically easy. Well, we got within a hundred yards and it sounded like a freight train and we knew we were in trouble, but it was too late, the current had its hold on us(later we were told these were converted by the storm to class V rapids). I had someone else's 7-year-old boy in my canoe and I just kept yelling 'remember what we talked about right… he said.. "pick my feet up and don't fight the current'. I forgot about the canoe and other contents and kept my eye on that child. When we approached the rapids, I realized the whirlpool we were going down into was about eight feet deep between several large boulders. I yelled 'hold your breath' and then that was it for a few seconds. I was underwater but kept my feet and butt up in the air. When I popped up I saw him just within reach (as well as some very random life jacket floating by). I grabbed him by the life jacket neck and lifted him up in the air and began a search for land. I saw some of our crew at a seventy-degree angle from the current but pulled him and me over to them. It never occurred to me that we were in danger. Just focused on the task that needed to get done. When we got to shore and did a head count I realized I had no idea where my own son was. I just watched him disappear on the back side of the rapids.*
>
> **DISASTROUS COPING STRATEGIES:**
> - **ANGER!**
> - **BLAME!**
> - **DEFEATISM!**
>
> …… can destroy a mission worse than the events that initiated the crisis. Giving in and giving up are all signs of focusing inward on one's peril when a leader needs to focus on his environment, the mission, and his team. Kolditz, *In Extremis Leadership.*

> **RESILIENCE**
> Ones' ability to respond well to a setback (failure) that is optimized through learned optimism and hardiness. Sweeney PJ, Matthews MD, Lester PB. *Leadership in Dangerous Situations.*

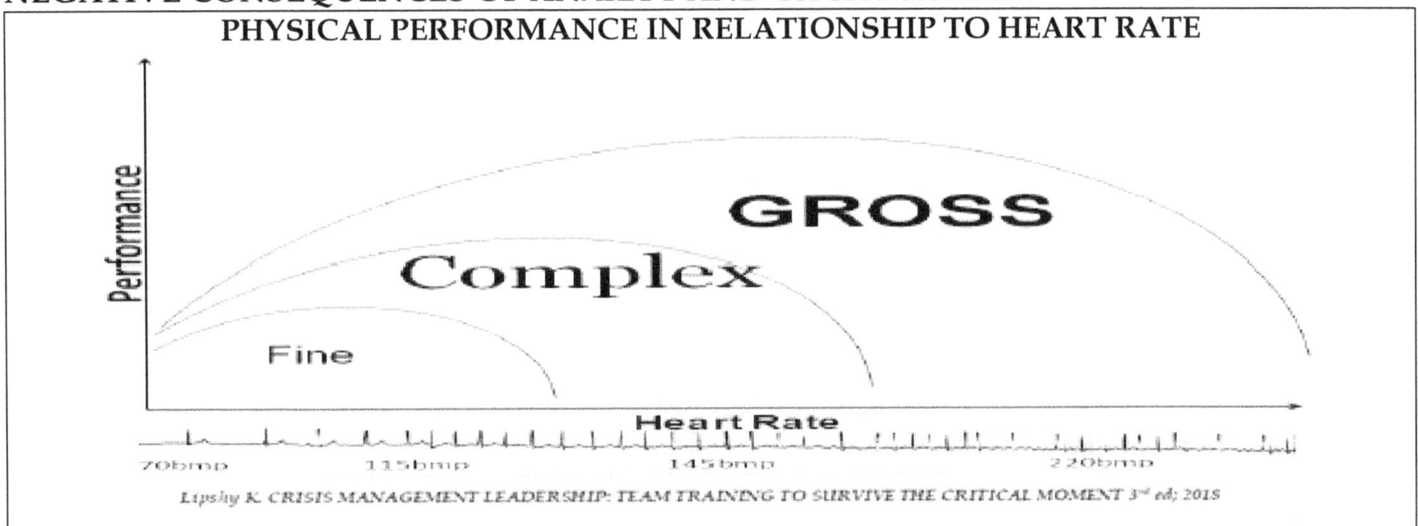

Bell-shaped curve seen when heart rate increases and motor skills are enhanced but then deteriorate. Adapted with permission from: Siddle B. *Sharpening the Warriors Edge: The Psychology and Science of Training*. 10th ed. Belleville, IL: PPCT Research publications; 2008 87

THE PHYSIOLOGY OF STRESS AND PERFORMANCE: THE YERKES–DODSON LAW IN ACTION

As previously discussed, **tachycardia** — an elevated heart rate — is an adaptive survival response. It enhances oxygen delivery, sharpens focus, and prepares the body for action. However, when heart rate rises beyond its optimal range, this adaptive response can quickly become **maladaptive and dangerous.**

The relationship between stress and performance has long been described by the **inverted U-shaped curve** known as the **Yerkes–Dodson Law.** Peter Nixon described this same respone in several papers in the 1970-80's. At one end of the curve, minimal stress produces **boredom, apathy, and slow response times**. At the other extreme, excessive stress leads to **anxiety, cognitive overload, and performance breakdown**. Between these two extremes lies the **optimal stress zone**, where arousal and focus are balanced, and performance peaks. Peter Nixon, *(Sincero, S.M")*

THE PHYSIOLOGIC "SWEET SPOT"

In most high-risk professions, optimal performance during stress corresponds to heart rates between **115 and 145 beats per minute (bpm)**. In *Sharpening the Warrior's Edge*, **Bruce K. Siddle** describes this as a **bell-shaped performance curve**, where performance improves with rising arousal up to a point — after which it deteriorates rapidly.

- Around **115 bpm, fine motor skills** (delicate finger movements) begin to decline.
- Between **145–175 bpm, complex motor coordination** (hand–eye tasks) progressively deteriorates.
- Beyond **175 bpm, gross motor control** — basic body movement — also breaks down.
- Above **220 bpm**, individuals may experience **perceptual narrowing, tunnel vision, or complete paralysis** of response. (Siddle)

For **athletes, soldiers, and tactical operators**, stress inoculation training enables them to function within a higher optimal range (up to 175 bpm) by automating their responses through **muscle memory and procedural rehearsal**. *(Grossman, On Combat)*

Unfortunately, the same physiologic escalation can prove **disastrous for surgeons, pilots, and healthcare professionals**, whose success depends on sustained fine and complex motor precision. Once the heart rate exceeds 145 bpm, performance rapidly degrades—hand tremors increase, visuospatial judgment falters, and decision-making becomes impulsive or erratic.

THE CASCADE OF COGNITIVE BREAKDOWN

When an untrained or unregulated individual encounters an unexpected threat, the perception of danger triggers a **sense of urgency**—the feeling that time is running out. This accelerates the heart rate further and deepens physiological arousal.

As heart rate climbs:

1. **Fine and complex motor skills deteriorate.**
2. **Perceptual distortion** and **information-processing delays** emerge.
3. **Cognitive tunneling** replaces situational awareness.
4. The body shifts fully into the **fight-or-flight response**, dominated by instinct rather than reasoning.

At this point, performance becomes erratic or paralyzed, and the individual's ability to lead, communicate, or perform critical technical tasks collapses.

Key Takeaway

Stress enhances performance only **to a point**. Beyond that threshold, the same physiologic mechanisms designed to save life can **compromise cognition, coordination, and judgment.** For the surgeon, pilot, or crisis leader, the art of mastery lies in **recognizing the physiological warning signs** and applying trained self-regulation—through controlled breathing, visualization, and deliberate focus—to remain within the optimal performance zone.

ORIGINATION OF MALADAPTIVE BEHAVIORS SECONDARY TO THE NATURAL FIGHT OR FLIGHT RESPONSE TO STRESS/TRAUMA:

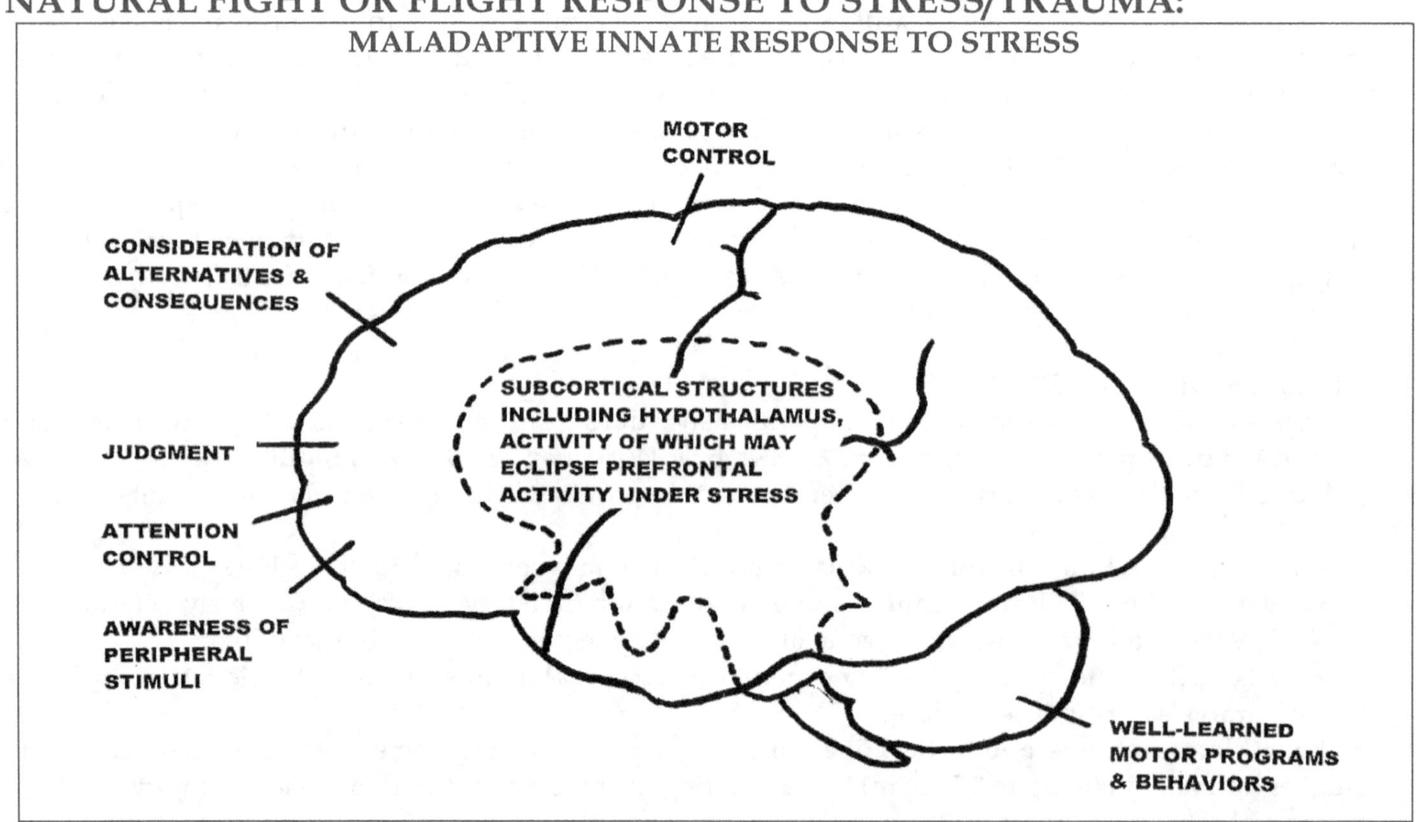

The Primordial Reflex: Fight, Flight, and the Collapse of Higher Reasoning

When anxiety triggers the **fight-or-flight response**, humans enter an **innate, primordial reflexive state**—a survival mechanism hardwired deep within our biology. As **Mathew Sharps** describes in his assessment of decision-making under stress among law enforcement officers, the **quality of human reasoning changes dramatically** when threat and urgency converge.

Under normal conditions, individuals rely on **higher-order problem-solving processes** that involve deliberate analysis, pattern recognition, and strategic reasoning. Even when faced with unexpected events, as long as there is adequate time and the situation is not perceived as life-threatening, decision-making remains thoughtful and rational.

However, once an individual perceives **threat, time pressure, and uncertainty**, the brain shifts abruptly to a **lower level of complexity**. This paradoxical regression—what Sharps calls the "reflexive override"—reflects a shift from cortical to **subcortical dominance**.

The Neurophysiology of Survival Reflexes

In primitive humans, acute stress triggered a cascade of subcortical responses that optimized survival. The **fight-or-flight instinct**, governed primarily by the amygdala and brainstem, redirected oxygen and blood flow **away from the cerebral cortex** (the center of judgment and reasoning) toward the **muscles and survival centers** needed for combat or escape.

This physiologic adaptation was vital in a hostile environment—it enhanced speed, strength, and instinctual reaction. Yet in modern complex settings, such as **surgery, aviation, or crisis command**, this same survival mechanism becomes **maladaptive**.

The result is a predictable degradation in cognitive performance, characterized by:

- **Impulsive, non-discriminatory behavior**
- **Diminished attention and situational awareness**
- **Reduced judgment and flexibility**
- **Perseveration** (repeating the same ineffective action)
- **Overreliance on habitual, instinctive reflexes**

In essence, the higher brain—the seat of logic and executive control—is **overridden** by primitive systems built for survival, not precision. While this reflex may save a life on the savannah, it can **endanger a patient on the operating table** or derail a team in crisis. *(Sharps M.; Grossman D.; Siddle B.)*

COMBATANT READINESS VS SURGEON READINESS:

Unlike surgeons, combatants work best during an adrenaline surge. As Rorke Denver explains in his book "at moments like these, the hair on the back of my neck always stands straight up. I was paying laser attention. My senses were almost tingling. I felt like I was somewhere back in the animal world." Rorke Denver

MALADAPTIVE BEHAVIORS SEEN IN RESPONSE TO STRESS / ANXIETY:

Several responses are seen by an observer when a person becomes stressed and anxious and enters a fight or flight mode. There are nine basic categories of maladaptive behavior seen:

- **Sound Anomalies**
- **Inability to speak**
- **Intrusive Thoughts**
- **Automatic Pilot**
- **Memory loss**
- **Sense of time deceleration**
- **Denial**
- **Tunnel Vision**
- **Panic**
- **Over-steering**
- **Dissociation / Paralysis**

SOUND ANOMALIES
- More common response seen with stress / anxiety
- Sounds subjectively diminished in volume (in some cases louder as the brain selects out specific foci).
- Loss of peripheral input

INABILITY TO SPEAK

INTRUSIVE THOUGHTS
- Mind drift - common occurrence under pressure.
- Thoughts enter subconscious
- Interferes with conscious efforts at resolving the current situation
- Loss of impulse control / lack of diplomacy in stressful situations.
- Random thoughts simply get blurted out.

SOUND ANOMALIES: Auditory exclusion also occurs under stress where your hearing is entirely focused on the subject that you are facing, to the obliteration of sounds from outside that venue. It is apparent that during stress, when you need more information, your body is shutting your sensory processes down, greatly narrowing your perspective. Again, that is fine if you are focused on your dinner, but not in the middle of a complex process that has gone awry when you must be able to take in conversations around you and gather important information from multiple resources. [Sharps]

INABILITY TO SPEAK: Complex motor coordination tends to decline after a heart rate of 130. One crisis response that deteriorates quickly during anxiety is the ability to speak. Dave Grossman explained to me in a personal conversation, that it is not uncommon for a person to not be able to talk when they become over-anxious. This is why he teaches people to train to say the message they expect they would need to communicate during an emergency, in a controlled environment (practice it over and over in a calm place). This way the message will come out automatically even if under duress.

> *One day in clinic, one of our PA's grabbed me and pushed me into a room. I looked at her as she tried to talk but nothing discernable came out other than 'HELP'. I quickly realized that a student was in trouble as I watched folks raising her legs and dropping her head. Afterwards, I joked about how she manhandled me in the hallway. She told me she simply could not talk. She wanted to speak but could not verbalize the words. It was as if her mouth would not cooperate with her brain. So, she just pushed me into the room.*

INTRUSIVE THOUGHTS: Mind drift is a common occurrence when one is under pressure. Your prefrontal inhibition allows a multitude of thoughts to enter your subconscious which then interferes with your conscious efforts to resolve the situation. This tendency is exactly what causes loss of impulse control and lack of diplomacy in some stressful situations. Your random thoughts simply get blurted out.

MALADAPTIVE REPONSES

AUTOMATIC PILOT:
- Habitual, perseveration behavior.
- Trained over and over to respond in a specific way to specific circumstances.
- Even if the situation has changed, response is unaltered.
- If the habit is recreated in the wrong scenario, it can be deadly.

MEMORY LOSS OR DISTORTION:
- Loss of memory during a stressful event is a common fact.
- We get stressed and can't 'think straight'.
- We are too rushed to find solutions or a way out.

SENSE OF TIME DECELERATION:
- Sense of time slowing down during stress.
- Perceived sense of speed in the presence of slow-moving surroundings, can lead to a false sense of security.

AUTOMATIC PILOT: Under stress, many resort unintentionally to habitual, perseverative behavior. They have been trained over and over to respond in a specific way to specific circumstances and even if the situation has changed, their response is unaltered. While typically this is a beneficial response, if the habit is recreated in the wrong scenario, it can be deadly. Sharps

MEMORY LOSS OR DISTORTION OF MEMORY: During a stressful event, memory loss or distortion is a common fact. We get stressed and can't "think straight." We are too rushed to find solutions or a way out. When one is a victim during a crisis, memory loss and distortion is even more profound. Sharps

SENSE OF TIME DECELERATION: Survivors report the sense of time slowing down during a crisis. The perceived sense of speed in the presence of slow-moving surroundings, can lead to a false sense of security. Sharps

DENIAL

- Ironic heuristic Fixation Response.
- In spite of obvious threats, victim continues on with current activities as if no threat exists.

DENIAL: Denial is a form of confirmation bias (heuristic response described earlier) that is often referred to as normalcy or complacency bias. Normalcy-bias is the situation where we react to the current situation utilizing past experiences with the assumption that this was the most appropriate (or normal) response to the situation in front of us; that is, you recall a certain set of actions or reactions previously utilized that were successful in scenarios seemingly similar to the one you are now facing. While this reaction may be acceptable in many circumstances, this can be a detrimental response. It is absolutely necessary to accept that an event is a crisis for a coordinated response to occur, yet frequently we waste valuable time in denial before we accept our fate. While on the surface it may seem very basic, participants observing an unfolding disaster first-hand must first persuade them-selves of the impending doom and then take on the task of convincing others. Unfortunately, on a basic level, we decide that everything was fine in prior experiences and therefore we must be "okay" in the current but dangerous situation. Sharps

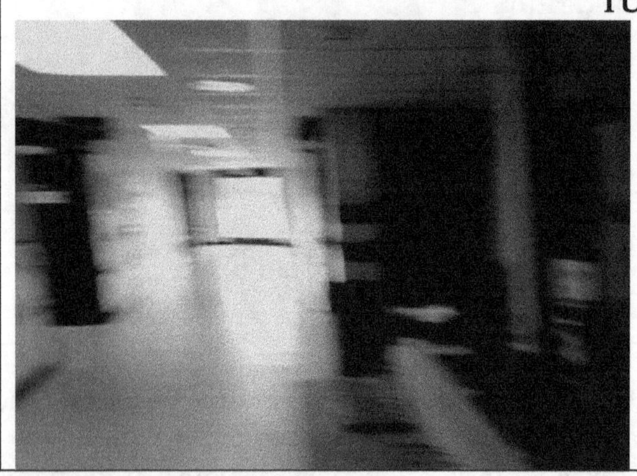

TUNNEL VISION

- Loss of situational awareness.
- 2nd most common phenomenon observed during stress.
- Instinctual response – Intense focus on target, ignoring invaluable peripheral stimuli.
- Focused on what is perceived to be the most important part of the scenario.
- Hyperfocus - centrally occupied, valuable information is lost.

This is why we ignore what is obviously in front of us or around us!

TUNNEL VISION: This is one type of loss of situational awareness. This turns out to be the second most common phenomenon observed during stress. This instinctual response allows the hunter to focus on his prey and ignore invaluable stimuli in the periphery. You become focused on what is perceived to be the most important part of the scenario. However, if you become hyper-focused, centrally occupied, valuable information may be lost. It is virtually impossible to lead a team through a crisis if one cannot gather details from the periphery. To make matters worse, this instinctual response is also what is responsible for one ignoring what is obviously in front of them. Missing a hazard in front, behind, or beside you can then be deadly to you and the rest of your team. It is vital that team members learn to speak up if it is apparent that another member has lost situational awareness.[Sharps]

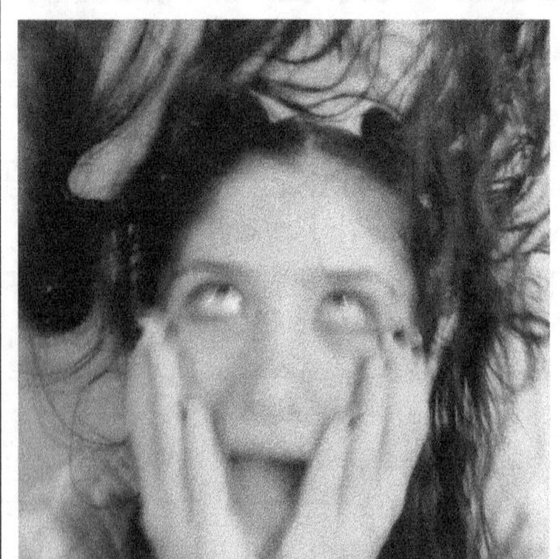

ANXIETY / PANIC!

- STATE vs. TRAIT ANXIETY*:
- <u>State anxiety-</u> response to particular event <u>Trait (resting) Anxiety-</u> individual personal characteristic- general tendency to see things as stressful.
- Surgeons and Anesthesia report *HIGHER* **trait anxiety** than nurses or techs AND Senior practitioners reported significantly *HIGHER* **trait anxiety** than junior practitioners.
- No difference in State Anxiety.
- **So..... by nature, we tend to be tightly wound and that may not be as conducive to learning as we think it is.**
[Phitayakorn R, et al]

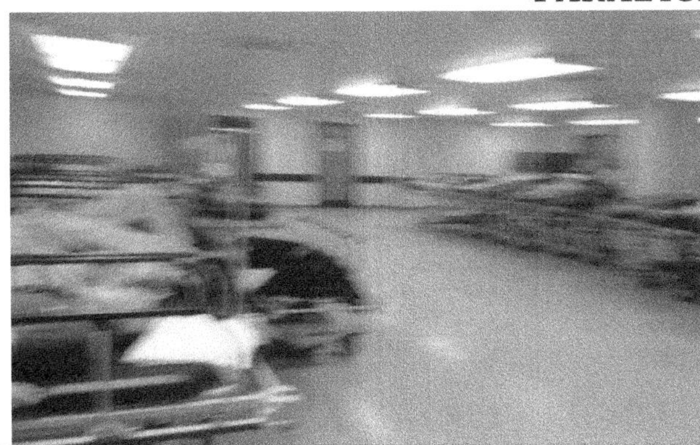

PARALYSIS (dissociation, milling)

- o More common than panic.
- o Amygdala response- when all hope is lost, when escape seems impossible and the situation unfamiliar to the extreme.

DISSOCIATION/PARALYSIS:

This is an extreme example of loss of situational awareness. Dissociation occurs when a person is clearly no longer a part of the immediate environment and functions totally independent to the region surrounding them. Both dissociation and paralysis are more common when individuals experience tachycardia above 170 beats per minute, secondary to cortical flow diversion and dysfunction. [Sharps]

> *"One night we had a placental abruption and the patient was hemorrhaging on the table. I walked into the room and the anesthesia provider was just staring into the air. I had to yell at him to think about intubating the patient and calling for blood and alert the blood bank about our problem. He was just starring off into nothingness, totally oblivious to what was going on."*

CAUSATION & OVER-STEERING

- ■ Under pressure, we apply OVERDOSES of established measures - making things worse.
- ■ We think in terms of <u>nonlinear</u> networks of causation rather than <u>chains</u> of causation.
- ■ Guided by the situation at each stage – we try to regulate the immediate situation
- ■ **THIS REACTION IS WORSENED BY ANXIETY!**
  a) When driving off the shoulder – one typically instinctively flings the car back onto the interstate often into the path of other cars.
  b) When we get lost **we keep wandering around getting more lost rather than stop and seek help!**
WE END UP ADOPTING AN OVER-RESPONSE TO AN EASILY FIXED PROBLEM!

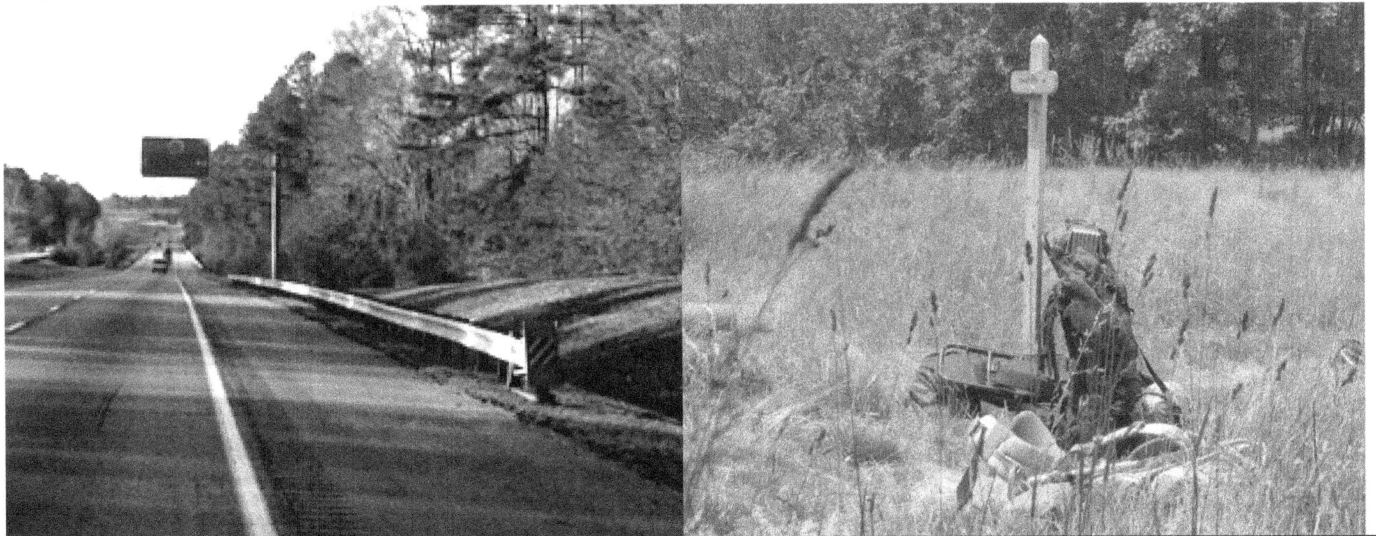

As Dörner (author of *Logic of Failure*) describes, "The tendency to over-steer is characteristic of human interaction in dynamic systems," meaning that we all too often guided by the situation at each stage and then try to over-regulate the situation.

This is similar to what happens when the average person drives off the shoulder and instinctively flings the car back into the path of other cars. The goal is to get back onto the freeway, but the usual startle response heightens that goal, instinctively causing most to overreact and over-steer in the direction they want to go.

We simply apply overdoses of established measures and make the situation worse, as in when one gets lost in the wilderness. As panic sets in, the tendency is to continue to try to make one's way to the point of origin and wander around as one becomes even more lost. It is rare for a lost hiker (or any health-care provider) to simply *stop* and go back to where they last knew where they were or to simply quit and wait for help. *But* that is what one needs to do when they find they are lost—*stop and seek help*. Dorner

THE CRITICAL MOMENT - SMOOTH CONTROLLED ORGANIZATIONAL PROCESS DURING THE DECISIVE MOMENT:

IV.G. ESTABLISHMENT OF LEADERSHIP / FOLLOWERSHIP/ MAINTAINING SITUATIONAL AWARENESS.

Transitioning from Recognition to Action: Establishing Leadership in Crisis

Once you have **recognized the problem**, **stopped all activity**, and **regained control of your team**, the next steps are critical. Above all, **someone must assume leadership.** Those who are not leading must consciously adopt the role of **followers**. From this point forward, **everything depends on precise communication and sustained situational awareness.** Without these, effective damage control, planning, and execution are impossible.

While general leadership principles are outlined in **Chapter II**, the principles in this section apply specifically to situations that have **escalated beyond routine operations into full-blown crisis.** These moments demand structure, clarity, and composure under pressure.

It is worth noting that leaders who practice **organized, decentralized command** in their daily operations—where leadership and followership are grounded in **trust, honesty, explicit communication, and mutual respect**—find that transitioning from everyday leadership to **crisis leadership** is far less difficult. In essence, teams that communicate clearly and operate with shared purpose during calm conditions are the ones most capable of maintaining control and cohesion when the environment turns chaotic.

TEAM COMMAND AND CONTROLLED RISK MANAGEMENT

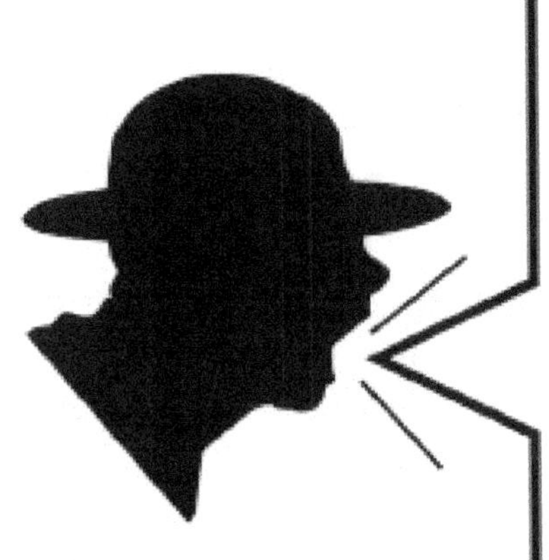

Lipsky K. CRISIS MANAGEMENT LEADERSHIP: TEAM TRAINING TO SURVIVE THE CRITICAL MOMENT 3rd ed; 2018

With permission from these sources Gaba, Okray, Crew Resource Management for the fire service, Crew resource management refresher Coast Guard

Taking Command: Leadership in Crisis

In a crisis, **someone must take command—take charge—and make a plan to get out alive.** Every team in chaos instinctively looks for direction. Leadership must emerge quickly and decisively to prevent confusion, duplication of effort, or paralysis.

In most organizations, **crisis leadership is pre-established by hierarchy**—the most senior or highest-ranking individual assumes command. However, in the **modern healthcare environment**, leadership is often **distributed across multiple, overlapping layers**—attending physicians, nursing supervisors, residents, and administrative leaders—each with independent spheres of responsibility. This can easily create confusion or even anarchy if **realms of authority** are not clearly defined. Before a crisis occurs, teams must clarify **who is in charge of what** and how command transitions if that individual becomes unavailable.

The Commander's Role: Lessons from the Coast Guard and Fire Service

Drawing from **Coast Guard Command and Control** and **Fire Service Incident Command** protocols, the effective crisis commander must fully understand and execute several key roles:

1. **Develop and lead the plan** to overcome the crisis while maintaining cognitive control under pressure (see *Risk Management* below).
2. **Exercise authority with respect.**
3. **Model calmness.** No yelling, no panic—emotional control sets the tone for the team.
4. **Use clear, concise communication** (see section on Communication).
5. **Be inclusive of team input.** Seek input but retain decisional authority.
6. **Prioritize and define tasks** clearly. Set achievable goals and time-sensitive benchmarks.
7. **Assign roles and distribute workload** evenly and appropriately. Avoid over-tasking individuals or assigning duties beyond their capability. Beware the "I can do anything" mindset. In the 1990s, Dr. Robert Helmreich's studies on commercial airline pilots revealed that many believed they were immune to cognitive overload. Under stress, however, performance declined sharply, and many failed to recognize they were overwhelmed and making critical mistakes.

8. **Manage resources effectively.** Declare emergencies early and call for assistance promptly. Key players should not leave the operational area.
9. **Monitor and manage team stress, conflict, and panic.** Use active listening, maintain composure, and stay mission-focused.
10. **Control followership.** Effective leaders ensure that followers understand their roles, communicate clearly, and execute instructions while remaining capable of independent thought and adaptation.

A team is composed of a leader who provides clear direction and followers who both think and act with disciplined initiative.

— Adapted from U.S. Coast Guard CRM and Fire Command principles – crew resource refresher coast guard, Okray, Gaba, Crew Resource management for the fire service.

Clarifications and Core Concepts

1. Authority with Respect

Effective leaders practice what the U.S. Coast Guard defines as **"authority with participation, assertiveness with respect."** This means leading decisively while maintaining courtesy and composure. Disrespect, criticism, or shouting only magnify stress and undermine confidence.

2. Respectful, Clear Communication

Respectful command is not passive humility—it is **assertive clarity**. Communication must be **direct, structured, and purposeful**, beginning with a concise statement to capture attention and followed by actionable directives. Ambiguity breeds confusion.

3. Inclusion of Team Input

Leaders must create an environment where every team member feels responsible for the outcome. Encourage expression of **"owned emotions"**—concerns voiced as personal observations, not accusations. When problems are raised, acknowledge whether they are **real or perceived**, propose immediate potential solutions, and seek quick consensus or course correction. Above all, **say what needs to be said—clearly and succinctly.**

<table>
<tr><td>

"CALM IS CONTAGIOUS" / MANAGING STRESS

One of leader's main responsibilities is to restore order.

- Leaders should evaluate the context within which units are operating and manage the physical and psychological aspects of the environment.
- Leader's focus should be **managing perceptions of stressors** by engendering attributions to make sense of the circumstances via:

a. education

b. cohesion

c. promoting coping strategies

d. instilling sense of commitment, control and challenge.

Sweeney PJ et al *Leadership in Dangerous Situations*

</td></tr>
</table>

<table>
<tr><td>

STOICISM-KEEP A STIFF UPPER LIP

side note regaring inappropriate management of excitement

Contrary to popular belief, a hyper-enthusiastic screaming commander is counterproductive in the midst of a crisis. Calm and level-headed leaders get the job done and keep their team members OUTWARD FOCUSED and situationally aware. Screaming only serves to intensify the emotions of team members who are already likely struggling to keep it together. Be the example; if you want them calm, you have to stay calm. NO YELLING! Kolditz, *In Extremis Leadership*.

The commander with a stiff upper lip who is not over-reactive to every small problem they face is more respected by their subordinates than those who lose their cool over everything. You must learn to

</td></tr>
</table>

remain calm in the heat of battle. Leadership models are passed onto those around us just like our children. They pick up our bad habits. _{Lt col Dave Grosman}

STOIC V.S. SCREAMING LEADERSHIP:

"I worked for two different cardiac surgeons.

I remember after one just finished an aortic bypass operation, the area around the repair just started to bubble and hiss loudly. He looked up at the monitor and asked if the anesthesia provider saw what was happening. The provider was extremely nervous and said he gave the patient a vasopressor because the pressure dropped when the clamps came off but the blood pressure was now extremely high. The surgeon just calmly said that he was now going to have to reinforce the anastomosis and that the anesthesia provider should have taken some time and talked with him before giving the pressors. He never lost his cool.

While working with another cardiac surgeon, the surgeon pulled the sternal saw through the patient's previous bypass graft. The patient started deteriorating fast as blood was spewing everywhere and just pouring out of the chest. As the patient started to die he just looked over the screen and started yelling profusely at the chief of anesthesia that they were killing his patient. He never let up. He just kept yelling. That just made everyone even more nervous."

It was clear that while both surgeons were respected, it was a different type of respect. One was respect based on pure fear the other was based on admiration.

CREW RESOURCE MANAGEMENT LEADERSHIP IN THE FIRE SERVICE
TYPES OF LEADERSHIP EXEMPLIFIED DURING A CRISIS:

- <u>Formal leaders</u>: as dictated by the organizational structure.
- <u>Informal leaders</u>: someone volunteered to lead.
- <u>Situational leadership</u>: someone was spontaneously called to duty.

WHAT DOES A LEADER NEED TO DO? (LESSONS LEARNED FROM FIRE CHIEFS)

- Lead People / Manage Things.
- Be confident but NOT ARROGANT!
- Risk calculations.
- Team building- shared mental models, clear direction, consistency, rewards. "The greater the fire-crew's cohesion the fewer the accidents".
- Team performance control.
- Everyone goes home safe.
- Worry about the "what ifs".
- Assure technical proficiency.
- Keep SA- Don't go into the thick of the situation. STAY BACK and keep an eye on things. Don't pick up the chain saw to clear cut a pathway.
- Solicit feedback.
- Debriefs after the event. _{Okray,Lubnau}

BRIEFINGS AND EXPECTATION MANAGEMENT

- For teams to be effective, the team as a whole must be knowledgeable in what their duties are for their own task, to the strategy, to the operation as a whole and to other teams.
- To do this they must be briefed.
- In a NASA study of 7500 flight crews they determined that the effectiveness of CRM depended on the Captain providing a thorough briefing and the subordinates making inquiries and advocating their position.
- "You don't know what you don't know and what you don't know could kill you".
- <u>Expectations</u>: Briefings manage expectations!
- We assume that a lot of factors will be in play BECAUSE they are supposed to happen that way.
- <u>Responsibilities</u>: there will be times when the exact responsibilities of teams and individuals will not be apparent to everyone. A briefing makes this clear. Okray, lubnau

RESOURCE MANAGEMENT AND BRIEFINGS:

To be prepared for complex crisis situations, leaders need to emphasize:
a. communication, b. inventory, c. mobilization of available resources when needed, as well as d. continued monitoring and cross-checking of all data. This is best accomplished in advance of a crisis using preemptive briefings involving the entire team. These concepts on team management have been instituted worldwide but acceptance and validation are lagging. Okray

MEMORY

- Humans function w/ two basic degrees of memory:
- <u>Short-term</u> or working memory and <u>long-term memory</u>.
- Stress shifts your focus AWAY from the group and back to you as an individual.
- When we panic, we can't remember anything recent, but we tend to remember remote memories – that is short term memory is diminished but long-term memory is enhanced.
- To help someone under duress, minimize the short term / working memory load by only dishing out 3-4 bits of information at a time.
- **Increasing memory: strategies for improvement:**
  - •Chunking: clump information in relational groupings rather than spreading them out individually.
  - •Visual Reminders- Associate verbal / auditory information with visual clues.
  - •Training in context- i.e. train like you play! Okray,Lubnau

The best time to improve team memory response is BEFORE these events occur! Practice on a day to day basis on improving your team's response to memory requests.

WORDS OF WARNING!

EMOTIONAL INVOLVEMENT: REMEMBER! THE NOOSE ALWAYS FEELS MUCH TIGHTER WHEN IT'S AROUND YOUR OWN NECK!

- Are you "EMOTIONALLY Involved"? Did you create the crisis?
- Beware of anxiety clouding your judgment.
- Think twice about running the team crisis management!

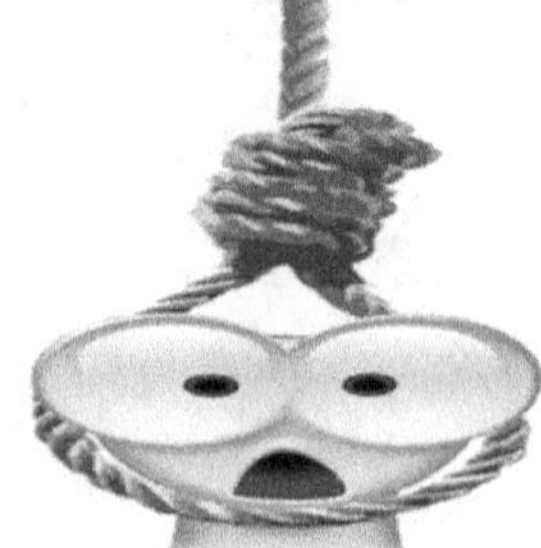

If the crisis was created by your own error, give a lot of thought whether you should be commanding. Think very hard about turning over the command to another experienced person if you sense your judgment is clouded by your own anxiety.

> *I was doing a really difficult hernia and ended up in the bladder. I wanted to just repair it and watch the patient but felt I was "emotionally involved" so got the opinion of several others to assure my judgement was not clouded.*

ERROR MANAGEMENT:

The commander must remain cognizant of, and manage errors. Minimization of further errors is a key role of leadership and crew during a disaster. This occurs through:

☐ Following *tried and true* standard SOP's and crisis checklists. This takes the guesswork out of many steps and eliminates arguing over protocols. Pilots who ignored an SOP are 1.6 times more likely to commit a second error.

☐ Minimizing distractions.

☐ Asking before all actions if that step makes sense.

☐ Controlling fixations errors such as:

    1. <u>One goal-one solution error</u>- The misbelief that "there has to be only one problem."

    2. <u>Exclusion error</u>- "It has to be anything but this."

    3. <u>Denial</u>- "Everything is fine." Gaba Okray, Crew Resource Management fire service, Crew Resource Management Coast Guard

☐ Maintaining situational awareness.

IV.H. TEAM LEADER MUST MAINTAIN TEAM SITUATIONAL AWARENESS!

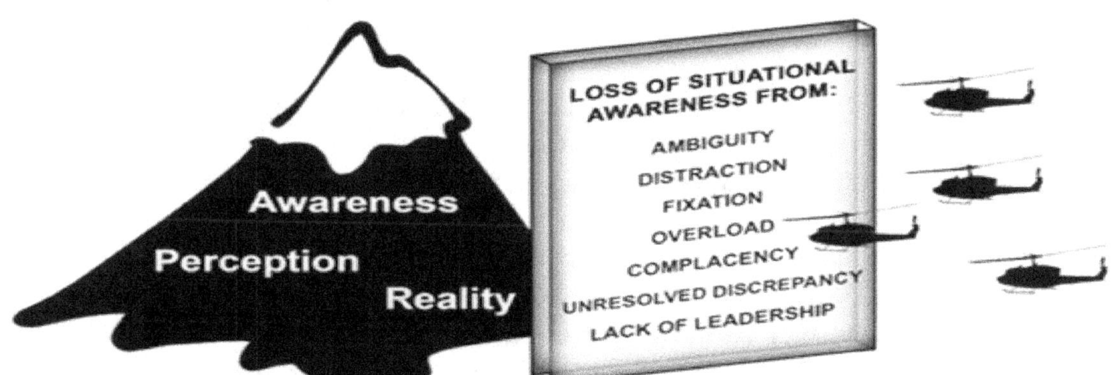

Gaba, Okray, Crew Resource Management for the fire service, Crew resource management refresher Coast Guard

SITUATIONAL AWARENESS

- WHAT IS SA: SA is the skill of becoming aware of the situation as it actually exists.
- Typically, there is a large variance between what actually exists and what we perceive to exist.
- <u>Skills involved</u>:
  - Monitoring.
  - Evaluation of information.
  - Anticipation of developments.
  - Consider contingencies.
  - Thinking ahead.
  - Focus on what is right and not who is right. Okray

Situational awareness (SA) simply put is knowing what is going on around you *and* knowing what is important based on the operator's occupational goals and decision task.

This is a continual process that starts with the perception of elements in the environment followed by the comprehension of the current situation. According to Mica Endsley (Chief Scientist of the US Air Force Pentagon, via personal communication), 88% of aviation accidents involving human errors were associated with poor SA. Seventy-six percent of SA errors occur in pilots due to ***problems in perception of needed information***, secondary to either failure in the system or cognitive processes. Twenty percent of SA errors occur at the ***level of comprehension***. Comprehension involves the integration of multiple pieces of information and a determination of relevance to the person's goals. The final stage of SA is the ***projection of this information into a forecast of future events and dynamics***.

SA alone will not guarantee the correct strategy choice. It is possible to have total awareness of the situation, but make a wrong decision based on that information. In a review of aircraft accidents, 26.6% involved poor decision making ***in spite of obvious appropriate awareness of the situation***. In turn, it is possible to be lucky and make a great decision in spite of being totally unaware of the situation surrounding you. This cannot be a passive process whereby one receives information yet is not actively involved. After information is processed, the recipient must act upon this in whatever role they are expected to have in a given situation. _{Endsley, Okray, crew resource management for fire service.}

CAUSES FOR LOSING SITUATIONAL AWARENESS

A. Fixation and tunnel vision: Commanding officers who get wrapped up in the minutiae and not the overall picture rapidly lose SA.

    To avoid fixation leaders, need to:
1. Designate at scene safety officers who manage the minutiae and relay reports back.
2. Allow for fixed time points to reassess the situation and stop activity to remain fully aware of everything going on around them.

B. Overconfidence: belief that one knows exactly what is happening and in absolute control.

C. Distraction: To reduce distractions, team leaders need to:
1. Maintain sterile cockpit (keeping distraction to a minimum while communicating vital information).
2. Train everyone to recognize the distractions.
3. Develop standardized protocols and checklists.

D. Information overload: To minimize information overload, leaders need to train staff to over learn particular skills. By over-training / over-learning tasks beyond the level of initial proficiency this allows for 65% fewer errors compared to simply aiming for an initial proficiency.

E. Communication deficiency.

F. Low stress level: not on our guard.

G. High Stress level.

H. Lack of experience.

I. Fatigue / Illness.

J. Reliance on machines.

K. Unresolved discrepancies.

L. Professional attitude: overconfidence; 'I Can do it!'; machismo. _{Okray,Lubnau}

OVERALL STRATEGIES FOR MAINTAINING SITUATIONAL AWARENESS

- Maintain control- keep a global perspective, step back, gather information, and shed unnecessary tasks.

- Continually gather information, monitor the results- "if you have been doing something for a minute without any results, do something different."
- Looking for ghosts- always remember to look for what "isn't there".
- Gut feeling- Pay attention to that nagging feeling that something is not right- even if you cannot pin it down.
- **<u>Things to help prepare you in advance to maintain SA:</u>**
  - Experience and training- preplan for these events.
  - Professional attitude.
  - Emotional / Physical stability. ^{Okray}

PERSON IN CHARGE SHOULD HAVE FULL PERSPECTIVE AND NOT BE PRE-OCCUPIED

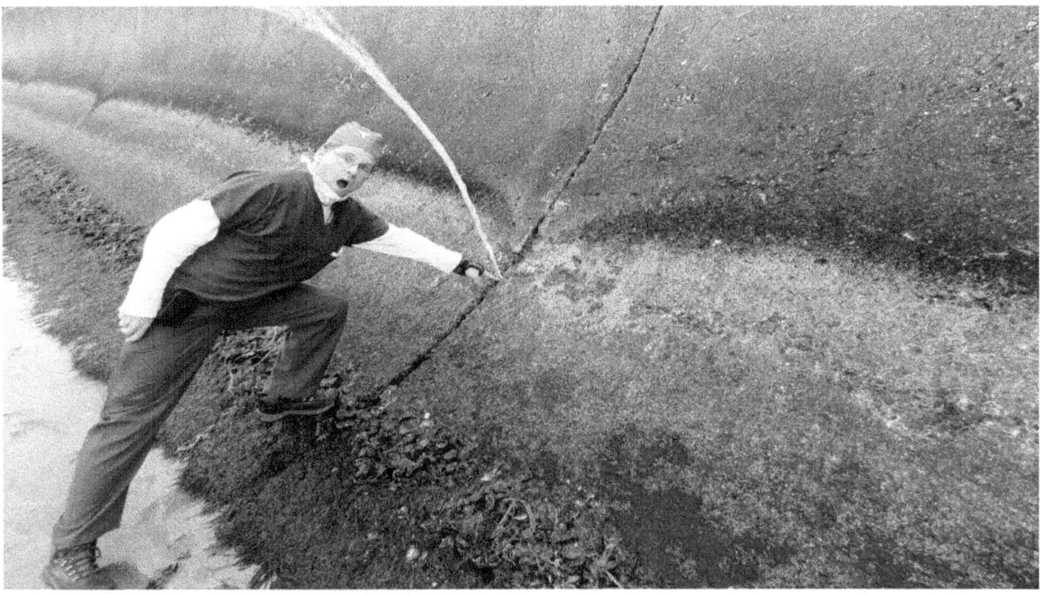

The commander cannot be preoccupied with every detail or very specific aspects of the event or he will be unable to maintain total control over the situation (with loss of SA).

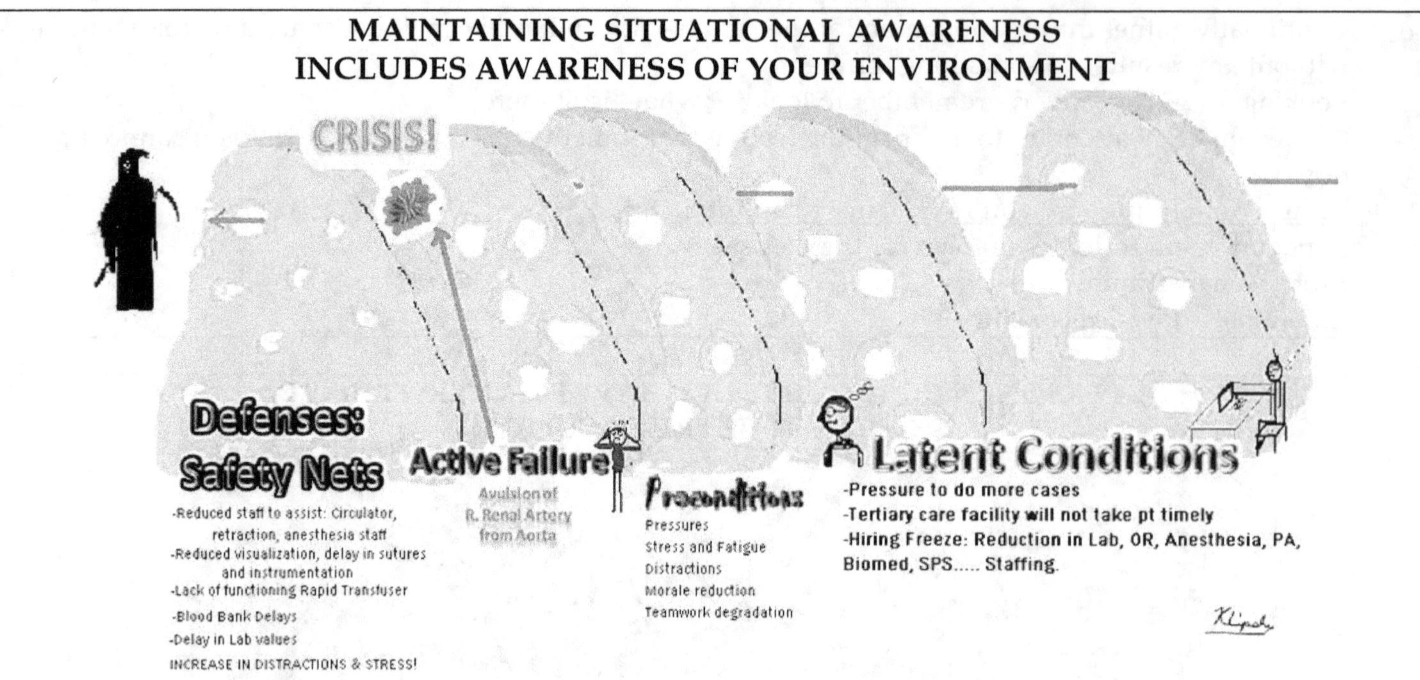

Use of Reason's System Model to explain transition from a difficult procedure to a crisis (misadventure or other unexpected event) to a disaster (death in the O.R.).

Latent conditions are brought about by administrative pressure to do more cases, lack of ability to transfer difficult cases to higher level center, recent release of staff or hiring of cheaper, less experienced staff.

Preconditions exist for years and include fatigue, stress, ambivalence, lack of knowledge, reduction in resources followed by teamwork and communication degradation.

System Safety nets are then discovered to be absent leading to propagation of a misadventure or other unexpected event into a patient care disaster. Safety nets typically revolve around lack of resources thought to exist but in actuality are absent (staff, training, supplies, equipment, etc.) as well as distractions created by inefficiencies elsewhere in the organization. Gordon Dupont Systems Safety Services

One aspect of maintaining situational awareness includes being aware of your working environment and system problems. While it is better to know this before an event occurs, you rely on your team to tell you when there are systemic problems that break down your safety nets increasing the risk of failure. This topic is covered in section *IV.CONCLUSION HEALTHY ORGANIZATIONAL SAFETY CLIMATE* and in even more detail in *Crisis Management Leadership in the Operating Room*, so it will not be replicated here.

IV.I. FOLLOWERSHIP, TEAMS and TEAMWORK!

AS A "FOLLOWER" I RESOLVE TO MAINTAIN:

- Respect for authority
- Establishment of assertiveness / authority balance
- Personal safety
- Safety of fellow followers and leaders
- Acceptance that authority goes with responsibility
- Knowledge of the limits of your own authority
- The desire to make the leader succeed
- Possession of good communication skills
- Development of positive learning attitude
- Ego balance and check
- Communication to assure I have clear assignments
- Acceptance of direction and information as needed
- Reporting of any personal mistakes
- Constant reports of work
- Flexibility

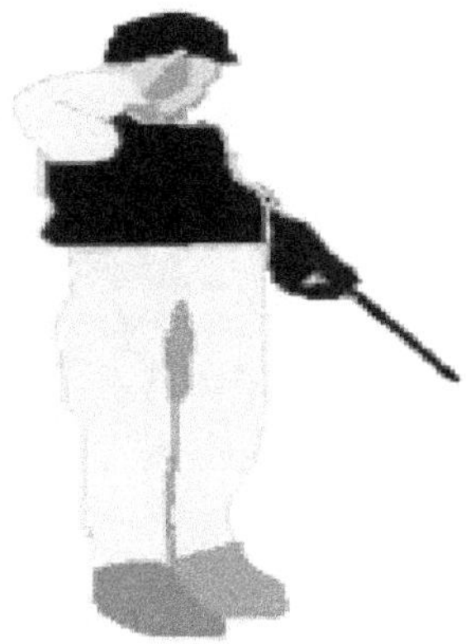

Lipsky K. CRISIS MANAGEMENT LEADERSHIP: TEAM TRAINING TO SURVIVE THE CRITICAL MOMENT 3rd ed; 2018

Gaba, Okray, Crew Resource Management for the fire service, Crew resource management refresher Coast Guard

FOLLOWERSHIP-
WHY DO FOLLOWERS FOLLOW:

1. They do not know any better and feel compelled to do so either emotionally or by organizational hierarchy.
2. They do know better through training / experience but still feel compelled to do so either emotionally or by organizational hierarchy.
3. They have faith in their leadership thru history.

DUTIES OF FOLLOWERS

- Contribute to the task and goal accomplishment.
- Understand environmental cues and communicate those cues in a respectful manner back to the leadership. ***70% of followers will not question a leader's point of view even when they believe the leader is about to make a serious mistake.***
- All successful leaders have CRITICAL FOLLOWERS.
- Remember to advocate your point but RAISE YOUR HAND FIRST!
- Constructive Criticism- "nothing fails like success. You never learn from it".
- Train.
- Help the leader lead- often times that means taking over duties so the leader can step back and maintain SA.
- Respect authority- Refrain from insubordination: Remember that not everyone is the chief. The goal of Crew Resource Management is to assure that everyone communicates effectively, but that does not imply that everyone is the chief.
- Be the safety eyes.
- Remember that PANIC & CALM is Contagious. Okray

TEAMWORK:

ESSENTIAL CHARACTERISTICS OF EFFECTIVE TEAMWORK

- Effective Communication
- Shared Mental Model
- Clear Roles & Responsibilities
- Mutual Trust
- Team Orientation-Briefing
- Mutual Performance Monitoring
- Backup Behavior
- Adaptability
- Team Leadership

Weller, Boyd. <u>Making a Difference Through Improving Teamwork in the Operating Room: A Systematic Review of the Evidence on What Works</u>; Patient Safety in Anesthesia. 4:77–83, (2014);

HALLMARKS & CRITICAL ESSENTIALS OF AN EFFECTIVE TEAM

Aside from consistent trustworthy leadership, Team Members in an effective team have:

A

- Aptitude and attitude- your attitude should be that you are ready and willing to do your best to succeed.
- Accountability
- Adaptive-flexible-resilient
- Autonomy with guidance- unhealthy autonomy = acting on one's own without seeking another's counsel. "Hierarchy that promotes isolationism is nothing more than taking and then reinforcing a closed-off shelter".

B

* Brand- what they are about

C

* Communication-transparent which provides for acknowlegment of receipt, comprehension and completion or problem achieving completion of task
* Conflict Resolution is the norm, assuring that the focus is on the situation and not the individuals; good conflict leads to creativity and avoids stagnation.
* Commitment- must be self motivated; individuals must take responsibility for knowlege and skills they require to perform their job effectively on the team.
* Collaboration, Cooperation and coordination- you cannot work in a silo in a complex system.
- Caring
- Consistency - for the team to be functional they need dependable consistent leadership.
- Constructive criticism
- Community- committed sense of community
- Cohesiveness
- Climate -fear and blame free
- Closeness

D

* Dependability: ability to count on one another to do their best quality work (Google)
- Direction- leadership; teams require clear direction. Ambiguity or lack of information can be disastrous for morale.

E

* Empowerment- the team must support its members and encourage discussion and participation to perpetuate collaboration.

- * Emotional intelligence- our ability to recognize, understand and manage our emotions along with our ability to recognize, understand and manage the emotions of others. This requires self-awareness, self-regulation, empathy and motivation.
- Empathy
- Expectations
- Education

F

- * Flexibility and resourcefulness- the members and team must be resilient and adaptable; the must be resourceful.
- Failure - deal w failure
- Focus- Lack of distraction

G

- Goals
- Genuine- no presences straightforward
- Guidance

H

- Humility accept an acknowledge error or failure
- Honesty
- Hazardous attitudes lacking: anti-authority, impulsivity, invulnerability, machismo, resigned, loner

I

- Interact and communicate
- No Incivility
- Inquiry- we need to be able to ask question, speak up
- Interpersonal risk by sharing mistakes
- Improving-desire to do better
- Interdependence- individuals can achieve mission goal only by working w others - i am depending on u to do your job for me to succeed. you cannot work in a silo in a complex system.

J

- Justice
- No jumping to conclusions

K

- * Knowledge KSA- The entire team is as strong or weak as the memberships' knowledge base of their primary responsibilities. If One member is struggling to do their own duty due to a knowledge deficit then the rest of the team will lag as well as they attempt to overcompensate, accommodate that members functions or to teach that member how do succeed.

L

- * Listening- Active Listening on behalf of the sender and receiver with assurance that the message is clear and comprehensible
- Leadership
- Leeway to make decisions
- Learn from past mistakes

M

- * Motivation- the team is motivated to do their best; does the work have meaning and is personally important to each member? Does what we do really matter? (Google).
- Mission
- Milestones
- Mutual learning

N

O	

* Norm- safety norm works best

* Opportunity to succeed

P	

* Psychological Safety -ability to take risks without feeling insecure or embarrassed (google).
* Passion to succeed – it has been said before that when the passion to succeed wanes, so will performance.
* Physically and mentally fit- cannot be fatigued.

Q	

* Quirks - no one is perfect

R	

* Responsible -Does their own duty flawlessly before casting doubt or criticism on others
* Resilient
* Respect- non-dismissive
* Rules-SOPs - takes guesswork out
* Responsibility
* Rewards
* Remember the goal of crew resource management is NOT to teach everyone to be the chief; the goal is to teach teams to communicate effectively to each other and to the chief.

S	

* Structure and Clarity- assurance that the goals, roles and execution plans are clear.
* Shared Vision Shared Mental Model- by Sharing ideas, sharing information the team has a shared mental model of the organizational goals and how they support these goals.
* Synergy-the need for things to work well. "minimum effort results in cooperative and effective action". Positive action of different individuals.
* Synchrony
* Simbiosis
* Safety- everyone gets home safely
* Seeking help and seeking feedback
* Sensitive to data- not everything IS measurable but no matter what we try to say we do care what the data says.
* Situational awareness
* Serendipity- turning misfortune into good luck. Making the best of a bad situation.
* Systems thinking rather than blame-oriented

T	

* Trust- see leadership; "when the chips are down and a snap decision must be made   Your team will have an synergy when reacting to an urgent command" if trust is in their foundation. (Okray and lubnau)
* Teaming-dynamic activity dominated by consistent mindset and practice of teamwork utilizing collaboration and coordination. you cannot work in a silo in a complex system. Requires communication, trust, willingness to reflect, cooperation, awareness and communication. (Edmondson)

U	

* Unified
* Ulterior motives - none
* Understanding- understand that teamwork is complex
* Acknowledge uncertainty
* Uncertainty is ok- WHEN you trust your team and leadership.

<table><tr><td>V</td></tr></table>

- Vision

<table><tr><td>W</td></tr></table>

- Winning attitude
- Work to make the team work
- Willingness to reflect.

WARNING SIGNS OF DYSFUNCTIONAL TEAMS (OKRAY LUBNAU)

- Team breaking into several smaller groups as the norm rather than the exception
- Frequent disagreements and arguments
- Personal matters brought into professional discussions
- Open disrespect for team members their values and / or possessions
- Observed lack of teamwork and support
- Organizational inaction towards necessary SOPs, meeting standards etc
- Tardiness and absences
- Destructive behind the scenes gossip

- Siebert A. The survivors personality. Penguin. New York NY. 2010.
- Edmondson AC. *Teaming: How Organizations Learn, Innovate, and Compete in the Knowledge Economy. John Wiley & Sons 2012.*
- Okray R, Lubnau T. *Crew Resource Management for the Fire Service.* Tulsa, OK: PennWell Press; 2004.
- M. Teamworks: Transforming Health Care's Error-Prone culture. Creative Team Publishing. San Diego CA. 2013.
- Davey Edward 5 essentials of great teamwork; http://www.tips4teamwork.com/5-essentials-of-great-teamwork.htm
- Productive Team Blog https://productiveteams.io/5-essentials-highperformance-team/
- Rozovsky J Five keys to a successful Google team (and why this is MORE imprtant than who you hire)
  https://rework.withgoogle.com/blog/five-keys-to-a-successful-google-team/
- How to build a strong team- on the tour de France; http://www.industryweek.com/corporate-culture/8-essentials-building-strong-team

- Mariotti C. Essentials of Teamwork (https://livology.com/teamwork-essentials/

IV.J. THE ART OF COMMUNICATING DURING A CRISIS: LESSONS FROM HIGH RISK FIELDS:

TWO WAY, CLOSED LOOP COMMUNICATION WITH A WARM HANDOFF = THE RIGHT MESSAGE TO THE RIGHT PERSON THE RIGHT WAY EVERY TIME!

SPEECHLESS UNDER FIRE

Speech is a fine-motor skill. As noted, when the heart rate begins to climb, fine-motor skills are the first to go. The average person cannot dial a phone when they are scared due to the inability to use fine-motor control. The same is true when under fire; the typical person becomes anxious and cannot talk clearly. When we need to communicate during a crisis, it turns out that we communicate our worst. Knowing that in advance provides an opportunity to rehearse critical communication BEFORE an incident occurs, increasing the likelihood that that skill will be automated when it is needed in a crisis. Grossman D. *On Combat:*

KEY ASPECTS OF COMMUNICATION ERRORS DURING CRISIS AND SELECTIVE FILTERS DURING INTERPRETATION

ACCURATE COMMUNICATION:

- Controlled! Steady! Calm!
- Accurate! Bold! Clear! Concise! Precise!
- Addressed to specific staff- NO GLOBAL COMMANDS
- Closed loop communication with feedback
- Open inclusive exchange
- Focus on WHAT is right and NOT WHO is right!

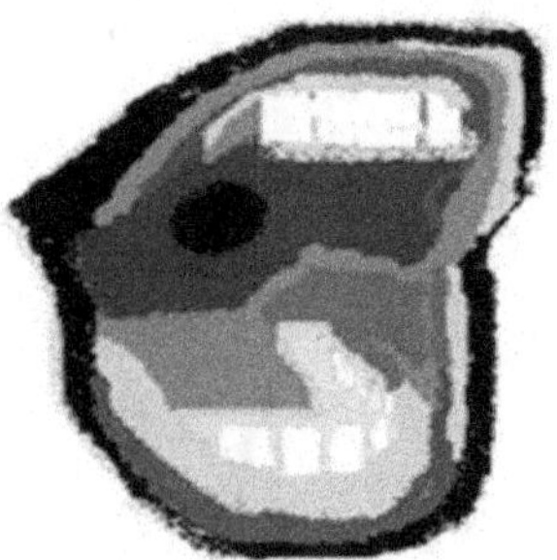

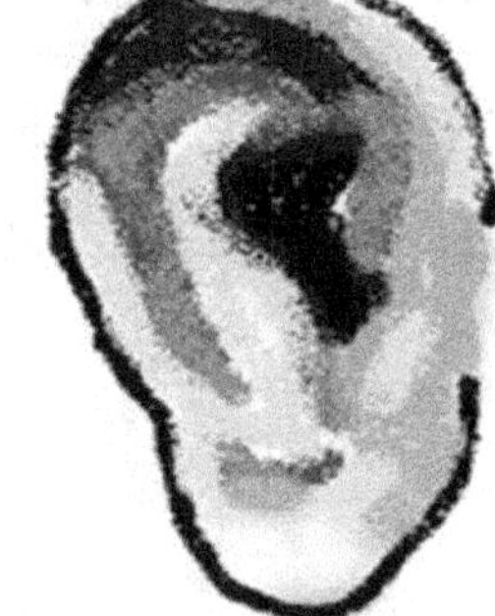

SENDER ERRORS:

- Not establishing a frame of reference
- Omission
- Biased-weighted information transmitted
- Forgetting body language is important
- Forgetting to repeat
- Disrespectful

RECEIVER ERRORS:

- Biased-preconceived notions
- Not consciously ready
- Thinking ahead of the sender
- Extrapolating the information based on biases
- Missing non-verbal signals
- Not asking for clarification
- Disrespectful

Lipsky K. CRISIS MANAGEMENT LEADERSHIP: TEAM TRAINING TO SURVIVE THE CRITICAL MOMENT 3rd ed; 2018 ITICAL MOMENT 3rd ed; 2018

Gaba, Okray, Crew Resource Management for the fire service, Crew resource management refresher Coast Guard

---

IN THE SITE OF THE CRISIS, COMMUNICATION MUST REMAIN *ACCURATE*:

- Controlled: voices should remain calm, steady, loud enough to be heard but without shouting.
- Commands need to be accurate, bold, clear, concise, and precise.
- Addressed to specific staff, not global commands.
- Close looped communication — needing constant feedback. Ask, "Does everyone understand me?" Open-ended questions function even better. Ask, "What did you understand I said?" or "What did you hear me say?"
- Open, inclusive exchange.
- Focused on what is right and not who is right

DURING A CRISIS, COMMUNICATION MUST NOT BE *ERRONEOUS.*

Examples of error in communication:

- **Sender Error:**
  - Not establishing a frame of reference: receiver is not on the same page as you.
  - Omitting information.
  - Providing biased–weighted information.
  - Forgetting that body language is important.
  - Forgetting to repeat — We normally talk about 125 words a minute and think at 500-1000 words a minute.
  - Giving disrespectful communication.
- **Receiver Error:**
  - Listening with bias, preconceived notions.
  - Poorly prepared to receive information, not consciously ready.
  - Thinking ahead of the sender, extrapolating the information, finishing sentences.
  - Missing non-verbal signals.
  - Not requiring clarification.
  - Disrespectful.
    Unfortunately, selective filters frequently occur during transition of information from the sender to the recipient's cognitive processing. These filters can easily distort the information resulting in misleading or erroneous interpretations, quickly resulting in inappropriate or dangerous actions on behalf of the recipient.
- **Filters to be aware of:**
  - Confirmation bias-resistance to change opinion, even when there is no support.
  - Defensive stature.
  - Blaming others.
  - Halo effect: the infallible one must be right, or "I am right; I am the infallible one."
  - "Odd man out" — "I just don't fit in." or "He does not fit in."
  - Fatigue.
  - Complacency.
  - Recklessness.
- **Other communication issues to be aware of:**
  - Inquiry: Are you asking the right question, in the right manner of the right person?
  - Advocacy: Are you an advocate of your team, mission, and position?
  - Listening: Were you really listening? Did he really hear me?
  - Conflict resolution: What is right, not who is right.
  - Feedback: to confirm understanding.   Gaba, Okra, CRM fire service, CRM coast guard

COMMUNICATION:

- FAA data suggests that in over 70% of aircraft incidents, errors in the transferring of information directly contributed to the cause of that incident.
- In 37% of incidents, there was a failure to initiate the information transfer process- that is the information was there but not made available to those who needed it the most.
- In the other 37% the information was provided in a useless manner (ambiguous, garbled, incomplete, and inaccurate).

USE MORE THAN ONE TYPE OF COMMUNICATION!

- Verbal (significant pitfall in that under duress we speak without actually thinking about what we are saying).
- Written. ■Non-verbal. ■Symbolic.

<u>**EFFECTIVE COMMUNICATION:**</u>

- More than one type of communication must be utilized (verbal, written, symbolic etc.) as people respond effectively in a different manner and one type may not be as effective.
- Be aware of Filters: Both the sender and receiver recognize that perceptions, influences, situations and filters affect the message.
- Require active listeners and comprehension.
- Require continuous loops of communication sending, reception and feedback, as staff are usually NOT listening to you. This has been validated in some studies where, **"videotaping the OR environment revealed how often individuals were not paying attention, despite their impression otherwise."** This attitude appeared to have occurred during critical event phases as well.

Okray; Bowermaster R, Eghtesady P, et al Application of the aviation black box principle. 'With approval'

REALITIES IN HUMAN COMMUNICATION:

- We protect ourselves when we communicate.
- We defend ourselves against looking ignorant.
- We wish to maintain consistency and support our own opinion even if we know that it may not be totally correct.
- We always wish to feel valued.
- The reality of the situation is always of secondary importance to our perception of the situation.
- We behave according to our perceptions.
- Emotions always overshadow everything.
- People always have their own motivation. okray

BEWARE OF "MITIGATED SPEECH"

- *"Mitigated speech"* describes our typical attempt to downplay or sugar coat the meaning of what is being said. We mitigate when we are being polite, or ashamed, or embarrassed or being deferential to authority.

  There are six ways to attempt to convince someone to change course and avoid a bad situation:

  1. **Command**- most direct way of making a point imaginable- zero mitigation "do this now".

  2. **Crew obligation statement**- request is much less specific and softer "I think we need to do this, this way".

  3. **Crew suggestion**- implicit statement- "let's do this, this way".

  4. **Query**- requesting to alter course, softer conceding you are not in charge, "which way do you want to deviate course?"

  5. **Preference**- note your preferred deviation route "I think we should go this way".

  6. **Hint**- "boy that looks bad over there" -most mitigated of all.

Gladwell M. *Outlier*

For a disastrous and deadly example of use of mitigated speech, look at the crash of the Columbia Avianca Flight 052, Jan 1990 in which a 707 enroute from Columbia South America to Kennedy Airport was forced to circle the northeast for an hour and a half before losing both engines due to lack of fuel.

Copilot to ATC: "That right to one-eight-zero on the heading and… ah… we'll try once again… We're running out of fuel…"

IMPROVING COMMUNICATION SKILLS:

- **Inquiry**: always ask for clarification if the order was not perfectly clear. Be respectful. If you need an answer to a question, ASK! Admit if you are confused or may have misunderstood direction.
- **Be Explicit**: Communication should be explicit, clear and NOT utilize implied instruction. Explicit communication does NOT assume everyone understands background information. Implying that the information is assumed can be dangerous. See details above about realities of communication. Even if we don't fully understand the information, we will not ask for clarification to protect ourselves and avoid appearing less knowledgeable.
- **Advocate for your team or mission**: A NTSB review of air carrier accidents from 1978-1990 revealed that 84% of the incidents were due to communication errors- usually in monitoring and challenging orders. 75% of those were due to external operational and organizational influences.
- **Advocacy** can be done in a respectful manner especially if you offer up solutions or alternate actions. Don't just throw up your hands when you don't get the answer you were hoping for. If someone dies it is just as much your fault.
- **Monitoring**: monitor the effects of your communication and actions.
- **Listen**: be patient and listen.
- **Watch out** for filters.
- **Resolve conflicts** immediately.
- Ask for feedback.
- **SUMMARY**: 8 of 10 subordinates would not question an officer even if they suspected there might be a danger in the current conditions and orders. ^{Okray}

DOES TEAMWORK & COMMUNICATION HAVE A BEARING ON PATIENT OUTCOME?

- Kaiser Permanente preformed a study in 2009, assessing intraoperative communication / teamwork behavior in 293 operating room procedures.
- Intraoperative observation of:
  a. Induction Phase
  b. Intraoperative Phase
  c. Handoff Phase
- Assessing:
  a. Briefing
  b. Information sharing
  c. Inquiry
  d. Vigilance.
- Followed by a review of 30-day outcomes data: Mortality and Morbidity
- **Conclusion: When surgical teams exhibited less teamwork, patients were at higher risk for death or complications even after risk adjustment for ASA category.**

Mazzocco K et al Am Jnl Surg; 2009. 197:678-685

EFFECTIVE COMMUNICATION LESSON

You are a resident seeing a patient in the endoscopy unit who hospitalized for severe diverticulitis several months ago.
The attending on record scheduled this patient for a colonoscopy several months after that episode because the patient is passing ribbon shaped stools and imaging stated there is a possibility of the patient having partial colon obstruction due to neoplasm. When the patient was scheduled for the procedure, he was totally asymptomatic for several months.
You assess the patient the morning of the procedure and the patient says he was seen by his primary care provider for another bout of diverticulitis a couple of weeks ago. Over the past two days he has been without any pain.
You call the attending to relay that the patient just finished his antibiotics just a few days ago and is currently pain free.
You explain that there was a CT scan that confirmed diverticulitis just two weeks ago.
The attending says that he will proceed with the endoscopy.

WHAT SHOULD YOU DO?

RECOMMENDATION: *While the attending is the person in charge, it is your obligation to assure that all the information you provided was received and understood. You can politely express your reluctance to proceed and ask to understand the attending physician's rational for proceeding under those circumstances.*
Odds are that he did not fully listen to you or that your information was not provided in a succinct and comprehendible method so you should try again.

EFFEECTIVE COMMUNICATION LESSON

You are a resident performing an endoscopy on a patient.
The procedure becomes very difficult so the attending takes over.
As he is performing the procedure the patient suddenly has a bradycardia rhythm in the 30's. Simultaneously his blood pressure is 70/50. The patient is suddenly totally unresponsive to any stimuli.
The attending immediately aborts the procedure and begins to withdraw the scope. The patient has a persistent bradycardia 30 seconds after the episode began and the blood pressure does not rise so the attending asks the staff to give him atropine. The heart rate immediately goes back to a rate in the 60s and the blood pressure 90 seconds after this episode began is in the 120/80 range.
In spite of this he remains completely unresponsive to deep stimuli.
He was only given 4mg of versed and 50 mcg of Fentanyl and was talking non-stop just prior to this; to be cautious he is given Flumazenil and Narcan but remains completely unresponsive to deep stimulation.
The endoscope is still inside the patient as the attending is slowly withdrawing the scope (he thought all was resolved when the heart rate and pressure were normal).
During this process multiple staff are coming into and out of the room and several conversations are going on simultaneously.
You realize that you remember that the patient was on a new seizure medication and it is clear that the leader is not aware of this situation.

WHAT WOULD YOU DO?

You should not withhold information that may be vital to this event, just because you are not sure if it is pertinent.
After 120 seconds into this episode a clear change of direction is needed.
No leadership is evident in the first 120 seconds of this scenario and the team has not paused to discuss likely theories as to what has occurred nor potential resolution.
The leader needs to completely stop the procedure and gain control at this point.

For an interview with Seon Jones and Gordon Wisbach on communication in severe conditions, refer to
"TEAM ORGANIZATION IN TRAUMA IN AN AUSTERE ENVIRONMENT: TRAUMA AND EMERGENCY SURGERY IN UNUSUAL SITUATION" in Appendix C at the back of the book

IV.K. THE CRITICAL MOMENT: RISK MANAGEMENT- TIME CRITICAL DECISION MAKING: (DAMAGE CONTROL FOLLOWED BY RISK ASSESSMENT, Containment, Risk Management, Planning, Execution, and Reassessment

We are now in the **risk-management and planning phase** of crisis control — the point where the leader must make the hardest call:

"Do I engage now and act, or do I pause for more information?"

This is the point when anxiety and second-guessing peak: *Will someone be hurt or die? If I act now, will I be criticized? If I hesitate, will I miss something important?* Too often leaders respond in one of two maladaptive ways:

- **Rush to action** (jump to conclusions, act hastily), or
- **Freeze or procrastinate** (over-gather information and fail to act).

You've already done the critical early work: you recognized the problem, stopped activity, regained control, and established command. Now you must move from containment into **measured action** — and that can usually be accomplished in **60–180 seconds**. Experienced teams and leaders do this faster; novices may need more structured support.

Reality check: Some situations require immediate, reflexive action (active shooter, catastrophic hemorrhage, airway obstruction). Those are obvious exceptions. In clinical crises, however, truly instantaneous reactions are uncommon — and a short, organized pause to gather critical information is often the safer route.

A practical, repeatable approach (60–180 second sequence)

Use this quick loop to move from analysis to action without losing time or composure:

1. **Quick Recon (10–30 s)**
   - Ask: *What just changed? Who is at immediate risk?*
   - Get 1–2 rapid objective data points (vital signs, major bleeding, airway patency, equipment failure).
   - Declare any immediate safety needs (e.g., call for help, apply a tourniquet, secure airway).
2. **Inventory & Assign (10–30 s)**
   - Identify available people and key resources.
   - Assign 1–2 clear, specific tasks (e.g., "Nurse A: place central line. Nurse B: get blood. Resident: prep airway.").
   - Keep assignments simple and matched to skill level.
3. **Formulate a Short Plan (20–60 s)**
   - Choose a **single, workable plan** (not the perfect plan). Use mental simulation: *Will this likely stop deterioration?*
   - Set a short timeline and decision points (e.g., "If no response in 2 minutes, convert to X.").
4. **Execute (10–60 s)**
   - Voice the plan clearly and once: brief the team, then act.
   - Use closed-loop communication: orders acknowledged and confirmed.
5. **Reassess & Iterate (continuous)**
   - Watch for effect; gather new data; be ready to abandon the plan if it's not working.
   - If the plan fails, switch to the next most plausible workable option.

Key principles to guide the decision

- **Workable solution beats perfect solution.** In time-compressed situations, choose the option that is most likely to stabilize the patient now.
- **Limit cognitive load.** Reduce choices to 1–2 options; eliminate irrelevant discussion.
- **Prioritize safety.** If immediate harm is likely, act first; if not, gather targeted information.
- **Use the team.** Delegate quickly. Don't try to solve everything yourself.
- **Time-box decisions.** Give yourself clear short windows (e.g., 30–90 seconds) to decide and act.

- **Anticipate next steps.** While one group executes, another should prepare resources for the likely second move.

Common errors to avoid
- **Over-information:** Asking for every possible data point before acting.
- **Over-confidence:** Assuming a plan must be perfect or that you alone can carry it out.
- **Multitasking without delegation:** Doing many small tasks yourself instead of coordinating the team.
- **Failure to call for help early:** Don't wait until failure is obvious to escalate.

Closing thought
The transition from recognition to action is not a single heroic maneuver — it's a disciplined, repeatable process. Train the team to run this 60–180 second loop until it becomes automatic: quick recon, assign, plan, act, reassess. In a crisis, a little structure saves time, reduces anxiety, and massively increases the probability of a good outcome.

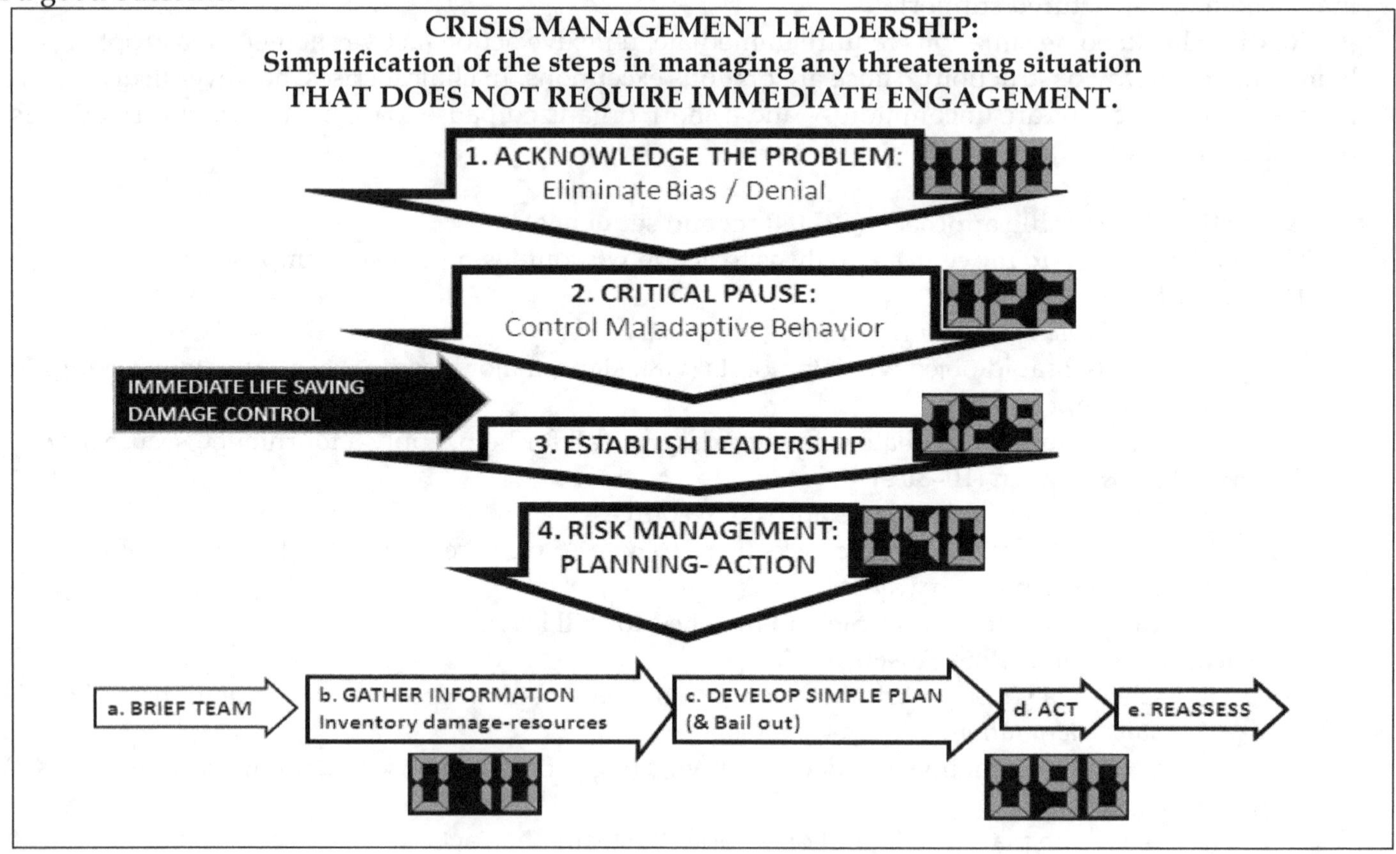

We previously discussed the S.T.O.P method for organizing one's thoughts during a crisis. It is now time to work out the details as to how the team leader organizes the planning process. We are now at the risk management stage where the team needs to perform the analysis, planning, action, and reassessment stages. This is predominately the role of the team leader, the commander. It is his or her job to move the team past the early checkpoints (noted above) surrounding early containment of the crisis and move the team forward through the decision making processes while under tremendous pressure, often with minimal information, minimal resources immediately available and as rapidly as possible. There are a multitude of methodologies (and mnemonics) available to describe this process, but the following five simple steps should be committed to memory so you can break things down when under fire. As in the **STOP** mnemonic, this may sound simple till you are under pressure.

USING THE S.T.O.P MNEMONIC WE REMEMBER TO:
a) **SIT**: STOP everything! Control anxiety, fear, panic and dissociation.
b) **THINK**: Get organized. Set up manageable tasks.
c) **OBSERVE**: Inquire. Get Information from your teammates.
d) **PLAN**: Organize a plan of action and then Act!

FIVE SIMPLE STEPS TO SUCCESSFULLY LEAD THRU ANY COMPLEX CRISIS SITUATION?
To get thru this organizing and planning process if you remember these five simple steps to successfully lead through a complex situation crisis you should do fine: [23]
a) **DEFINE THE SITUATION**: Define the situation. Stay simple and begin with very simple steps. Do not attempt to be too complex. It is not always immediately obvious what you want to achieve, so let the team know what you need from them now.
b) **DEVELOP A MODEL AND GATHER INFORMATION**: Make an *inventory* of damage and resources. In a crisis, the gathering of information may be limited but it is extremely vital to avoid failure. Take a few seconds to find out what is going on around you.
c) **PROGNOSIS/PREDICTION AND EXTRAPOLATE**: Use information gathered to determine potential for success of goals. What can we expect the outcome to be? Should we follow established practice or strike out in new direction?
d) **PLANNING OF ACTIONS AND *EXECUTION***: Use simplest possible steps to obtain goals and be alert for biases. Prioritize. Task delegation. Confirmation of comprehension.
e) **REASSESSMENT AND REVISION OF STRATEGY**: Review effects and revision of strategy planning.

PROGNOSIS/PREDICTION: RISK MANAGEMENT ASSESSMENT
During a disaster, the act of generating a prognosis or prediction is a component of risk management assessment. This process involves:
a) Sizing up the situation, i.e. the probability of successful or poor outcomes.
b) Assessment of the severity of failure.
c) Assessment of risk exposure to team, equipment, others in the vicinity (patient).
d) Assessment of the risk to the mission.

SEAL RULE OF COMBAT LEADERSHIP:
"Your team needs you to take control! Make a call and move forwards." Rorke Denver

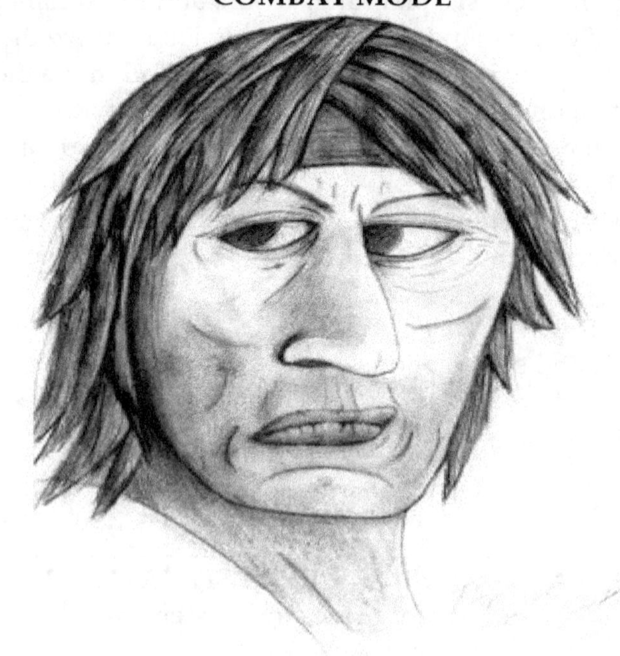
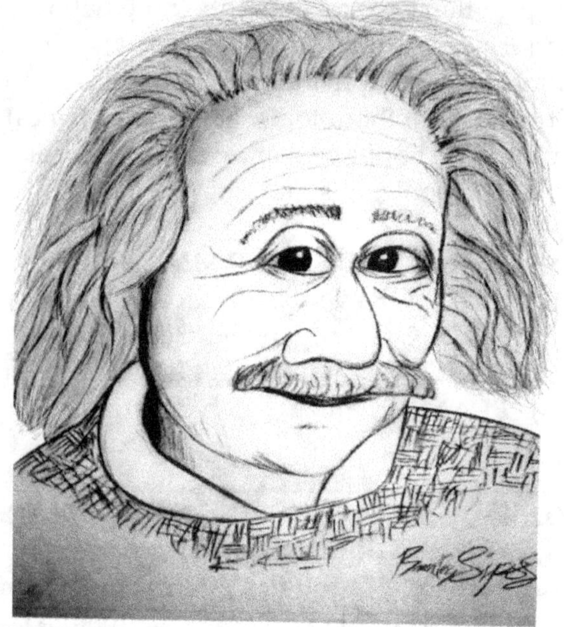

Drawings by Bradley Lipshy

Two Processing Speeds During Crisis: Engagement vs. Rational Decision Making

In any crisis, leaders operate within one of **two general processing modes**:

1. **Engagement Mode** — also known as *tactical* or *combat* mode
2. **Rational Decision-Making Mode** — also known as *strategic* or *analytical* mode

Which mode is most effective depends on several situational factors:

- **Threat Level:** Is the threat *immediate and life-threatening* (e.g., an active shooter, a patient hemorrhaging on the table), or *non-immediate* (e.g., a common bile duct injury discovered intraoperatively)?
- **Response Time:** Do you have *seconds* to act, or *minutes* to plan?
- **Authority and Experience:** Are you a seasoned leader with a vast experiential library capable of acting on intuition (while guarding against bias), or a novice who must pause for more information?
- **Information Available:** Do you have sufficient situational data, or are you operating in uncertainty?
- **Proximity to the Threat:** Are you *on the front line* — with no time or distance buffer — or *removed enough* to analyze and delegate?

These modes were described to me by **Mathew Sharps**, author of *Processing Under Pressure*, and by others studying human performance in extremis.

1. Engagement / Tactical / Combat Mode

This is the **fast, instinctive**, and **highly focused** response mode. It relies heavily on automatic, trained reactions and minimal deliberation. Information gathering stops; commands are issued and executed without debate. This mode can be essential in situations where seconds determine survival.

As **Dr. Daved Van Stralen** describes, experienced emergency medical services (EMS) providers often excel in this mode. Upon arriving at a chaotic scene, they immediately act: extract victims, stabilize them, and coordinate efforts in a fluid, almost automatic rhythm. Years of repetition, team familiarity, and muscle memory allow them to respond effectively without hesitation.

However, this mode has limits. **Combat-style engagement works best** when:

- The mission and environment are clearly defined.
- The threats are anticipated.
- The leader and team have trained extensively for those exact scenarios.

For **novices**, or in **unfamiliar, ambiguous crises**, tactical engagement without assessment can be disastrous. Acting on impulse without adequate understanding risks compounding the problem.

2. Rational Decision-Making / Strategic Mode

This mode is **slower, deliberate, and information-driven.** The leader observes, gathers input, analyzes data, and develops a plan before execution. Communication is open and collaborative, focused on verification, clarity, and collective situational awareness.

The same EMS providers who can perform instantaneously in tactical mode also know when to **shift gears** — when the scene is stable, when there is time to think, and when the situation benefits from dialogue. They transition into a **strategic decision-making mode**: asking questions, obtaining history, explaining plans to the patient, and coordinating the team toward a joint decision.

In medicine, most crises actually lend themselves to this second mode. Unlike combat, where immediate reaction may save lives, clinical scenarios typically allow **a few seconds to minutes** for assessment, delegation, and deliberate action.

3. Training the Switch

Commanders must learn **when to act and when to think.** The most common pitfall — especially among inexperienced leaders — is the "**Rambo reflex**," the urge to rush into action before understanding the situation. This is often fueled by adrenaline, ego, or fear of inaction.

Fire service research provides a valuable analogy: experienced fire chiefs train their teams to recognize that, in most scenarios, they have **at least ten seconds** to assess, plan, and act. Truly instantaneous emergencies are rare. Yet, **human nature** drives us to seize the first apparent solution, often mistaking speed for competence.

The key is **discipline under pressure** — the ability to control emotion, slow cognition just enough to think critically, and then act with purpose. This is not innate behavior; it must be learned, rehearsed, and reinforced until it becomes second nature.

Lesson: Speed without structure leads to chaos. Structure without adaptability leads to paralysis.

The expert crisis leader masters both — knowing exactly when to shift from rational analysis to tactical execution.

NOVICE LEADERSHIP V.S. EXPERIENCED COMMANDERS

What is the difference between an experienced commander and a novice leader when that critical moment occurs?

EXPERIENCED COMMANDERS:

Maintain a vast library of past experience to rely upon.

Utilize <u>Impulse</u> and <u>Intuition</u> to develop an initial plan of action immediately after the situation has changed. (see **III A. Phase one: recognition that there is a problem**)

DO NOT ACT ON THAT IMPULSE right away but instead take a few seconds to rely upon their observations, their followers and other information to assess the viability of that plan of action. This process takes only a few seconds in their hand.

If that plan is viable, they act.

If it is not, they discuss a different course of action (keep it simple).

They act.

They reassess.

NOVICE LEADERS:

Do not have a large library of experience and take much more time to sort out what is in front of them. They may either act on impulse, panic and immediately take action without further information or take longer to assess the situation to determine a series of multiple possible solutions and become paralyzed.

Michael D. Matthews, former law enforcement officer, professor of engineering psychology, West Point, Past president of American Psychological Asso. Society for Military Psychology. Fellow, Strategic Services Office of the Chief of Staff of the Army.

Immediate Engagement vs. Rational Decision Analysis During Crisis: Which Is Right for You — Right Now?

In the 1980s, Kenneth Hammond described decision-making as a continuum that ranges from intuitive to analytical thinking (later expanded by Gary Klein). Successful commanders rarely rely exclusively on one or the other; instead, they skillfully combine intuition and rational analysis.

Through intense training and accumulated experience, seasoned leaders learn to rapidly size up a situation and generate an instinctive, experience-based plan of action. Rather than acting blindly on that impulse, they pause briefly to assess risk, evaluate alternative actions, and then decide whether to engage or gather more information. This is the hallmark of expertise: the ability to switch between instinct and analysis, almost seamlessly.

The more experienced the leader, the faster this process occurs. They are able to draw from a deep library of prior experiences, filter relevant cues, and assess options one at a time rather than being overwhelmed by too many simultaneous scenarios.

By contrast, less experienced leaders tend to make one of two common errors:

A. Acting too quickly, without enough information to proceed safely, or

B. Overanalyzing and freezing, paralyzed by the inability to commit to a single course of action.

As Sweeney, Matthews, and Lester note in *Leadership in Dangerous Situations*, adaptability — knowing when to engage and when to pause — is the defining difference between novice and expert leadership.

The Balance Between Intuition and Analysis

In *Blink*, Malcolm Gladwell explores the psychology of snap decisions under extreme pressure. Two principles from his work, echoed by Lt. Gen. Paul Van Riper (USMC, Ret.) during our breakfast conversation, are essential for understanding leadership in crisis:

1. **Too Much Information Can Be Detrimental**

    At times, *too much data* is often worse than not enough. When overwhelmed by information, the subconscious becomes flooded with competing possibilities, leading to indecision.

    In truly high-intensity environments — battlefields, trading floors, mass casualty scenes — experienced leaders rely on pattern recognition and instinctive responses developed through

135

training. These leaders don't compare every possible option; they act on the most plausible one and adjust as needed. As Gladwell writes, "spontaneity is not random."

2. **"Spontaneity Is Not Random"**
    Rapid decisions that appear spontaneous are, in fact, the product of structured, repetitive, and high-pressure training.
    Special Forces units, emergency response teams, and trauma surgeons rehearse countless "what if" scenarios so that, when crisis strikes, their responses are nearly automatic. Through deliberate practice, these individuals build an extensive "mental library" of stored experiences. When faced with unexpected events, they instinctively retrieve and apply the most fitting model from prior experience.

However, one must also recognize human cognitive limits: fluid intelligence — the ability to solve novel problems — declines with age, while crystallized intelligence, the repository of experience, grows. Building that mental library early in one's career is essential.

Application to Medicine and Other High-Stakes Fields

Fortunately, few situations in medicine demand true *split-second* reactions. Most emergencies allow at least 60–120 seconds for focused analysis and structured decision-making.

Examples of genuine instantaneous-action events (such as catastrophic hemorrhage from penetrating trauma) are rare. In most critical situations — whether it's a difficult airway, a deteriorating vital sign, or a surgical complication — there is usually time to pause, gather essential data, and act deliberately.

This concept is not unique to medicine. As Representative Lubnau, a veteran of the fire service, observed: "Even in firefighting, you usually have ten seconds to think — ten seconds that can save your life."

Military leaders including Rorke Denver, Patrick Sweeney, Mike Matthews, and Tom Kolditz echo this principle: even in combat, when time permits, successful commanders take a brief pause to assess, orient, and plan.

The same pattern is observable in emergency medicine. Skilled paramedics arriving on scene immediately triage — stabilizing life threats — while simultaneously performing a methodical risk assessment. They confirm information, verify scene safety, and avoid assumptions — even when given guidance by physicians.

As Dr. Pat Croskerry emphasizes, this vigilance is critical: clinicians must build "defense systems" to prevent premature closure and resist the instinct to assume that the current scenario matches one previously encountered.

Putting It All Together: When to Engage, When to Think

So how do successful commanders know, instinctively, which approach is appropriate?

In a personal conversation, Lt. Gen. Paul Van Riper, USMC (Ret.), explained this elegantly over breakfast as he described the model he uses to teach officers at Quantico Marine Headquarters.

Imagine, he said, a simple scenario — one that civilians can also relate to:

You're driving on the interstate with a van full of children. Suddenly, you see steam rising from under the hood, and a warning light flashes "Check Engine."

Your pattern recognition triggers a familiar memory: this could be overheating, a common and manageable issue. You slow down, assess your options, and plan to pull over — rational decision mode. But then you notice flames, smell electrical fumes, and feel the engine fail. Instantly, you shift into engagement mode. There is no time for further analysis — only immediate, decisive action. You guide the van safely to the shoulder and order everyone out, calmly but firmly, on the side opposite the traffic.

This is precisely the mental shift that experienced commanders master: knowing when there is time to think and when there is no time to delay.

The same logic applies to medical and emergency settings:

- During the Boston Marathon bombing, responders had to act instantly—apply tourniquets, control bleeding, and move casualties—without deliberation.
- In the operating room, when a patient "codes," there is no discussion—airway, breathing, circulation take precedence immediately.
- In contrast, during less acute crises, leaders can—and should—pause to gather critical data before proceeding.

Experienced emergency responders, paramedics, and clinicians are capable of quickly discerning whether immediate engagement or rational analysis is appropriate. They do this by *subconsciously* performing rapid risk and time assessments while processing the situation through their trained cognitive frameworks.

Key Takeaway:
Effective crisis leadership is not about always acting fast or always thinking deeply. It's about knowing *when* to switch between the two—engaging when the threat is immediate, analyzing when there's time to think, and doing both with clarity, control, and confidence.

1. IMMEDIATE INNATE INFORMATION PROCESSING, PROBLEM RECOGNITION, THREAT ASSESSMENT…… SIZING UP THE SITUATION.

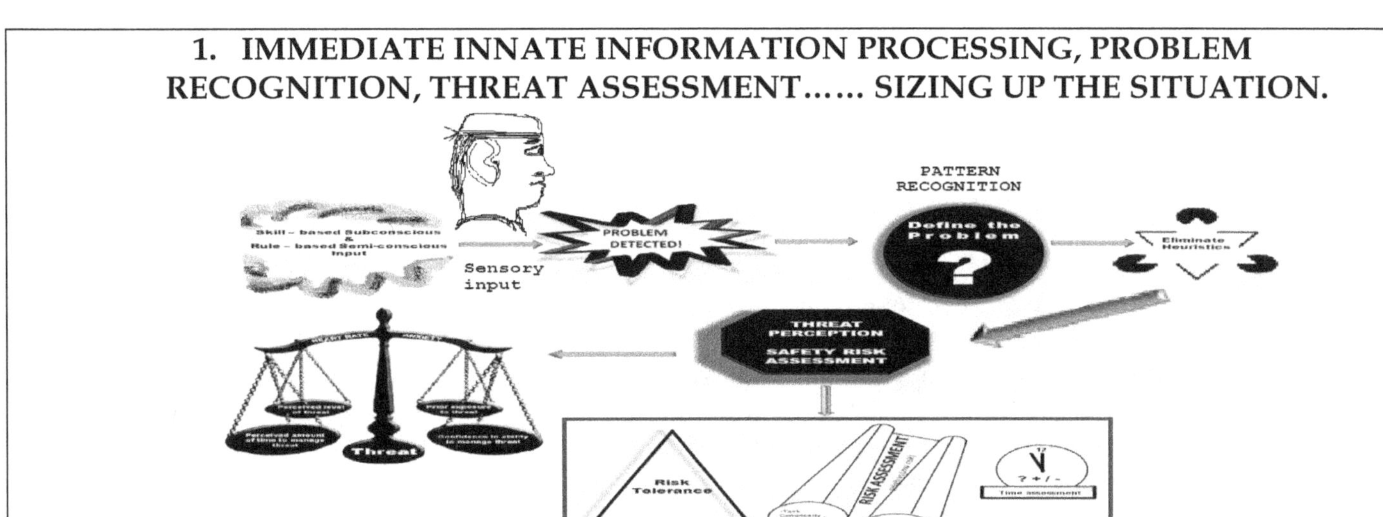

2. UTILIZATION OF MENTAL AND MUSCLE MEMORY

**LIBRARY AND SKILLS FROM
REAL LIFE EXPERIENCE, BOOKS, PLANNING, TRAINING/REHEARSAL**

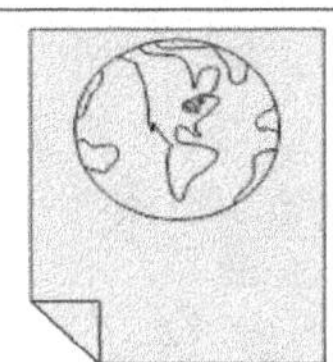
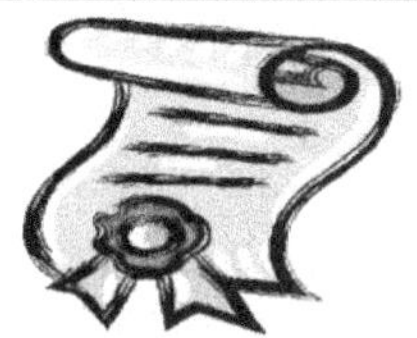

3. CREATING A PICTURE…A STORY…. YOUR MENTAL MAP….

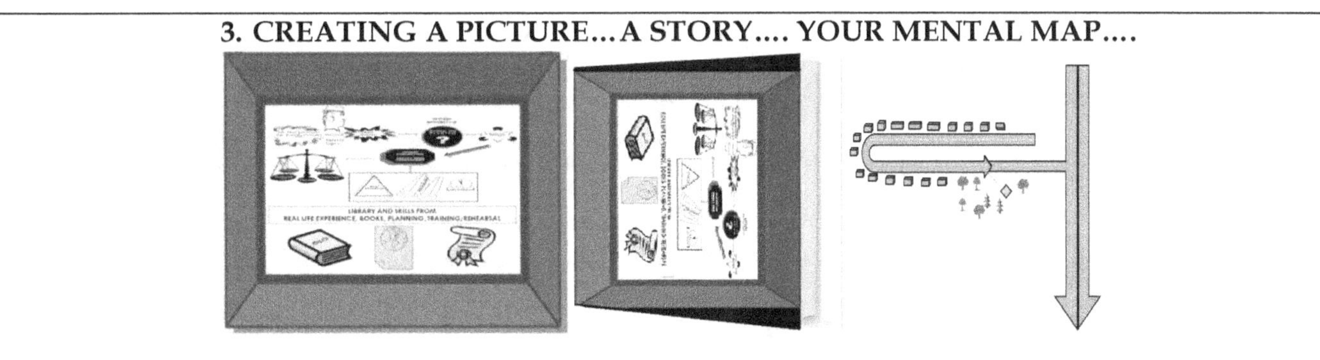

4. USING YOUR MENTAL MAP, STORY, PICTURE ALONG WITH INTUITION / TRAINING (in the span of a fraction of a second or so) TO DETERMINE IF YOU NEED TO ENGAGE OR PERFORM RATIONAL ANALYSIS.

A. ENGAGEMENT:
1. I HAVE TO REACT NOW!!!
2. I HAVE ENOUGH EXPERIENCE TO HANDLE THIS SITUATION

B. RATIONAL DECISION MAKING:
1. I HAVE SOME TIME
2. THE THREAT IS NOT IMMEDIATELY LIFE THREATENING IN THE NEXT 60 SECONDS

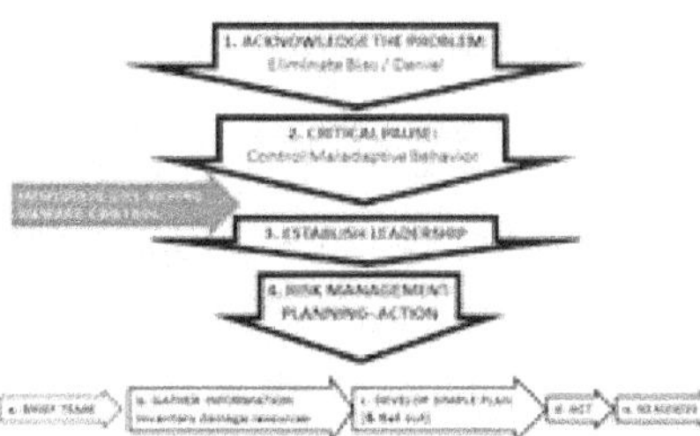

PARALYSIS – INDIVIDUAL or PLEURALISTIC INACTION
It is all too common that commanders get bogged down into planning and just do not make a decision and act. JUST MAKE A DECISION. Paralysis during decision making is all too common. As Rorke Denver told me, commanders frequently gather information make a plan but do not follow thru and act. You have to *"do something!" "a bad call is better than no call" "Make the call then adjust"*. In some cases, this becomes a group-wide ailment known as dilution of responsibility or pleuralistic inaction, where everyone simply sits around and waits for someone to take control.

TIME RELAVANCY- How much time do we have?
As we discussed, when under duress, time frames are not very clear. We want to act quickly but take a moment to gather the information before acting too hastily.
So, what do time frames really look like? In football after 30 seconds of huddling and setting up the line, a quarterback then has between 2-5 seconds after the hike to decide whether to pass, run or hand off the ball- it seems much longer when watching the game. The margin between a success and failure is within fractions of a second. A punt or kickoff return of 100 yards takes about 10 seconds. A fast break in the NBA takes approximately 3-5 seconds. A double play in MLB, takes about 4-5 seconds after the ball hits the bat. Most crises in medicine do not require split second precise decisions, but 30-60 seconds is a very long time and you can accomplish a lot in that time period.

KEEP IT SIMPLE!

Always keep it simple. The more options you have the longer it will take to make a decision, so keep it simple. Avoid paralysis. _{Lt Col Dave Grosman.}

TASKING YOUR FOLLOWERS ELIMINATES INWARD FOCUSING

While we are used to making decisions by committee, when all hell breaks loose people just want someone to make a decision. People are task focused and when crises happen, authoritarian leadership works best because they are tasked. **Thomas Kolditz, Author of *In Extremis Leadership*. Professor and head of the department of behavioral sciences and leadership, US Military Academy at West Point.**

How do we work through a complex situation and is there a point in our lives where we lose the ability to deal with a novel situation? For a discussion with Randall Engle see the appendix at the back of this book.

SO, WHAT WOULD THIS LOOK LIKE IN REAL LIFE?
*An experienced vascular surgeon takes a patient to the operating room for a carotid endarterectomy. The plan is to perform the procedure under a field block with the patient awake using a clamp and sew technique (no shunt). He has a new tech scrubbed in. After the proximal and distal Carotid artery and branches have been exposed and controlled, the surgeon places a shunt on the drapes and explains to the team his process for using the shunt should it be needed in an emergency. He assures the entire team is familiar with this process and their individual roles should this occur. The patient is awake and cooperative at this time. The patient's inflow is clamped and the vessel opened and plaque removed. Prior to application of a patch the patient becomes restless. Anesthesia suddenly reports that the patient has bradycardia to 30 and then intermittently very long pauses (he is still talking albeit with obvious confusion). They treat the patient with Atropine. The experienced surgeon **PAUSES** the case and asks if there is any doubt whether this is due to lack of perfusion of the patient's brain due to the bradycardia or the obstruction of Carotid inflow. He explains to anesthesia that if they have any question as to the stability of the patient, anesthesia would need to let the team know so that the procedure can now be stopped and a shunt inserted as rehearsed previously. The anesthesia team suggests that that would be a good idea at this time. The shunt is inserted and the patient responds well. This entire scene takes place over approximately 90 seconds.*

IV.L. MORE WORDS OF WARNING FROM EXPERIENCED CHIEFS!

THE MOST DANGEROUS PERIODS DURING A CRISIS:
1. INCEPTION.
2. TRANSITION PERIOD.
3. AFTER THE VICTORY.
4. RECOVERY PERIOD.

<u>INCEPTION PERIOD:</u> As discussed, at the instant a crisis occurs there is frequently a delay in recognizing that things have changed.

<u>TRANSITION PERIOD</u>: The transition period occurs when the incident has become too large for "local" resources or has lasted too long for those resources. It is a transition to a larger attack and a change in strategy. The most dangerous period during a crisis is when the crisis event and the team are in transition at the same time. At that moment, everyone is at maximal risk. ^{Okray}

<u>AFTER THE VICTORY:</u> Known in the military as the consolidation and reorganization phase, teams are most vulnerable after they sense the danger is over, when in fact they may not be completely safe. It is also at this time that their adrenaline surge in response to the event may be falling. ^{Lt Col Dave Grossman, On combat}

<u>RECOVERY-TRAUMATIC MEMORY-TIME OFF AFTER THE DISASTER:</u>
One small caveat about maladaptive responses. After a particularly threatening, highly emotional event, it appears that the prefrontal cortex is suppressed by activation of the amygdala and subsequently the hippocampus. The effect is that memory is enhanced making this event and cues immediately preceding the event, the sole focus of attention (aka weapons focus). Recovery is suppressed for several minutes and new memory formation is suppressed during this refractory period. Full recovery can take hours or days. The importance is that
1. The victim must be relieved of responsibility immediately
2. Victim should be off duty for at least 24 hours until memory is restored to normal.

_{Sweeney PJ, Matthews MD, Lester PB. *Leadership in Dangerous Situations*.}

> *"I remember being on call and having a delivery at 3am that had a complication in which the mother did not survive. I wish I could have gone home but had to work till 8am until the end of my16 hour- shift instead. It was emotionally draining and clearly the worst day of my life."*

THE IMPACT OF A CATASTROPHE:
2012 AMERICAN SOCIETY OF ANESTHESIOLOGISTS SURVEY

A perioperative catastrophe may have a profound and lasting emotional impact on the anesthesiologist involved and may affect his or her ability to provide patient care in the aftermath of such events. 84% of Anesthesiologists were involved in at least one unanticipated death or serious injury of a perioperative patient over the course of his/her career. 70% experienced guilt, anxiety, and reliving of the event (88% requiring time to recover emotionally & 19% never fully recovered, 12% considered a career change) 67% believed that their ability to provide patient care was compromised in the first 4 hours subsequent to the event. 7% were given time off. [3]
(repeated twice in this guide for enhancing the point)

FOR FIRST HAND ACCOUNT ON VULNERABILITY read *"VULNERABILITY AND RESILIENCY- A LESSON ON HUMANITY FROM TIM LEEUWENBURG ("rural proceduralist"- Kangaroo Island, Australia) At the end of this book*

DEATH BY ASPIRATION:
One week out from a colectomy our patient (BMI 45) had an episode of vomitus. An NGT was discussed with the patient and the nurses attempted to place it, but he was not able to tolerate insertion at all. The next day his abdomen was worse but he did not want the NGT placed without sedation. His iv fell out overnight and peripheral access was not successful. By this point we determined we he would be best served with a central line in the OR and while sedated, place the NGT. The NGT went in easily. The central line did not and patient said he had enough after 20 minutes. On the way to the unit, the NGT "fell out". I asked to let us replace it and the patient said "no". I kept thinking maybe I should have pushed further but he said he did not feel like he was going to vomit, so…. The next am, I checked on him and the same response was given-"will you let me put in an NGT to keep you from vomiting and breathing in the vomitus?"… "NO". Three hours later he vomited, aspirated and arrested, and did not recover. Yes, I was distraught, "I should have pushed more"…. I went back to work as if nothing had happened. I slept poorly that night. I went to work as usual the next day, but was still thinking about this as I am pushing through a regular work day. Am I distracted? Obviously. Have we discussed the case as a team… of course not. Did we provide consoling discussions to those involved.. no……

EVERY MAN FOR HIMSELF

Two hunters are being chased by a bear when one hunter stops to put on a pair of running shoes.
"What are you doin"! asks the other hunter, "you can't outrun a bear"!
"I know" says his friend, "I just need to outrun you!"
*Rorke Denver former head of basic and advanced SEAL training and author of **DAMN FEW: MAKING THE MODERN-DAY SEAL WARRIOR***

LEADERS BEWARE OF THE FIGHT OR FLIGHT INSTINCT:
Beware of the reactive need to "go it alone"- "when really bad things happen and it's a life or death situation, humans tend to react in predictable manners. They resort to prior, over-learned behavior, they lose the mental capacity for creativeness and cognitive processing and they tend to separate from the group and attempt to save themselves on their own."

HUMAN ERROR AND NOVICE TENDENCIES:
1. We jump to drastic conclusion early in the decision-making process.
2. We then wait to act upon observed situational changes, when we should be moving.
3. And then we do not use the time available to attempt any corrective action.

■ ERRORS OF COMMISSION: 60% of the mistakes we make when we are in a hurry are errors of commission where we carry out a task incorrectly.

■ ERRORS OF OMMISSION: 40% of the time our errors are one of omission where we neglected to carry out a task element. okray

HOW RELIABLE ARE WE AT REPORTING MISTAKES?
➤ 33% of hospital staff reported that errors are handled appropriately.
➤ 33% of intensive care staff did not acknowledge that they make errors.
➤ 50% of intensive care staff reported that they find it difficult to discuss mistakes.
Sexton, Thomas, Helmreich

MANAGING CONFRONTATION WITH STYLE!
Turning an Argument into a Partnership!

KENNETH A. LIPSHY, MD, FACS

HAVE YOU BEEN DIRECTLY CONFRONTED IN AN UNCIVIL MANNER OR WITNESSED THIS OCCURRING TO ANOTHER PERSON?

HOW WELL DID THAT GO? DID ALL PARTIES PART TENSION-FREE COMPARED TO WHEN THE CONFRONTATION STARTED?

GROUP CONFLICT IS HEALTHY BUT INCIVILITY IS DISRUPTIVE!

YOUR *PERCEIVED* THREAT LEVEL DETERMINES YOUR RESPONSE!

FACTORS THAT WEIGH INTO HOW MUCH YOU FEEL THREATENED

- WITNESSED VS *TARGETING* YOU!
- Attack on you *DIRECTLY* (your skills / performance/ beliefs) vs *GENERIC* attacks
- *SURPRISE* VS FORECASTED ATTACK

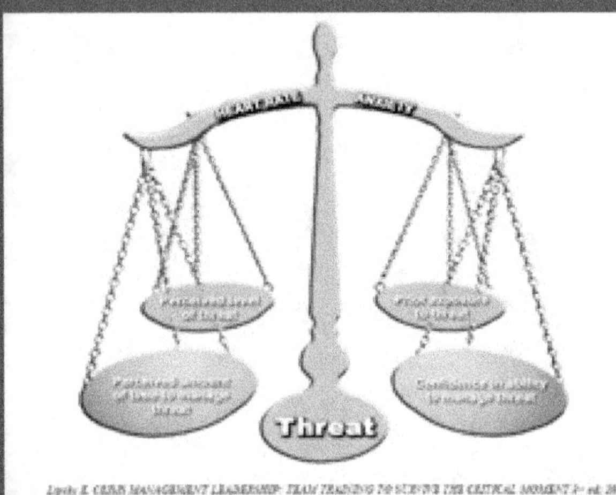

Lipshy K. CRISIS MANAGEMENT LEADERSHIP: TEAM TRAINING TO SURVIVE THE CRITICAL MOMENT 1st ed. 2018

HIGHEST PERCEIVED THREAT LEVELS:

TARGET OF ATTACK

ATTACK IS PERSONAL

ATTACK IS UNEXPECTED

UNFAMILIARITY NO PRIOR EXPOSURE

DISTRACTED/FATIGUED/STRESSED

IMMEDIATE RESOLUTIONS REQUIRED

ZERO CONFIDENCE IN SUCCESS

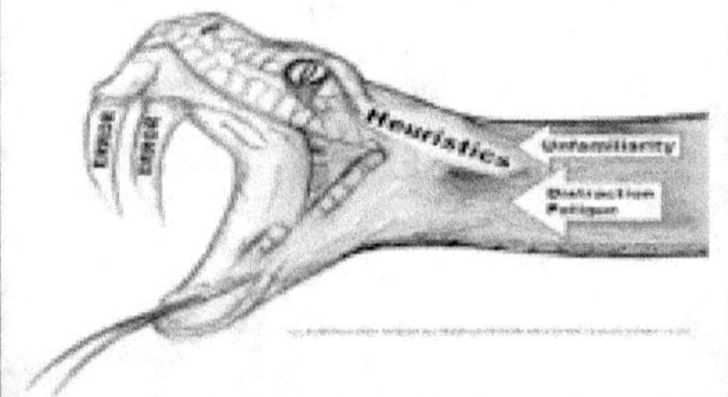

You are more susceptible to make a mistake when you encounter a situation that you are unfamiliar with or when you are distracted, fatigued, or stressed.

BEFORE YOU ENGAGE, GUAGE YOUR MENTAL STATE WHEN YOU ARE SURPRISED!

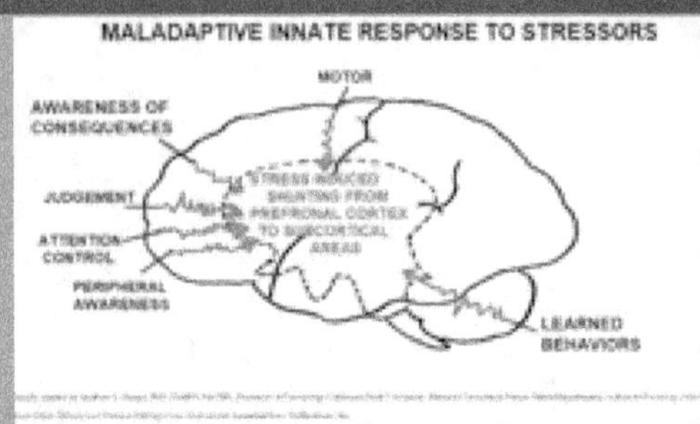

FIGHT OR FLIGHT!

INSTINCTUAL FIGHTING BACK OR AVOIDANCE ......

Not helpful when the goal is to resolve a problem!

WHAT'S WRONG WITH "REACTING IN KIND"?

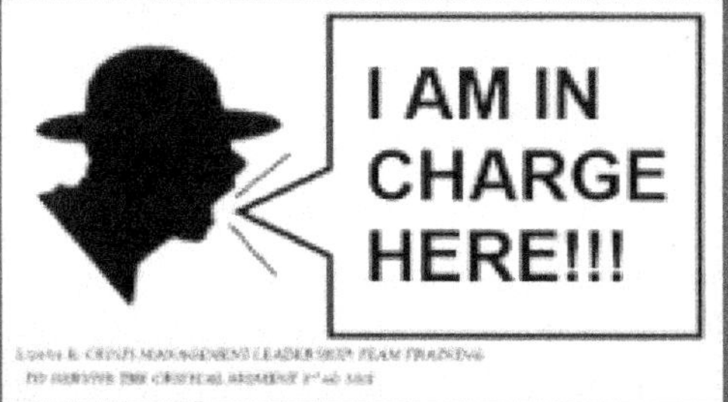

THE LEADER'S GOALS: DEESCALATE, MAINTAIN RESPECT, RETAIN TEAM STRUCTURE. **AVOID** "RETURNING FIRE" WHICH DISTRACTS, CREATES DISCOMFORT AND "US AGAINST THEM", CAUSING DISENGAGEMENT AND INEFFECTIVE TEAMWORK.

SHOULD YOU ENGAGE OR SHOULD YOU TAKE SOME TIME TO ANALYZE THE SITUATION BEFORE RESPONDING?

IF YOUR PERSONAL SAFETY IS NOT AT RISK, AND YOU CAN SUCCESSFULLY USE THE RESPONSE MANAGEMENT TECHNIQUES BELOW YOU MAY FEEL CONFIDENT YOU CAN ENGAGE THE CONFRONTOR WITHOUT AGGRAVATING THE CIRCUMSTANCES

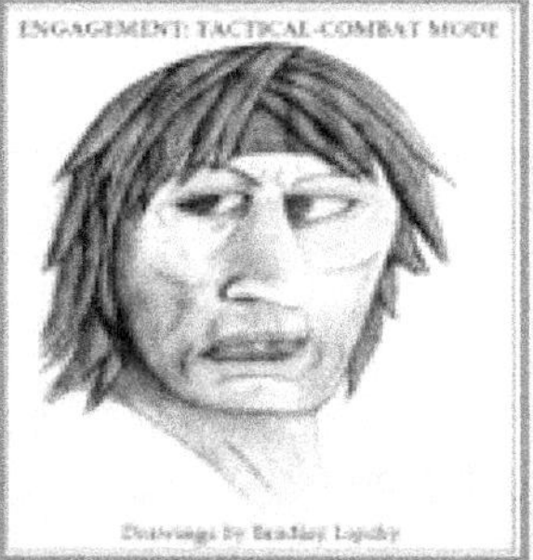

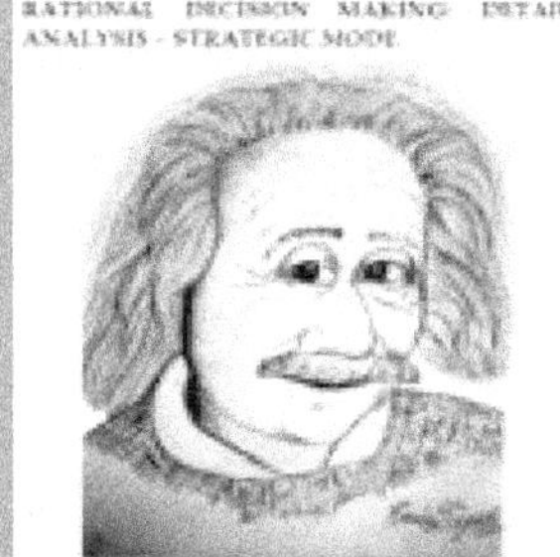

IF YOU HAVE THE EMOTIONAL INTELLIGENCE TO KNOW YOU ARE NOT MENTALLY EQUIPPED TO MANAGE THE SITUATION EFFECTIVELY, OR IF YOU FEEL YOU NEED PROFESSIONAL ASSISTANCE (POLICE) THEN DEFERRING THE DISCUSSION UNTIL LATER MAY BE THE BEST OPTION

IF YOU DECIDE YOU CAN ENGAGE WHAT STEPS CAN YOU TAKE TO AVOID EXACERBATING THE CONFLICT?

STRESS THERMOMETER: Recognized your personal stress threat level and if high, use combat breathing. If you find that is not working then defer the contact- take a break by asking to resume the confrontation later at a scheduled time (if you are tense).

BODY LANGUAGE: Control your body language and voice tone. Keep an open relaxed posture, maintain eye contact, and avoid distracting facial responses. This relaxes you and helps you focus.

EMPATHY: Picture yourself in their shoes as that validates your concern for their emotions and it helps your decision-making process... it WILL help avoid a costly mistake. Don't Judge! Remember that we all have bad days and we don't know the emotions or stressors that were behind the person's loss of control.

RESPECT: be respectful, don't be threatening, don't provoke the situation. Never tell someone "you need to calm down"... No One likes that.

- **LISTEN**: listening shows the assailant you do care, you are not threatened and gives you time to relax and try to understand the situation, avoiding any embarrassment in misinterpreting what was going on and making a mistake.
- **FOCUS ON ISSUE NOT PEOPLE**: if you focus on the issue and avoid focusing on the person, you both will feel less threatened.
- **SOLUTION FOCUSED**: Focus on a solution and working together. Be positive. Move forwards. Don't be drawn into personal issues. Address the concern with a solution in mind that is agreeable. No one wants to walk away empty handed.
- **APOLOGIZE**: If you recognize an error was made or you realize you are rude / inappropriate.
- **RECAP**: Summarize what you discussed, Reflect back on the conversation. Shows you are listening and trying to resolve the situation that began the confrontation.

FIVE D'S OF CONFLICT MANAGEMENT

- **DIRECT**- Use above concepts to be direct with all parties. Be Civil and use the words "I" and "We" to show
- **DISTRACT**-Shift the focus and try to de-escalate by asking the victim or the aggressor for something to divert their attention while you assess the situation and make a plan to address the concerns, try to shift to a neutral topic.
- **DELAY/DEFER**- If the situation is volatile, don't tackle the aggressor head on, try to be supportive. Assure the recipient is safe. Assess escape routes.
- **DELEGATE**- Engaged trained professionals if needed- i.e. Police or other skilled intermediary.
- **DOCUMENT**- Follow up confrontational events with reports to superiors.
- **SUPPORT THE VICTIMS**.

* 5D's in By-stander intervention by C. Blakeman, Association of Surgical Education, Dealing with Microaggressions in Surgical Learning Environments A Cooper, K Lipsky DIO and Faculty Development; accessed on April 14 2023

• Lipsky K. CRISIS MANAGEMENT LEADERSHIP: TEAM TRAINING TO SURVIVE THE CRITICAL MOMENT 3rd ed; 2018

IV.M. DEBRIEFING – AFTER THE DUST SETTLES

AFTER ACTION REPORT (AAR) : DEBRIEFING

(All untoward / adverse events should have group discussion by those involved as quickly as possible to assess for opportunities for improvement)

- A. Case scenario- succinct synopsis, objectivity only
- B. Background- brief history of similar situations- how often, past experiences
- C. Expectations- What should have happened. What was the intent. Ideally, what should have occurred in chronological order. Objective only.
- D. Situation - What actually occurred-chain of events- steps along the way in chronological order. Subjective comments allowed in this step- but require validation if needed/able.
    1. Was communication clear
    2. Were roles and responsibilities clear
    3. Was situational awareness maintained
    4. Was workload distributed equitably
    5. Errors
    6. Resources available or a hindrance
    7. Doctrine / Policy / procedural issues- help or hinder
    8. Sustainment: Three ups- record positive actions and response here- what went right; commendations; heroic efforts.
    9. Improvement: Three downs- ways to be better next time (team, system)
- E. Improvement/ Solutions offered: Items for team. Items for command structure to process. (command relationships, triage and treatment plans, focal points for train)
    4. Specific areas to discuss for the future-
    5. What is being proposed as potentially able to prevent future occurrences
    6. Opportunities for training

Adapted from (Sweeney, et al

FULL DESCRIPTIVE DEBRIEFING LIST AVAILABLE AT THE END OF THIS GUIDE.

DO'S AND DON'TS OF DEBRIEFING:

- DO: Set the expectations (above).
- DO: Facilitate the debriefing to meet its objectives.
- DO: Keep the crew level-headed.
- DO: Obtain participation of EVERYEONE including, reluctant speakers/participants.
- DO: Get thru all the steps above.
- DO: Expand on instructional points.
- DO: Make note of all positive aspects .

- *DO NOT LECTURE.*
- *DO NOT OVERANALYZE.*
- *DO NOT INTERRUPT.*
- *DO NOT CUT THE SESSION SHORT.*
- *DO NOT GIVE THE IMPRESSION YOU KNOW ALL THE ANSWERS.* Okray

    A key component to remember is that as soon as possible after a crisis is resolved, the team must sit together and review the positive and negative aspects of the case. The debriefing is a vital step which precedes the investigational team that will follow. Facts tend to be twisted and vary as time progresses and an individual's impression and responses will be clearer immediately after the incident than it is after time inputs thoughts from others. This makes it more difficult to understand what the participants were thinking during the incident and difficult to make changes to prevent the accident from occurring in the future. Once the retrospective nature of a subsequent investigation takes over, it is more difficult to know exactly what definitively was going on when the incident occurred. [142]

CHAPTER IV CRISIS MANAGEMENT LEADERSHIP REFERENCES

- Bowermaster R, Miller M, Ashcraft T, Boyd M, Brar A, Manning P, Eghtesady P. Application of the Aviation Black Box Principle in Pediatric Cardiac Surgery: Tracking All Failures in the Pediatric Cardiac Operating Room. *J Am Coll Surg* 2015;220:149-155.
- Cristancho SM, Apramian T, Vanstone M, Lingard L, Ott M, Forbes T, Novick R. Thinking like an expert: surgical decision making as a cyclical process of being aware. Am Journal Surgery 2016. 211(1):64–69.
- Cristancho S, Apramian T, Vanstone M, Lingard L, Ott M, Novick R. Understanding Clinical Uncertainty: What Is Going on When Experienced Surgeons Are Not Sure What to Do? Academic Medicine 2013. 88(10)1516–1521.
- Cristancho S, Vanstone M, Lingard L, LeBel M, Ott M. When surgeons face intraoperative challenges: a naturalistic model of surgical decision making. Am Journal of Surgery 2013. 205(2):156–162.
- Dörner D. *The Logic of Failure: Recognizing and Avoiding Error in Complex Situations*. Reading, MA: Perseus Books; 1996.
- Endsley, MR, Garland DJ. *Situation Awareness Analysis and Measurement*. Mahwah, NJ: Lawrence Erlbaum Associates; 2000.
- Endsley, M. R. (1995). Toward a theory of situation awareness in dynamic systems. Human Factors, 37(1), 32–64.
- Gaba DM, Fish KJ, Howard SK. *Crisis Management in Anesthesiology*. New York, NY: Churchill Livingstone; 1994.
- Gazoni FM, Amato PE, Malik ZM, Durieu ME. The impact of perioperative catastrophes on anesthesiologists: results of a national survey. *Anesth Analg*. 2012;114(3):596–603.
- Gladwell M. *Blink, the power of thinking without thinking*. New York: Little, Brown and Company; 2005.
- Gonzales L. *Deep Survival: Who Lives, Who Dies and Why*. New York, NY: WW Norton; 2003.
- Grossman D. *On Combat: the psychology and physiology of deadly conflict in war and in peace*. US. Warrior Science Publications; 2008.
- IAFC. Crew resource management: a positive change for the fire service. Fairfax, VA: International Association of Fire Chiefs. http://www.iafc.org/files/1SAFEhealthSHS/pubs_CRMmanual.pdf. Accessed February 18, 2013.
- Jones, D. G., & Endsley, M. R. (1996). Sources of situation awareness errors in aviation. Aviation, Space and Environmental Medicine, 67(6), 507–512.
- Klein G. The sources of power, how people make decisions. Cambridge: MIT Press, 1999.
- Klein G. Naturalistic Decision Making. Human Factors: The Journal of the Human Factors and Ergonomics Society. **2008;**50(3):**456-460.**
- **Klein G, Pliske R, Crandall B, Woods DD. Problem Detection. Cogn Tech Work. 2005;7:14-28.**
- Kolditz TA. *In Extremis Leadership: Leading As If Your Life Depended On It*. San Francisco, CA: Jossey-Bass; 2007.
- Mazzocco K, Petitti DB, Fong KT, Bonacum D, Brookey J, Graham S, Lasky RE, Sexton JB, Thomas EJ. Surgical Team Behaviors and Patient Outcomes. *Am Jnl Surgery*. 2009; 197:678-685
- McGreevy JM, Otten TD. Briefing and debriefing in the operating room using fighter pilot crew resource management. *J Am Coll Surg*. 2007;205(1):169-176.
- Nixon PG . The human function curve - a paradigm for our times.Act Nerv Super (Praha). 1982;Suppl 3(Pt 1):130-3.PMID: 7183056
- Nixon PG. The human function curve. With special reference to cardiovascular disorders: part I. Practitioner. 1976 Nov;217(1301):765-70.PMID: 995833 No abstract available.
- Nixon PG. The human function curve. With special reference to cardiovascular disorders: part II. Practitioner. 1976 Dec;217(1302):935-44.PMID: 796840 Review. No abstract available.
- Nixon PG. Stress and the cardiovascular system. Practitioner. 1982 Sep;226(1371):1589-98.PMID: 6890677 No abstract available.
- Northouse PG. Leadership: Theory and practice. 6th ed. Los Angeles. Sage. 2013.
- NTSB: Loss of Control on Approach Colgan Air, Inc. Operating as Continental Connection Flight 3407 Bombardier DHC-8-400, N200WQ Clarence Center, New York http://www.ntsb.gov/investigations/AccidentReports/Reports/AAR1001.pdf#page=176
- NTSB: http://www.ntsb.gov/news/events/Pages/Loss_of_Control_and_Impact
- Okray R, Lubnau T. *Crew Resource Management for the Fire Service*. Tulsa, OK: PennWell Press; 2004.
- Phitayakorn R, Minehart RD, Hemingway MW, Pian-Smith MC, Petrusa E. Relationship between physiologic and psychological measures of autonomic activation in operating room teams during a simulated airway emergency. *Am J Surg*. 2015;209(1):86-92.
- Rao A, Tait I, Alijani A. Systematic review and meta-analysis of the role of mental training in the acquisition of technical skills in surgery. Am Journal Surg 2015;210(3):545-553
- Ripley A. *The Unthinkable: Who Survives When Disaster Strikes and Why*. New York, NY: Three Rivers Press; 2000.
- Siddle B. *Sharpening the Warriors Edge: The Psychology and Science of Training*. 10th ed. Belleville, IL: PPCT Research publications; 2008.
- Sincero SM. How does Stress Affect Performance? Feb 2012. Retrieved Mar 07, 2015 from Explorable.com: https://explorable.com/how-does-stress-affect-performance
- Sweeney PJ, Matthews MD, Lester PB. *Leadership in Dangerous Situations*. Annapolis, MD: Naval Institute Press; 2011.
- USCG. Crew resource management refresher. United States Coast Guard. 2002. http://www.uscg.mil/safety/docs/PPTs/CRM_Refresher2002.ppt. Accessed February 2, 2013.
- Weller, Boyd. Making a Difference Through Improving Teamwork in the Operating Room: A Systematic Review of the Evidence on What Works; Patient Safety in Anesthesia. 4:77–83, (2014);

V. CONCLUSION

- **Healthy Organizational Safety climate**
- **Error, Stress and Burnout**
- **Teamwork**
- **Summary**

HEALTHY ORGANIZATIONAL SAFETY CLIMATE

HEALTHY ORGANIZATIONAL CLIMATE:

Healthy Organizations are composed of:
- Members who are committed to common values;
- Leaders who exemplify those values by setting the example through personal behaviors consistent with those values;
- Members who feel free to communicate concerns to others in the organization;
- Leaders who are open and responsive to concerns raised by its membership.

Sweeney PJ, Matthews MD, Lester PB. *Leadership in Dangerous Situations.*

- How people respond during a disaster tends to be a reflection of their organization.
- How they react entirely depends on their relationship with their supervisor and the organization.
- Where there is lack of trust, teams break down rapidly.

Kolditz, *In Extremis Leadership.*

BE AWARE OF YOUR WORKING ENVIRONMENT!
DON'T WORK IN A SILO!

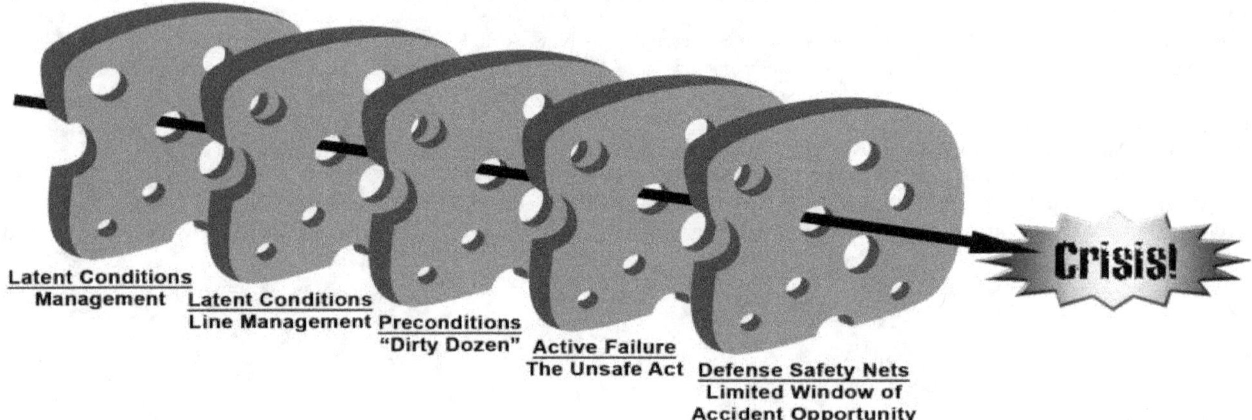

Use of Reason's System Model to explain transition from a difficult procedure to a crisis (misadventure or other unexpected event) to a disaster (death in the O.R.).

Latent conditions are brought about by administrative pressure to do more cases, lack of ability to transfer difficult cases to higher level center, recent release of staff or hiring of cheaper, less experienced staff.

> **Preconditions** exist for years and include fatigue, stress, ambivalence, lack of knowledge, reduction
> in resources followed by teamwork and communication degradation.
> **System Safety** nets are then discovered to be absent leading to propagation of a misadventure or
> other unexpected event into a patient care disaster. Safety nets typically revolve around lack of
> resources thought to exist but in actuality are absent (staff, training, supplies, equipment, etc.) as well
> as distractions created by inefficiencies elsewhere in the organization. Adaptation From Reason and
> w permission Gordon DuPont

Systems Theory and Situational Awareness

As discussed earlier, one essential component of **situational awareness** is an understanding of the **systems**
in which we operate. In complex environments such as healthcare, aviation, or the military, problems rarely
arise from a single event or individual action. Instead, they evolve from a web of interdependent
components within a system that is itself inherently fragile.

Systems Theory holds that in complex organizations, *errors are not random or isolated*. Rather, they are
inevitable byproducts of people doing their best within systems that contain multiple, subtle
vulnerabilities. Each visible error is a **symptom of deeper systemic issues**, not merely the result of
individual failure.

"Events, objects, locations, and methods do not exist independently, but rather are intertwined as
interdependent components of complex systems. Complex systems also incorporate multiple layers of
seemingly unrelated issues — including social, legal, cultural, and economic factors — which ultimately shape
the system's final form. If an alteration occurs in any one of the components making up a complex system,
its effect ripples throughout the entire system."

— **J. Calland, 2002**

This systems-based understanding is crucial for leaders seeking to recognize latent hazards before they
culminate in crises.

Latent Conditions

Latent conditions are **hidden vulnerabilities** embedded within an organization long before a crisis
emerges. They often arise from high-level administrative or policy decisions — pressures to increase
productivity, budget cuts, understaffing, or hiring of less experienced personnel. These decisions may
appear benign in isolation but can **erode resilience** across the system.

Examples include:

- Production pressure to increase case volume or turnover speed
- Limited capacity to transfer complex patients to higher-level centers
- Inadequate staff training or retention due to financial constraints
- Failure of leadership to correct communication, behavior, or process deficits

These conditions form the "holes" in James Reason's **Swiss Cheese Model**, through which multiple small
vulnerabilities can align to produce a catastrophic event.

Preconditions

Preconditions are the *recognized but unaddressed* factors that predispose individuals or teams to active
failure. They exist in the operational environment for months or years, often normalized as part of "the way
we do things."

Common examples include:

- Fatigue and workload imbalance
- Chronic stress and burnout
- Ambivalence or complacency
- Knowledge gaps and inadequate supervision
- Decline in teamwork and communication as resources thin

While preconditions do not directly cause harm, they **lower the threshold for error**. Proper **human factors and systems training** can mitigate most of these risks if addressed proactively.

Active Failures

Active failures are the visible unsafe actions — errors or violations — performed by individuals (the surgeon, nurse, pilot, or technician). These are the "sharp-end" manifestations of systemic vulnerability.

While active failures are often the focus of investigations, they are only the **final step** in a long chain of events that includes system design flaws, communication gaps, and latent organizational pressures.

Absent Safety Nets

Finally, when errors occur, **system safety nets** — the redundant layers designed to prevent harm — are often missing, inadequate, or falsely presumed to exist. These may include:

- Shortages in critical staff or equipment
- Gaps in training or credentialing
- Inefficient processes that create cognitive overload and distraction
- Absence of cross-checks or feedback mechanisms

When these safety nets fail, isolated errors propagate unchecked, transforming minor process deviations into full-blown patient care disasters.

Key Insight

True situational awareness extends beyond one's immediate environment to include an understanding of the **organizational ecosystem** — its strengths, weaknesses, and hidden interdependencies. The effective leader not only manages the crisis at hand but also recognizes and addresses the latent, predisposing, and systemic factors that allowed it to occur in the first place.

<table>
<tr><td align="center">SYSTEMS ISSUES CAN BE VERY SUBTLE: JACK SCREW EXAMPLE

As incidents decline, awareness to known safety precautions tend to lapse. When this occurs, governing bodies begin to allow less stringent maintenance requirements to take effect. On the other extreme, when a disaster occurs, overly stringent regulations tend to occur, that have unintended downstream effects that potentially can create a situation worse than the one the regulation was designed to prevent. Some systems problems are so subtle, they may not be recognized until the disaster that revealed the problem, occurs. In 2000, an Alaskan Airways Flight 261 crashed into the Pacific after losing control due the loss of Jack Screw functioning. NTSA investigation revealed that a FAA regulation had allowed less frequent lubrication based on lack of evidence that less frequent lubrication was dangerous.

Samuel Elfassy Senior Director, Corporate Safety, Environment & Quality at Air Canada.

NTSB: http://www.ntsb.gov/news/events/Pages/Loss_of_Control_and_Impact_with_Pacific_Ocean_Alaska_Airlines_Flight_261_McDonnell_Douglas_MD-83_N963AS_about_2.7_miles_no.aspx accessed July 15 2015</td></tr>
</table>

Never forget that everything in the organization is interconnected but potential problems remain seemingly hidden till everything times itself perfectly at the instant the disaster occurs. Lapses, missteps, slips, corner cuts seem to be preceded by equipment failures and supply reductions which were preceded by multiple preconditions, seemingly brought about by short staffing in equipment repair and supply services, compounded by new poorly trained staffing hires and increased workload brought about by staffing shortages that came about by budget cuts and production increase pressures.

Don't take it for granted that everything is there to protect your team when a crisis develops

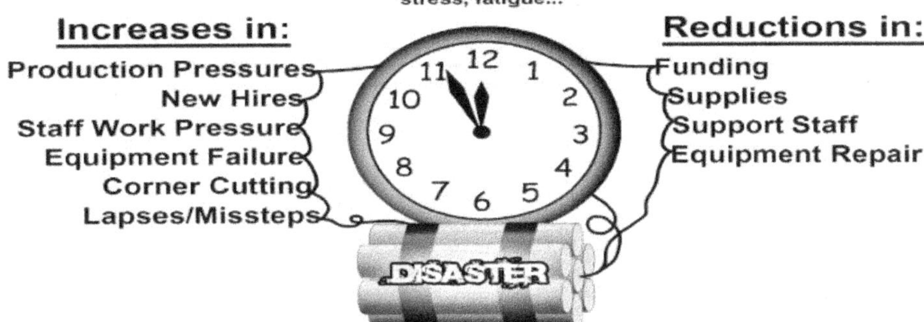

Ticking Time Bomb: How everything in the organization is interconnected but seemingly hidden till everything times itself perfectly at the instant the disaster occurs. Lapses, missteps, slips, corner cuts seem to be preceded by equipment failures and supply reductions which were preceded by multiple preconditions, seemingly brought about by short staffing in equipment repair and supply services, compounded by new poorly trained hires and increased workload brought about by staffing shortages that came about by budget cuts and production increase pressures.

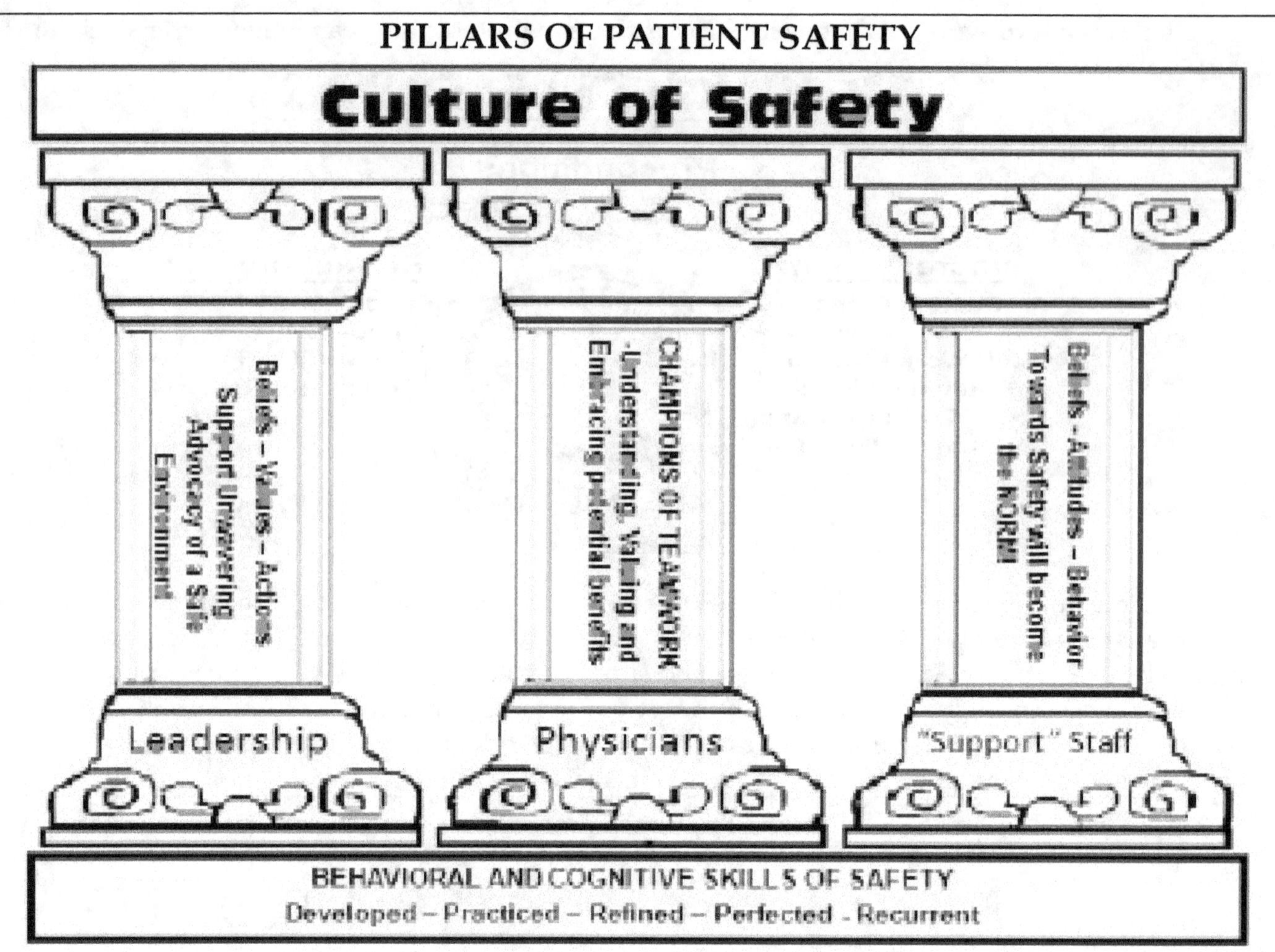

Lipsky K. CRISIS MANAGEMENT LEADERSHIP: TEAM TRAINING TO SURVIVE THE CRITICAL MOMENT 3rd ed; 2018

A change in patient safety philosophy can only be brought about by a change in the healthcare facility patient safety culture. For a cultural change to occur, facility leadership, physicians and "support" staff need to have their priorities aligned.

Leadership must show that they have a) beliefs, b) values, and c) actions to support their unwavering advocacy of a safe environment.

They must assure that their values and philosophy toward patient safety are perceived by their employees as consistent, intense, and they have been accepted through consensus by all staff.

Facility employees must be continually informed of this value system through communications that are credible, consistent, and salient as well be provided with or offered a reward system that promotes safety (in lieu of punishing violations).

Physicians must support this philosophy verbally and by their actions in public, otherwise the remaining staff will not view this culture as being one designed by consensus. For this to occur, they must be actively involved in the construction of patient safety measures and monitoring.

Once the first two pillars are solidified, the support staff will understand that safety culture is the norm for everyone and employees' beliefs and attitudes, and behaviors towards safety will become the norm.

Pillars of Patient Safety-Adapted with permission from:
Reason J. *Managing the Risks of Organizational Accidents*. Burlington, VT: Ashgate; 1997. 53

Weick KE, Sutcliffe KM, *Managing the Unexpected: Resilient Performance in an Age of Uncertainty.* San Francisco, CA: John Wiley; 2007. 88
Salas E, Wilson KA, Murphy CE, King H, Baker D. What crew resource management training will not do for patient safety: unless…?. *J Patient Saf.* 2007;3(2):1-3. 150 salas weick Reason

Pillars of Patient Safety

A sustainable transformation in **patient safety philosophy** begins with a transformation in **organizational culture**. True safety is not achieved through checklists or policies alone — it requires a collective shift in mindset across the entire health-care facility.

For this cultural shift to occur, **leadership, physicians, and all supporting staff** must be aligned in both their priorities and their purpose. Safety cannot be delegated — it must be lived, modeled, and reinforced at every level of the organization.

1. Leadership Commitment

Leadership establishes the tone and direction of the safety culture. To be credible, leaders must demonstrate through **beliefs, values, and actions** an unwavering advocacy for a safe environment.

- **Beliefs:** Leaders must openly convey that patient safety is the organization's highest priority — above production quotas, convenience, or cost savings.
- **Values:** Safety must be embedded in the organization's core values, consistently reinforced through decisions and policies.
- **Actions:** Leaders must act in visible, consistent ways that demonstrate their commitment — attending safety briefings, supporting transparent reporting, and backing staff who speak up about hazards.

Leadership's credibility depends on alignment between their **stated philosophy** and their **observable behaviors**. Employees must perceive that the commitment to safety is not merely rhetorical but *genuine, consistent, and enduring.*

2. Consensus and Communication

A culture of safety cannot exist without **collective ownership**. The organization's philosophy toward patient safety must be accepted **through consensus** by *all staff* — clinical and non-clinical alike. This requires ongoing, clear, and credible communication that:

- Reinforces the organization's safety priorities,
- Demonstrates leadership transparency, and
- Maintains salience — messages must be meaningful and relevant to daily work.

Safety values should be continually communicated through a **variety of channels**: staff meetings, performance reviews, safety huddles, and institutional storytelling. These reinforce the idea that *everyone* has a role in maintaining and improving patient safety.

3. Motivation Through Reward, Not Punishment

A truly mature safety culture moves beyond punitive responses to errors. Instead, it promotes **learning, accountability, and improvement**.

Staff should be encouraged to report near-misses and unsafe conditions without fear of retribution. Recognition and reward systems — formal or informal — should emphasize **proactive safety behaviors**: vigilance, teamwork, and transparency. Punishment, when necessary, should be reserved for willful negligence or reckless disregard for safety, not for human error in a flawed system.

4. Physician Engagement

Physicians hold a unique and powerful role in shaping safety culture. Their **visible endorsement** and **behavioral modeling** strongly influence how seriously others perceive institutional priorities.

When physicians **speak and act consistently** in support of safety—adhering to protocols, encouraging reporting, and collaborating across disciplines—the message is clear: safety is everyone's responsibility. Conversely, visible physician disengagement or cynicism can rapidly undermine years of cultural progress. For this reason, physicians must be **actively involved** in the design, implementation, and monitoring of safety measures. Participation in these processes not only improves systems but also reinforces their ownership of safety as a professional and ethical imperative.

Key Insight

Patient safety is not a program—it is a philosophy lived through culture.

Its pillars—leadership commitment, shared values, open communication, just reward systems, and physician engagement—form the foundation of a resilient, high-reliability organization where every action reflects the collective will to prevent harm.

CREW RESOURCE MANAGEMENT (CRM)

EFFECTIVE CRM FOCUSES ON:
1. TEAM TRAINING.
2. SIMULATION.
3. INTERACTIVE GROUP DEBRIEFINGS.
4. MEASUREMENT AND IMPROVEMENT OF AIRCREW PERFORMANCE. Cooper

The Reluctant Birth of Crew Resource Management—and the Lesson for Medicine

A decade after United Airlines first introduced its **Crew Resource Management (CRM)** program, **Alan Diehl**, a world-renowned aviation safety investigator, presented a seminar at the **International Society of Air Safety Investigators**. Despite ten years of successful CRM implementation and mounting data demonstrating its effectiveness, many aviation leaders remained skeptical. They questioned whether there was enough evidence to justify mandatory CRM training across the industry.

A full decade later, **controversy and resistance persisted**.

In a personal conversation with me, Dr. Diehl described those years as *"extremely frustrating times."* Needless disasters and near misses continued to occur—even when data clearly showed that they were preventable through structured teamwork and communication training. Today, Diehl is rightly regarded as an aviation safety pioneer. Back then, however, he often faced opposition from within his own community.

In his report, Diehl analyzed **28 National Transportation Safety Board (NTSB)** accident reviews and **169 U.S. Air Force** accident investigations from 1987 to 1989. His conclusion was striking:

24 of the 28 NTSB accidents and **113 of the 169 Air Force accidents** involved **aircrew error** as a primary factor.

Moreover, units that had implemented **Cockpit Resource Management** demonstrated a **36–86% reduction in accidents** compared to untrained groups.

The lesson remains timeless—**training alone is not enough**. Even the most data-supported initiatives cannot succeed without a **parallel cultural transformation**.

"Without a culture change, no change will be possible."

The resistance faced by aviation in embracing CRM mirrors the challenges medicine continues to face today in fully institutionalizing **team training, communication, and systems-based safety thinking**. Both fields demonstrate that human error is inevitable—but its consequences are not. Sustainable improvement begins not with more rules or technology, but with a collective commitment to change how we think, communicate, and lead.

SIMULATION AND SAFETY CULTURE

- **Lessons about Human Factors / CRM:**
  - It is normal for people to summarily dismiss new information they think will never work in their particular area; i.e., any change in the status quo.
- **Barriers to implementation of a culture of safety in any organization:**
  - The biggest barrier to implementation of a culture of safety is the **power structure** in the organization itself.
  - The 2nd factor preventing the adoption of a safety culture is **operational inertia**. Questioning the rationale behind operational SOP's is difficult. Changing the routine takes a lot of energy.
  - The 3rd barrier is the **budget**. In the 1980's the airline industry faced the same issue of training all their staff "will simply cost too much," but found in the end that an 80% reduction in incidents, injuries, lawsuits, death, and bad publicity made it worth it.
- **Creating a safety culture takes:**
  - Trust in its membership.
  - Non-punitive policies.
  - Willingness to reduce error in the system.
  - Provision of training in error avoidance, detection and maintenance.
  - Training in the evaluation and reinforcement of error avoidance. [Okray]

Lessons from Aviation: The Debate Over Crew Resource Management- Human Performance, Burnout, and the Cost of Error

Balch et al. reported that **burnout and other measures of surgeon distress** correlate directly with excessive workloads—specifically, more than **eighty hours per week** and **more than two nights on call per week** among American surgeons. Their findings were sobering:

"When physicians are in distress, their performance in delivering care can be suboptimal."

This impairment not only compromises patient safety but also increases the risk of **home–work conflict** and **lapses in professional judgment**. [Balch]

In the world of patient care—particularly in **surgery**—there is a pervasive expectation of **unbroken success**. As **Charles Bosk** observed in his classic work *Forgive and Remember: Managing Medical Failure*, the first question asked after any complication or adverse outcome is too often, *"What did you do wrong?"* [Bosk] This culture of blame fosters maladaptive behaviors, especially during times of stress, failure, or major change.

A **recent American College of Surgeons (ACS) survey** on burnout further underscores this danger. The study revealed a strong association between **medical errors** and **stress, fatigue, burnout, alcohol misuse, and suicidal ideation**. Notably, **8.9% of surgeons** reported committing a medical error within the preceding three months, most of which were attributed to **lapses in judgment, fatigue, or distraction**. Even more concerning, a **prior medical error** was found to be **independently predictive of heavy alcohol use and suicidal ideation**—a stark reminder that medical errors affect not only patients, but also the clinicians involved. [Bosk, Shanafelt]

Comparable findings have been observed in anesthesia. A **2012 American Society of Anesthesiologists (ASA)** study similarly documented the psychological and behavioral toll of adverse outcomes on anesthesia providers. [Gazoni]

The **University of Toronto group**, led by **Bernstein et al. (2015)**, explored how residents learn to recover from emotionally traumatic clinical events during training. Their findings confirmed that most residents remain deeply affected by these experiences and that few programs offer formal mechanisms for recovery.

In other words, the concept of supporting the **"second victim"** — the clinician involved in or affected by a medical error — is still not universally embraced across institutions. [Balogun et al]

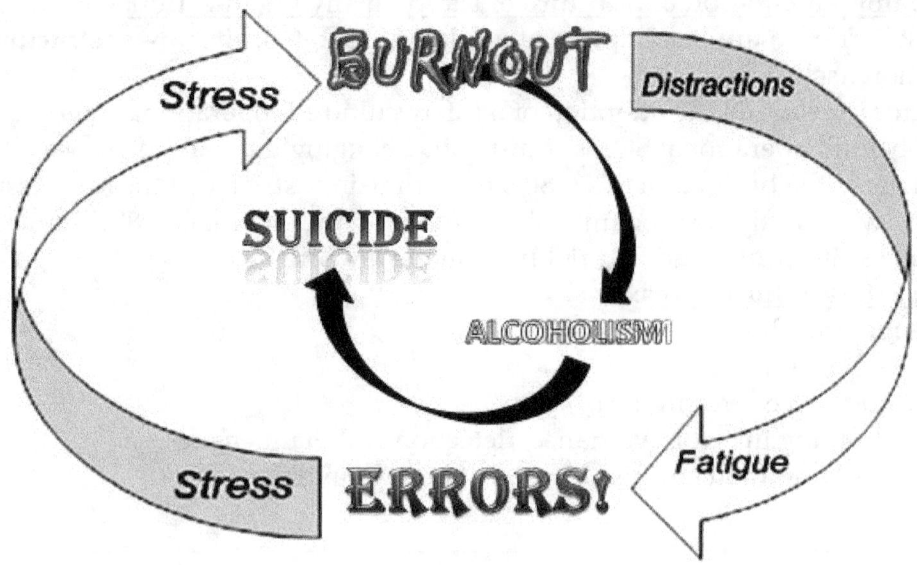

A recent American College of Surgeons Survey on burnout revealed a tight relationship between causing a patient error and stress, fatigue, burnout, alcoholism, and suicidal ideation. The only sure-fire way to cut the cycle is to reduce the stress induced by creating an error. [156-161 Shanafelt, shanafelt shanafelt, shanafelt Campbell, Oreskovich]

The Leadership Imperative

The implication for leadership is clear:

Anything that **reduces error, mitigates fatigue**, and **minimizes distraction** simultaneously enhances **patient safety** and **team well-being**. The leader's role is not only to prevent mistakes but also to create a culture where clinicians can recover, learn, and grow from them.

A safe environment is one where the system anticipates human fallibility, supports its members when errors occur, and continually reinforces the link between **psychological safety** and **patient safety**.

IMPACT OF PERIOPERATIVE CATASTROPHES-
2012 AMERICAN SOCIETY OF ANESTHESIOLOGISTS SURVEY:

- 84% experienced more than 1 unanticipated death or serious injury over career.
- **70% experienced guilt, anxiety, and reliving of the event (88% requiring time to recover emotionally & 19% never fully recovered, 12% considered a career change).**
- 67% believed that their ability to provide patient care was compromised in the first 4 hours subsequent to the event.
- **Only 7% were given time off.**
- CONCLUSION: A perioperative catastrophe may have a profound and lasting emotional impact on the anesthesiologist involved and may affect his or her ability to provide patient care in the aftermath of such events. [Gazoni]

YES this is repeated for a purpose- IT IS ALL TOO OFTEN IGNORED!

DURING DOD TRAUMA SURGEON SIMULATION, HEALTH-CARE PROVIDERS TEND TO BE OPTIMISTS REGARDING THEIR OWN ANTICIPATED PERFORMANCE

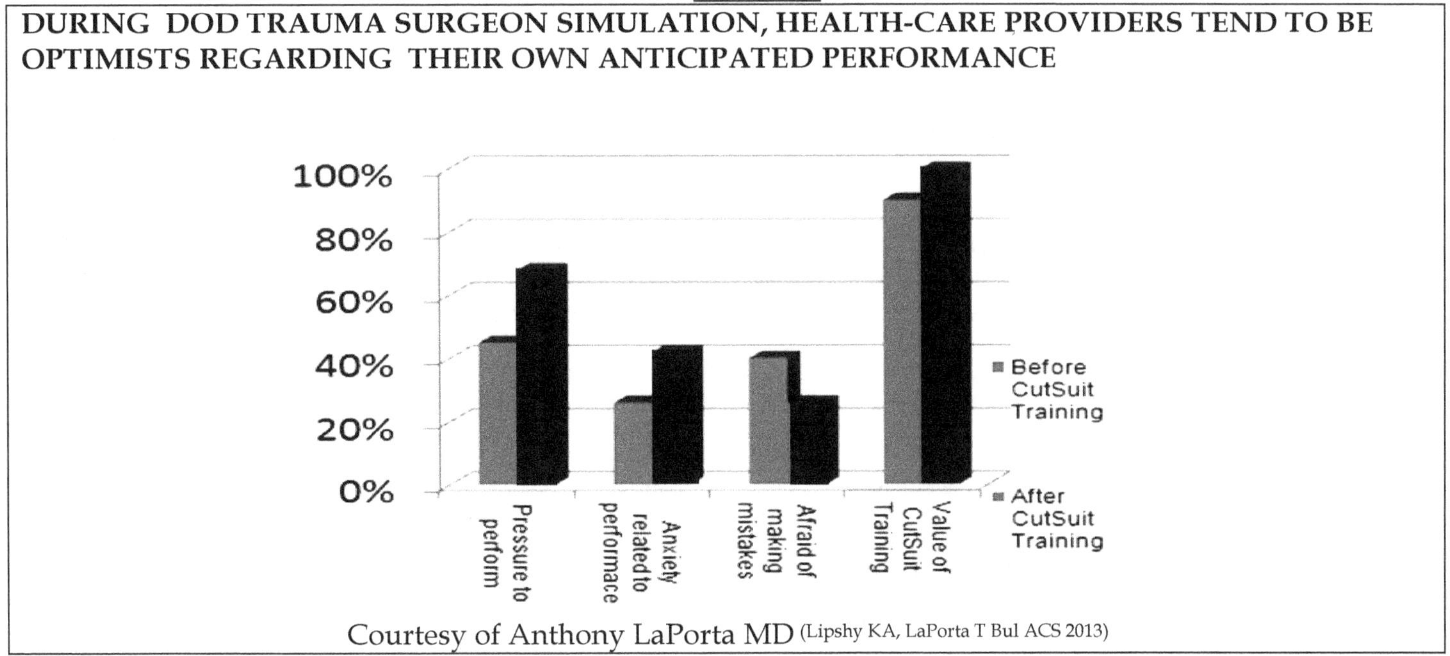

Courtesy of Anthony LaPorta MD (Lipshy KA, LaPorta T Bul ACS 2013)

Participants in a DOD trauma simulation were surveyed before and after the course. Pre-training surveys revealed providers were alarmingly overconfident in their skill levels and underestimated the degree of anxiety they expected to face in similar emergent traumatic experiences. During post-training, participants acknowledged that they faced more anxiety than they originally anticipated, but also said they realized that in the simulation environment they could make mistakes that they could not afford to make in real-life scenarios. (Hunt, LaPorta, Rush, et al)

OPTIMIST BIAS: "HEY! I'M A TEAM PLAYER!"
- Teamwork is in the Eye of the Beholder.
- Surgeons and Anesthesiologists rated teamwork within their own discipline the highest 85.2%.
- Surgeons perceive that everyone in the OR is doing a good job regarding teamwork (80% range).
- OR nurses rate teamwork as LOW with surgeons (48%) and Anesthesia (63%).
- Overall disparity in interpretation in communication on approachability, ability to express concerns, overall culture of safety. Makary MA, Sexton JB, Freischlag JA

TEAMWORK SELF-ASSESSMENT
- <u>**2007 Mayo Study**</u> -*"information conveyed in the OR is shared in a tense, ad hoc manner not conducive to comfortable communication"*.
- 59% of non-physician respondents thought that *"surgeon attitudes and personalities negatively impacted teamwork"*.
- **Pronovost-** Impression of teamwork amongst **ICU** RN's and MDs.
- MD's rated RN's at 90% rating for collaboration.
- RN's rated MD's at only 54%!

Makray, Pronovost Sexton

While on the surface this may appear subtle, this data would account for the disparity in interpretation in communication on approachability, ability to express concerns, and an overall culture of safety.

Pronovost discussed the same discrepancy when reviewing data regarding impression of teamwork amongst ICU RNs and MDs, where MDs rated the RNs at a 90% rating for collaboration, but RNs rated the MDs at only 54%. Pronovost

In an interesting study by Helmriech' s group, surveys were submitted to aviation and surgery teams. In their study, while pilots were least likely to deny the effects of fatigue on performance (26%), *70% of surgeons and 47% of anesthetists* denied the risks of those conditions. At the same time, while 97% of pilots and 94% of ICU staff rejected hierarchies where senior staff members were not open to input from junior members, only 55% of surgeons believed junior staff should have input. [Helmreich]

The more disparaging news was the discordance in the discernment of teamwork ability of surgeons whereby 73% of surgical residents, 64% of consultant surgeons, 39% of anesthesia consultants, 28% of surgical nurses, 25% of anesthetic nurses, and 10% of anesthetic residents felt the surgeons were team players.

Having said that, the most frightening aspect of the study was that only 33% of hospital staff reported that errors are handled appropriately, 33% of intensive care staff did not acknowledge that they make errors, and over 50% of intensive care staff reported that they find it difficult to discuss mistakes.[Sexton]

CHAPTER V CONCLUSION REFERENCES

- Balogun JA, Bramall AN, Bernstein M. How Surgical Trainees Handle Catastrophic Errors: A Qualitative Study. JSE 2015.72(6):1179-1184.
- Balch CM, Shanafelt TD, DyrbyeL, et al. Surgeon distress as calibrated by hours worked, and nights on call. *J Am Coll Surg*. November 2010;211(5):609-619.
- Bergs J, Lambrechts F, Simons P, Vlayen A, Marneffe W, Hellings J, Cleemput I, Vandijck D. Barriers and facilitators related to the implementation of surgical safety checklists: a systematic review of the qualitative evidence. Br Med J Qual Saf. 2015;24(12):776-86.
- Bosk CL. *Forgive and Remember: Managing Medical Failure*. 2nd ed. Chicago, IL: University of Chicago Press; 2003.
- Calland JF, Guerlain S, Adams RB, Tribble CG, Foley E, Chekan EG. A systems approach to surgical safety. *Surg Endosc*. 2002;16(6):1005-1014.
- Cook R, Rasmussen J. 'Going solid': a model of system dynamics and consequences for patient safety. Qual SAF health care. 2005;14:130-134
- Cooper GE, White MD, Lauber JK. Resource management on the flightdeck: proceedings of a NASA/ industry workshop. In: *NASA Conference Publication No. CP-2120*. San Francisco, CA: NASA - Ames Research Center; 1980.
- Dekker S. *Field Guide to Human Error Investigation*. Surrey, UK: Ashgate Press / TJ International Ltd; 2002.
- Diehl, A. *"Does cockpit management training reduce aircrew error?"* Proceedings of the Twenty-Second International Seminar of the International Society Of Air Safety Investigators. Canberra, Australia. November 4-7, 1991. *ISASI Forum*.1991;24(4):46.
- Edmondson AC. *Teaming: How Organizations Learn, Innovate, and Compete in the Knowledge Economy. John Wiley & Sons* 2012.
- FAA. *Human Factors Guide for Aviation Maintenance and Boeing Maintenance Error Decision Aid (MEDA) Users Guide*. http://www.hf.faa.gov/hfguide/07/07_methods.html. Accessed February 2, 2013.
- Gazoni FM, Amato PE, Malik ZM, Durieu ME. The impact of perioperative catastrophes on anesthesiologists: results of a national survey. *Anesth Analg*. 2012;114(3):596-603.
- Hunt B, Wall V, LaPorta AJ, Rush R, Moloff A, Schoeff JE, Tieman M, Lea M. New methods of early surgical training using the human worn partial task surgical simulator in scenario based stress immersion training. *MEdSim Magazine*. 2012;4(3):25-28. http://issuu.com/halldale/docs/medsim_3_2012. Accessed August 16, 2013.
- Kolditz TA. *In Extremis Leadership: Leading As If Your Life Depended On It*. San Francisco, CA: Jossey-Bass; 2007.
- Makary MA, Sexton JB, Freischlag JA, et al. Operating room teamwork among physicians and nurses: teamwork in the eye of the beholder. *J Am Coll Surg*. 2006;202:746-752.
- NTSB: http://www.ntsb.gov/news/events/Pages/Loss_of_Control_and_Impact_with_Pacific_Ocean_Alaska_Airlines_Flight_261_McDonnell_Douglas_MD-83_N963AS_about_2.7_miles_no.aspx accessed July 15 2015
- Pronovost P. Intensive care unit safety reporting system (ICUSRS). Reported in: *Safety and Medicine*. http://ocw.jhsph.edu/courses/patientsafety/PDFs/PS_lec4_Pronovost.pdf. Accessed February 12, 2013.
- Reason J. *Managing the Risks of Organizational Accidents*. Burlington, VT: Ashgate; 1997.
- Russ SJ, Sevdalis N, Moorthy K, Mayer EK, Rout S, Caris J, Mansell J, Davies R, Vincent C, Darzi A. A qualitative evaluation of the barriers and facilitators toward implementation of the WHO surgical safety checklist across hospitals in England: lessons from the "Surgical Checklist Implementation Project". Ann Surg. 2015 Jan;261(1):81-91
- Salas E, Wilson KA, Murphy CE, King H, Baker D. What crew resource management training will not do for patient safety: unless...?. *J Patient Saf*. 2007;3(2):1-3.
- Sexton JB, Thomas EJ, Helmreich RL. Error, stress, and teamwork in medicine and aviation: cross sectional surveys. *BMJ*. March 2000;320(7237): 745-749.
- Shanafelt TD, Balch CM, Bechamps G, et al. Burnout and medical errors among American surgeons. *Ann Surg*. 2010;251(6):995-1000.
- Weller, Boyd. Making a Difference Through Improving Teamwork in the Operating Room: A Systematic Review of the Evidence on What Works; Patient Safety in Anesthesia. 4:77–83, (2014);
- Weick KE, Sutcliffe KM, *Managing the Unexpected: Resilient Performance in an Age of Uncertainty*. San Francisco, CA: John Wiley; 2007.

SUMMARY

I. <u>**STEPS FOR EFFECTIVE DECISION MAKING AND COMMUNCATION PROCESSING DURING ANY SITUATION**</u>: (See Appendix A for details)

AFTER PROCESSING INCOMING SENSORY INPUT, UTILIZING YOUR AVAILABLE LIBRARY OF EXPERIENCE, AND CREATING A STORY CONSISTENT WITH A SCENE THAT DESERVES A RATIONAL DECISION MAKING PROCESS RATHER THAN IMMEDIATE ENGAGEMENT YOU DO THE FOLLOWING:

    A. <u>**INTRODUCTION/CRITICAL PAUSE**</u>: Team "Leader" creates a pause in the situation to calm / quiet team members down, gain control over the communication process and introduce their intent.

    B. <u>**BRIEFING**</u>: Team "leader" summarizes their personal assessment of their observation of known facts regarding the situation at hand (typically leaders propose a goal early on, but experts recommend withholding their recommendation until all the information has been gathered). *

    C. <u>**QUERY/CRITICAL PAUSE:**</u> Team "leader" pauses the process and queries team members about their knowledge of key components of the situation at hand creating an inventory of damage, resources, obstacles, potential solutions to their dilemma and safety to proceed.*

    D. <u>**PREDICTION, PLAN AND REASSESS**</u>: Team members assess their knowledge base as a whole and create a series of potential solutions with expected outcomes and "bail-out" plans should their expectations not be observed. To avoid information overload, experienced leaders attempt to propose one goal/solution/plan at a time. If concern is raised an alternate can be proposed at this point. Team specifies period of time for which they will reassess the situation to determine effectiveness of current plan.*

    *success depends upon the use of effective communication skills described throughout this training guide.

II. <u>***KEY COMPONENTS OF EFFECTIVE COMMUNICATION SKILLS:**</u>

    1. LISTENING: Everyone should be an active listener and acknowledge comprehension.

    2. CONTROL: Everyone should utilize controlled calm steady voices that are loud enough to be heard but without shouting.

    3. PRECISION: The team leader shall use commands that are accurate, bold, clear, concise, and precise.

    4. EXPLICIT: Communication shall be explicit, clear and NOT utilize implied instruction. Explicit communication does NOT assume everyone understands background information. Avoid mitigated speech!

    5. FEEDBACK: Communication requires continuous closed loops of communication sending and reception that requires constant feedback with open, inclusive exchange.

    6. FOCUSED: Speakers address communication to specific staff, not global commands.

    7. AWARENESS: All team members must recognize that perceptions, influences, situations and filters affect the message as well as the need to utilize more than one type of communication when possible (verbal, written, symbolic, non-verbal).

WHY SHOULD WE WORRY? HERE'S WHY:

1. These events are rare!

2. Experience does not prevent failure — senior providers make mistakes during crises!

3. Signs are frequently non-specific, resulting in a delay in the determination of the cause and appropriate corrective action, creating more team stress.

4. The team is usually forced to rely upon cognitive taking far beyond the information processing capacity of the human brain.

5. Only 10-20% of people have an ability to remain calm in a crisis situation!

LEADERSHIP STEPS TOWARDS STAFF EDUCATION

- Medical Team Training modeled after CRM.
- STOP THE DISTRACTIONS!
- Remember Briefing and Debriefings.
- Develop Crisis Checklists (but be aware of their pitfalls).
- Disaster / Crisis response training.
  a. Be aware of Heuristics and other mental miscues.
  b. Train Teams how to function effectively during the critical moment by taking the critical pause, assessing the situation, and being decisive.
  c. Train Individuals and Teams on how to lead during a crisis by defining goals, gathering information, planning and acting.

WHAT HAVE WE LEARNED:

Understand the key components of effectively preparing your team for and leading your team thru an unexpected threatening event where time-critical, rapid process decision making is required through:

1. Understanding what constitutes a "crisis".
2. Identifying routes that human error creates or perpetuates a crisis.
3. Understanding how other high risk professionals train to reduce errors & why.
4. Understanding how to curtail maladaptive behavior during a crisis.
5. Understanding the components of effective leadership during a crisis.

YOUR OWN WORST ENEMY:

"Complacency kills, as do poor planning, carelessness, and bad judgment.

While accidents do happen, we often have only ourselves to blame when we're in a pickle.

Sometimes you have to learn from your own mistakes, but a wise man learns from the mistakes of others.

IF YOU FAIL TO HAVE A PLAN, YOU PLAN TO FAIL!"

BEAR GRYLLS

REFERENCES

- ACGME and ABS. The General Surgery Milestone Project A Joint Initiative of The Accreditation Council for Graduate Medical Education and The American Board of Surgery July 2015.
http://www.acgme.org/Portals/0/PDFs/Milestones/SurgeryMilestones.pdf assessed 110616

- ACGME Holmboe ES, Edgar L, Hamstra S. The Milestones Guidebook Version 2016.
http://www.acgme.org/Portals/0/MilestonesGuidebook.pdf assessed 110616

- ACGME. The Six ACGME competencies: what the RC's expect from programs. New program directors Pre-course. 2008.
http://www.siumed.edu/resaffairs/pdfs/What%20the%20RRCs%20expect%20from%20the%20competencies%202008.pdf assessed 110616

- Ackoff RL. The Future of Operational Research is Past The Journal of the Operational Research Society Vol. 30, No. 2 (Feb., 1979), pp. 93-104

- AHRQ. TeamSTEPPS Pocket Guide – 06.136. The Department of Defense Patient Safety Program in collaboration with the Agency for Healthcare Research and Quality AHRQ. Revised March 2008 Version 06.1
http://teamstepps.ahrq.gov/abouttoolsmaterials.htm#TrainingMaterials Accessed March 1, 2013.

- The American College of Surgeons. Pellegrini CA. Addressing surgeon fatigue and sleep deprivation. *Bull Am Coll Surg.2015;100(8):72-74.*

- The American College of Surgeons. Statement on peak performance and management of fatigue. *Bull Am Coll Surg.2014;99(8):53-54.* Available at: bulletin.facs.org/2014/08/statement-on-peak-performance-and-management-of-fatigue/. Accessed Sept 18, 2015.

- American College of Surgeons. Non-technical skills matter too: Nation's doctors, payers and surgical stakeholders recommend teamwork, communication training and standardized processes to improve safety-
NEWS FROM THE AMERICAN COLLEGE OF SURGEONS AND THE AMERICAN ACADEMY OF ORTHOPAEDIC SURGEONS | FOR IMMEDIATE RELEASE. American College of Surgery Press release. Aug 5 2016.
https://www.facs.org/media/press-releases/2016/skills-080516

- Anton N, Montero PN, Howley LD, Brown C, Stefanidis D. What coping strategies are surgeons relying upon during surgery? Am Jnl Surg 2015. 210:846-851.

- The Arbinger Institute. The Outward mindset: how to change lives and transform organizations. Berrett-Koehler publishers. 2019

- Arora S, Sevdalis N, Nestel D, Tierney T, Woloshynowych M, Kneebone R. Managing intraoperative stress: what do surgeons want from a crisis training program. *Am J Surg.* 2009;197(4):537-543.

- Arora S, Hull L, Sevdalis N, et al. Factors compromising safety in surgery: stressful events in the operating room. *Am J Surg.* 2010;199:60–65.

- Arora S, Sevdalis N, Nestel D, et al. The impact of stress on surgical performance: a systematic review of the literature. *Surgery.* 2010;147:318–330.

- Arora S, Tierney T, Sevdalis N, et al. The Imperial Stress Assessment Tool (ISAT): a feasible, reliable and valid approach to measuring stress in the operating room. *World J Surg.* 2010;34:1756–1763.

- Arriaga AF, Bader AM, Wong JM, Lipsitz SR, Berry WR, Ziewacz JE, Hepner DL, Boorman DJ, Pozner CN, SminkDS, Gawande AA. Simulation based trial of surgical crisis checklists. *N Engl J Med.* 2013;368(3):246-253.

- Ashcroft DM, Morecrof C, Parker D, Noyce PR. Safety culture assessment in community pharmacy: development, face validity and feasibility of the Manchester Patients Safety Assessment Framework. *Qual Saf Health Care.* 2005;14(6):417-21.

- Babcock W. Resuscitation during anesthesia. *Anesth Analg.* 1924;3:208-213.

- Baden-Powell, Robert. *Scouting for Boys*: A handbook for instruction in good citizenship through woodcraft. *Campfire Yarn No. 3 - Becoming a Scout.* London, Windsor House, Bream's Buildings, E.C.: Horace Cox 1908.

- Balch CM, Shanafelt TD, DyrbyeL, et al. Surgeon distress as calibrated by hours worked, and nights on call. *J Am Coll Surg.* November 2010;211(5):609-619.

- Balogun JA, Bramall AN, Bernstein M. How Surgical Trainees Handle Catastrophic Errors: A Qualitative Study. JSE 2015.72(6):1179-1184.

- Banja J. The normalization of deviance in healthcare delivery. *Bus Horiz.* 2010 ; 53(2): 139.

- BargerLK, Cade BE, Ayas NT, Cronin JW, Rosner B, Speizer FE, Czeisler CA. Extended Work Shifts and the Risk of Motor Vehicle Crashes among Interns. N Engl J Med 2005; 352:125-134

- *Barnard, Chester I. (1938). The Functions of the Executive. Cambridge, MA: Harvard University Press. OCLC 555075.*

- Barry, E.S., & Grunberg, N.E., (2020). A conceptual framework to guide leader and follower education, development, and assessment. Journal of Leadership, Accountability and Ethics. 17(1), 127-134. https://doi.org/10.33423/jlae.v17i1.2795.

- Bergman JZ, Rentsch JR, Small EE, et al. The shared leadership Process in decision-making teams. J Soc Psychol 2012;152:17–42.

- Bergs J, Lambrechts F, Simons P, Vlayen A, Marneffe W, Hellings J, Cleemput I, Vandijck D. Barriers and facilitators related to the implementation of surgical safety checklists: a systematic review of the qualitative evidence. Br Med J Qual Saf. 2015;24(12):776-86.

- Blackbourne LH. *First to Cut Trauma Lessons Learned in the Combat Zone 1ST Edition, 2009* United States Army Institute of Surgical Research. San Antonio Texas. http://www.usaisr.amedd.army.mil/publications.html

- Bock M, Doz P, Fanolla A, Segur-Cabanac I, Auricchio F, Melani C, Girardi F, Meier H, Pycha A. A comparative effectiveness analysis of the implementation of surgical safety checklists in a tertiary care hospital. *JAMA Surg.* 2016;151(7):639-646

- Bosk CL. *Forgive and Remember: Managing Medical Failure.* 2nd ed. Chicago, IL: University of Chicago Press; 2003.

- Bowermaster R, Miller M, Ashcraft T, Boyd M, Brar A, Manning P, Eghtesady P. Application of the Aviation Black Box Principle in Pediatric Cardiac Surgery: Tracking All Failures in the Pediatric Cardiac Operating Room. *J Am Coll Surg* 2015;220:149-155.

- Brunicardi FC, Hobson FL. Time management: a review for physicians. J Natl Med Assoc. 1996 Sep;88(9):581-7.

- Butler F. Tactical Medicine Training SEAL Mission Commanders *Military Medicine.* 2001; 166(7):625.

- Butler FK, Hagmann JH, Richards DT. Tactical Management of Urban Warfare Casualties in Special Operations. *Military Medicine,* 2000; 165(S1):1-48.

- Butler FK, Holcomb JB. ***The Tactical Combat Casualty Care (TCCC) Transition Initiative.*** Army Medical Department Journal PB 8-05-4/5/6:33-37

- Butler FK. **Current State of Preparedness and Resilience.** Hartford Consensus IV 8 Jan 2016

- Butler FK, Blackbourne LH. Battlefield trauma care then and now: A decade of Tactical Combat Casualty Care. J Trauma Acute Care Surg. 2012;73(6S5):S395-402

- Butler FK. **Military History of Increasing Survival-***The U.S. Military Experience with Tourniquets and Hemostatic Dressings in the Afghanistan and Iraq Conflicts.* Journal of Special Operaations Medicine 2015; 15(4):149-152.

- Butler FK, Hagmann J, Butler EG. Tactical Combat Casualty Care in Special Operations. *Mil Med.* 1996;161(supp):1-16.

- Callahan CW, Grunberg NE. Military Medical Leadership in Fundamentals of Military Medical Practice. Schoomaker EB, Smith DC eds, Washington DC Borden Institute. 2017.

- Calland JF, Guerlain S, Adams RB, Tribble CG, Foley E, Chekan EG. A systems approach to surgical safety. *Surg Endosc.* 2002;16(6):1005-1014.

- Callison, D; Key Words, Concepts and Methods for Information Age Instruction: A Guide to Teaching Information Inquiry.

- Charuluxananan S, Punjasawadwong Y, Suraseranivongse S, et al. The Thai Anesthesia Incidents Study (THAI Study) of anesthetic outcomes: II. anesthetic profiles and adverse events. *J Med Assoc Thai.* 2005;88:Suppl 7:S14-S29.

- Chopra V, Bovill JG, Spierdjk J, Koornneef F. Reported significant observations during anesthesia: a prospective analysis over an 18 year period. *Br J Anaesth.* 1992;68:13-17.

- Clifton BS, Hotten WIT. Deaths associated with anesthesia. Br J Anaesth. 1963:35:250-259.

- Cristancho SM, Apramian T, Vanstone M, Lingard L, Ott M, Forbes T, Novick R. Thinking like an expert: surgical decision making as a cyclical process of being aware. Am Journal Surgery 2016. 211(1):64–69.

- Cristancho S, Apramian T, Vanstone M, Lingard L, Ott M, Novick R. Understanding Clinical Uncertainty: What Is Going on When Experienced Surgeons Are Not Sure What to Do? Academic Medicine 2013. 88(10)1516–1521.

- Cristancho S, Vanstone M, Lingard L, LeBel M, Ott M. When surgeons face intraoperative challenges: a naturalistic model of surgical decision making. Am Journal of Surgery 2013. 205(2):156–162.

- Cohen I. Improving time-critical decision making in life-threatening situations: observations and insights. *Decision Analysis.* 2008;5(2):100-110.

- Collyer S, Malecki G. *Tactical decision Making under stress: history and overview* in Cannon-Bower J and Salas E. Making Decisions under stress APA 1998.

- Conley DM, Singer SJ, Edmondson L, Berry WR, Gawande AA. Effective Surgical Safety Checklist Implementation. Journal of the American College of Surgeons. 2011; 212(5):873–879.

- Cooper JB, Newbower RS, Long CD, McPeek B. Preventable anesthesia mishaps: a study of human factors. Anesthesiology. 1978;49(6):399-406.

- Cooper GE, White MD, Lauber JK. Resource management on the flightdeck: proceedings of a NASA/ industry workshop. In: *NASA Conference Publication No. CP-2120.* San Francisco, CA: NASA - Ames Research Center; 1980.

- Cook R, Rasmussen J. 'Going solid': a model of system dynamics and consequences for patient safety. <u>Qual SAF health care.</u> 2005;14:130-134

- Covey SR. the Seven Habits of Highly Effective People: restoring the Character Ethic. New York NY. Free Press; 2004.

- Croskerry P. Cognitive Forcing Strategies in Clinical Decision-making. Ann Emerg Med 2003; 41(1):110-120.

- Croskerry P. Diagnostic Failure: A cognitive and Affective approach. *In Advances in Patient Safety: From research to Implementation (Vol 2:Concepts and Methodology.,* Henriksen K, Battles JB, Marks ES, Lewin DI. Rockville MD. Agency for Healthcare Research and Quality; 2005.

- Davis D, Mazmanian P, Fordis M, Van Harrison R, Thorpe KE, Math M; Perrier L. Accuracy of Physician Self-assessment Compared With Observed Measures of Competence A Systematic Review. *JAMA.* 2006;296(9):1094-1102.

- Dawson D, Reid K. *Fatigue, Alcohol and Performance Impairment.* Nature 17 Jul 1997. Vol 388, p23

- D'Angelo AL, Law K, Cohen E, Ray R, Shaffer DW, Pugh C. Error management: Do residents Identify Operative Errors as Reversible? Annual Meeting of the Association for Surgical Education Conference Dates: 12-16 April 2016 Location: Boston, Massachusetts.

- Dekker S. *Field Guide to Human Error Investigation.* Surrey, UK: Ashgate Press / TJ International Ltd; 2002.

- Denver R. Damn Few: making the modern SEAL warrior. New York, NY: Hyperion; 2013.

- Diehl, A. "*Does cockpit management training reduce aircrew error?*" Proceedings of the Twenty-Second International Seminar of the International Society Of Air Safety Investigators. Canberra, Australia. November 4-7, 1991. *ISASI Forum*.1991;24(4):46.
- Dismukes K, Young G, Sumwait R. Cockpit interruptions and distractions: effective management requires a careful balancing act. *Aviat Safety Rep Syst Directline*. 1998;10:4–9.
- DiTulio A, Steinemann S, Skinner A, et al. How to assess teamwork in the trauma bay? Introduction of a modified "NOTECHS" scale for trauma *Association for Surgical Education*. Boston, MA; 2011.
- Dörner D. *The Logic of Failure: Recognizing and Avoiding Error in Complex Situations*. Reading, MA: Perseus Books; 1996.
- Doty J, Doty C. Command Responsibility and Accountability. MILITARY REVIEW 2012 Jan-Feb:35-38.
- Doty J, Fenlason J. Its not about trust; its about thinking and judgment. Military Review 2015 Mar-Apr 149-154.
- Doty J, Sowden W. Competency vs Character? It must be both! Military review. 2009 Nov-Dec 69-76.
- Dripps RD, Lamont A, Eckenhoff JE. The role of anesthesia in surgical mortality. JAMA. 1961;178(3):261-266.
- Duhigg C. The power of habit: why we do what we do in life and business. NYNY random house. 2014.
- Duckworth AL, Seligman MEP. Self discipline outdoes IQ in predicting academic performance in adolescents. Psychological science. 2005. 16:939-944.
- Valentine MA, **Edmondson** AC .Team Scaffolds: How Mesolevel Structures Enable Role-Based Coordination in Temporary Groups. Organization Science. 2015; 26(2):405-422. http://dx.doi.org/10.1287/orsc.2014.0947
- Edmondson AC. *Teaming: How Organizations Learn, Innovate, and Compete in the Knowledge Economy. John Wiley & Sons 2012.*
- Edmondson AC. Framing for learning: Lessons in successful technology implementation. *California Management Review*.2003; 45 (2): 34-54
- Edmondson AC. Bohmer, R.M., and Pisano, G.P. Disrupted routines: Team learning and new technology implementation in hospitals. *Administrative Science Quarterly, 2001;*46: 685-716.
- Pisano G, Bohmer R, and Edmondson A. Organizational differences in rates of learning: Evidence from the adoption of minimally invasive cardiac surgery. *Management Science, 2001;*47 (6): 752-768.
- Edmondson A, Bohmer R, and Pisano G. Speeding up team learning. *Harvard Business Review,2001;*79 (9): 125-134.
- Edwards G, Morton HJV, Pask EA, Wylie WD. Deaths associated with anesthesia: report on 1000 cases. Anaesthesia . 1956;11:194-220.
- Endsley, M. R. (1995). Toward a theory of situation awareness in dynamic systems. Human Factors, 37(1), 32–64
- Endsley, MR, Garland DJ. *Situation Awareness Analysis and Measurement*. Mahwah, NJ: Lawrence Erlbaum Associates; 2000.
- FAA. *Human Factors Guide for Aviation Maintenance and Boeing Maintenance Error Decision Aid (MEDA) Users Guide*. http://www.hf.faa.gov/hfguide/07/07_methods.html. Accessed February 2, 2013.
- FAA Fact Sheet – Pilot Fatigue; http://www.faa.gov/news/fact_sheets/news_story.cfm?newsId=11857
- Fabri PJ, Zayas-Castro JL. Human error, not communication and systems, underlies surgical complications. Surgery. 2008;144(4):557-565.
- Feuerbacher RL, Funk K, Spight D, Diggs B, Hunter J. Realistic distractions and interruptions that impair simulated surgical performance by novice surgeons. *Arch Surg*. 2012;147(11):1026-1030.
- Flin R, Paterson-Brown S, Maran N, Rowley D, Youngson G, Macpherson S, Yule S; **The Non-Technical Skills for Surgeons (NOTSS) System Handbook** v1.2; University of Aberdeen ; 2006. http://www.abdn.ac.uk/iprc/notss; http://scholar.harvard.edu/files/ntsl/files/notss_handbook_2012.pdf;
- Flin R. Sitting in the hot seat: leaders and teams for critical incident management. Rhona Flin, John Wiley and Sons. 1996 & 2026.
- Fischer J. Editorial opinion: is damage to the common bile duct during laparoscopic cholecystectomy an inherent risk of the operation. *Am J Surg* 2009;197:829-832.
- Fisher, GH. Measuring ambiguity. *Am J Psychol*. 1967;80(4):541-557.
- Fioratou E, Flin R. No simple fix for fixation errors: cognitive processes and their clinical applications. *Anaesthesia*. January 2010;65(1):61-69.
- Fleming M, Wentzell N. Patient safety culture improvement tool: development and guidelines for use. *Healthc Q*. 2008;11(3):10-15.
- Gaba DM, Fish KJ, Howard SK. *Crisis Management in Anesthesiology*. New York, NY: Churchill Livingstone; 1994.
- Gawande A. *The Checklist Manifesto: How to Get Things Right*. New York, NY: Metropolitan Books; 2009.
- Kirby T. Atul Gawande — making surgery safer worldwide. Lancet.2010;376(9746):1045
- Garrard L, Chamorro-premuzic, T. The dark side of high employee engagement. HBR Aug 16 2016, Accessed Aug 16 2016) https://hbr.org/2016/08/the-dark-side-of-high-employee-engagement)
- Gazoni FM, Amato PE, Malik ZM, Durieu ME. The impact of perioperative catastrophes on anesthesiologists: results of a national survey. *Anesth Analg*. 2012;114(3):596–603.
- Ginter PM, Swayne LM, Duncan WJ Strategic management of Healthcare organizations. Blackwell business. Malden MA. 1999.
- Gillman L., Widder S. Trauma Team Dynamics - A Trauma Crisis Resource Management Manual Springer, Switzerland 2016, 2025
- Gladwell M. *Blink, the power of thinking without thinking*. New York: Little, Brown and Company; 2005.
- Gladwell M. *Outliers*. New York: Little Brown and Company; 2008.
- Goleman D. Leadership that gets results. Harvard Business Review. 2000;78:78-93

- Gonzales L. *Deep Survival: Who Lives, Who Dies and Why*. New York, NY: WW Norton; 2003.
- Gonzales L. *Everyday Survival: Why Smart People Make Dumb Mistakes*. New York, NY: WW Norton; 2008.
- Goleman D. Leadership That Gets Results. Harvard Business Review. March-April. 2000.
- Grantcharov T, Reznick R.TEACHING ROUNDS: Teaching procedural skills. *BMJ* 2008;336:1129-31.
- Greenberg CC, Regenbogen SE, Studdert DM, Lipsitz SR, Rogers SO, Zinner MJ, Gawande AA. Patterns of Communication Breakdowns Resulting in Injury to Surgical Patients. J Am Coll Surg 2007;204: 533–540.
- Greenfield KR, Palmer RR (ed) Army Ground Forces Study No 1. Ch II Administration of training under GHQ –p23 in The Army Ground Forces - ORIGINS OF THE ARMY GROUND FORCES: GENERAL HEADQUARTERS U.S. ARMY, 1940-1942 Study No. 1 Historical Section   •   Army Ground Forces. 1946 http://www.history.army.mil/books/agf/AGF001/ch02.htm ; http://www.history.army.mil/books/agf/AGF001/index.htm#Contents (assessed nov 8 2016)
- *Grunberg, N. E., Barry, E. S., Callahan, C. W., Kleber, H. G., McManigle, J. E., & Schoomaker, E. B. (2019). A conceptual framework for leader and leadership education and development. International Journal of Leadership in Education, 22(5), 644-650. https://doi.org/10.1080/13603124.2018.1492026*
- Grossman D. *On Combat: the psychology and physiology of deadly conflict in war and in peace*. US. Warrior Science Publications; 2008.
- Harrison TL, Shipstead Z, Hicks KL, Hambrick DZ, Redick TS, and EngleRW. Working Memory Training May Increase Working Memory Capacity but Not Fluid Intelligence. Psychological Science 24(12) 2409–2419.
- Harvard Business Review: On Leadership (Vol 2). Harvard Business School Publishing Cooperation, 2020
- Hassan I, Weyers P, Maschuw K, et al. Negative stress-coping strategies among novices in surgery correlate with poor virtual laparoscopic performance. *Br J Surg*. 2006;93(12):1554–1559.
- Hastie R, Dawes RM. *Rational Choice in an Uncertain World, the Psychology of Judgment and Decision Making*. Thousand Oaks, CA: Sage Publications; 2001.
- Hayward RA, Hofer TP. Estimating hospital deaths due to medical errors: preventability is in the eye of the reviewer. *JAMA*. 2001;286(4):415-420.
- Healey AN[1], Primus CP, Koutantji M. Quantifying distraction and interruption in urological surgery. Qual Saf Health Care. 2007 Apr;16(2):135-9.
- Healey AN, Sevdalis N, Vincent CA. Measuring intra-operative interference from distraction and interruption observed in the operating theatre. *Ergonomics*.2006;49:589–604.
- Helmreich RL, Schaefer HG; Team performance in the operating room. In: Bogner MS ed. *Human Error in Medicine*. Hillside, NJ: Lawrence Erlbaum; 1994.
- Helmreich RL, Merritt AC. *Culture at Work in Aviation and Medicine*. Aldershot, UK: Ashgate Press; 1998.
- Helmreich RL, Ashleigh CM, Wilhelm JA. Evolution of CRM training in commercial aviation. *Int J Aviati Psychol*. 1999;9(1):19-32.
- Helmreich RL. On error management: lessons from aviation *BMJ* 2000;320:781-785.
- Henrickson SE, Wadhera RK, El Bardissi AW, Wiegmann DA, Sundt TM. Development and pilot evaluation of a preoperative briefing protocol for cardiovascular surgery. *J Am Coll Surg*. 2009;208:1115-1123.
- Hermann CF. Some consequences of crisis which limit the viability of organizations. *Admin Sci Q*. 1963;8(1):61-62.
- Higgins RSD, Mathews JB, Rosengart TK, Wong SL. Surgical Chairs Playbook. ACS. 2023.
- Hoffman DD. *Visual Intelligence: How We Create What We See*. New York, NY: WW Norton and Co.; 1998.
- Hogarth RM. *Educating Intuition*. Chicago, IL: University Chicago Press; 2001.
- Howell AM, Panesar SS, Burns EM, Donaldson LJ, Darzi A. Reducing the Burden of Surgical Harm. A Systematic Review of the Interventions Used to Reduce Adverse Events in Surgery. AnnSurg 2014;259:630–641.
- Horn JL. Age differences in fluid and crystallized intelligence. Acta Psychologica. 1967;26:107–129.
- Hu YY, Henrickson Parker S, Lipsitz SR, Arriga AF, Peyre SE, Corso KA, Roth EM, Yule SJ, Greenberg CC. surgeon's leadership styles and team behavior in the Operating room. JACS 2016. 22(1):41-51.
- Hughes AM, Gregory ME, Joseph DL, Sonesh SC, Marlow SL, Lacerenza CN, Benishek LE, King HB, Salas E. Saving lives: A meta-analysis of team training in healthcare. J Appl Psychol. 2016; DOI: 10.1037/apl0000120 online first publication, June 16, 2016. http://dx.DOI.org/10.1037/apl0000120 accessed July 18 2016.
- Hughes, Daniel J. (ed.) *Moltke on the Art of War: selected writings*. (1993). Presidio Press: New York, New York. p. 45, 92.
- Hunt B, Wall V, LaPorta AJ, Rush R, Moloff A, Schoeff JE, Tieman M, Lea M. New methods of early surgical training using the human worn partial task surgical simulator in scenario based stress immersion training. *MEdSim Magazine*. 2012;4(3):25-28. http://issuu.com/halldale/docs/medsim_3_2012. Accessed August 16, 2013.
- IAFC. Crew resource management: a positive change for the fire service. Fairfax, VA: International Association of Fire Chiefs. http://www.iafc.org/files/1SAFEhealthSHS/pubs_CRMmanual.pdf. Accessed February 18, 2013.
- IBM. IBM 2010 Global CEO Study: Creativity Selected as Most Crucial Factor for Future Success-Fewer than half of CEOs Successfully Handling Growing Complexity; Diverging priorities in Asia, North America, and Europe. IBM Newsroom. May 18 2010 https://www-03.ibm.com/press/us/en/pressrelease/31670.wss
- Institute of Medicine, Committee on Quality Health Care in America. Crossing the Quality Chasm: A new health system for the 21st century. Committee on quality of health care in America. Washington, D.C.: National Academies Press; 2001.

- Jaeggi SM, Buschkuehl M, Jonides J, Perrig WJ. Improving fluid intelligence with training on working memory. Proc Natl Acad Sci USA 2008; 105(19):6829-6833.
- Jenkins M. Panic. There's a backcountry killer on the loose. *Backpacker*. December 2007;35(254:9):60-119.
- Jones, D. G., & Endsley, M. R. (1996). Sources of situation awareness errors in aviation. <u>Aviation, Space and Environmental Medicine, 67</u>(6), 507–512.
- Joseph B, Pandit V, Hadeed G, Kulvatunyou N, Zangbar B, Tang A, O'Keeffe T, Wynne, J, Green D, Friese R S, Rhee P. Unveiling posttraumatic stress disorder in trauma surgeons: A national survey. Journal of Trauma and Acute Care Surgery 2014;77:148-154.
- Kahneman D. *Thinking Fast and Slow*. New York, NY: Farrar, Straus and Giroux; 2011.
- Kahneman D, Tversky A. Prospect Theory:An analysis of Decision under Risk. Econometrica 1979;47(2):263-292.
- Kahneman D, Tversky A. Judgment under uncertainty: Heuristics and Biases. Science 1974;185:1124-1131.
- Kissable-lee NA, Yule S, Pozner CN, Smink DS. Attending surgeons' leadership style in the operating room: comparing junior residents' experiences and preferences. JSE 2016. 73(1):40-44.
- Klein G. The sources of power, how people make decisions. Cambridge: MIT Press, 1999.
- Klein G. Naturalistic Decision Making. Human Factors: The Journal of the Human Factors and Ergonomics Society. 2008;50(3):456-460.
- Klein G, Pliske R, Crandall B, Woods DD. Problem Detection. Cogn Tech Work. 2005;7:14-28.
- Klingensmith ME. Presidential Address: Leadership and followership in surgical education. Am Journal of Surgery. 2017.213(2):207-213.
- Kohn LT, Corrigan JM, Donaldson Ms, eds. To Err is Human: building a safer health system. Washington DC. National Academy press; 1999.
- Kolditz TA. *In Extremis Leadership: Leading As If Your Life Depended On It.* San Francisco, CA: Jossey-Bass; 2007.
- Kumar MM, Fish KJ. Anaesthesia crisis resource management training: an intimidating concept, a rewarding experience. *Can J Anaesth*. 1996;43:430-434.
- Lancaster LC, Stillman D: When Generations Collide: Who They Are. Why They Clash. How to Solve the Generational Puzzle at Work. New York, NY, HarperCollins Publishers, 2003
- Landers R. Reducing Surgical Errors: Implementing a Three-Hinge Approach to Success. AORN JOURNAL 2015; 101(6):657–665.
- LaPorte, TR, Consolini, PM. Working in Practice but not in theory: theoretical challenges of "high reliability organizations'. Journal of Public administration research and theory: J-PART 1991 1(1)19-48.
- La Porte, Todd R. "High reliability organizations: Unlikely, demanding and at risk." Journal of contingencies and crisis management 4, no. 2 (1996): 60-71.
- Latorella KA. Investigating interruptions: an example from the flightdeck. *Hum Fac Erg Soc P.* 1996;40:249–253.
- Lee L, Berger DH, Awad SS, Brandt ML, Martinez G, Brunicardi FC. Conflict resolution: practical principles for surgeons. World J Surgery.2008;32(11):2331-2335.
- Lipshitz R, Shaul OB. *Schemata and mental models in recognition-primed decision making.* In Zsambok, C. E. & Klein, G., Naturalistic Decision Making. Mahwah. NJ. Lawrence Erlbaum Associates, 1997. 293-304.
- Lipshy KA Crisis Management Leadership In The Operating Room: Prepare your team to survive any crisis. 2013 Creative Team Publishing. San Diego CA.
- Lipshy KA. Britt LD. How do we improve patient safety? A look at the issues and an interview with Dr. Britt. Bull Am Coll Surg. 2017 Feb;102(2):22-29.
- **Lipshy KA**. Invited response to Paull et al, errors upstream and downstream to the universal protocol associated with wrong surgery events. Am J Surg. 2016 Apr;211(4):827-9. doi: 10.1016/j.amjsurg.2015.07.035. Epub 2016 Feb 23.
- **Lipshy KA**, LaPorta TA. Operating Room Crisis Management Leadership Training: Guidance for surgical team education. Bulletin Amer Coll Surg 2013;98(9):24-33.
- **Lipshy KA,** Feinleib J, Trainer B; Abbreviated in-situ inter-professional debriefing simulation training in peri-operative care environments: Minimizing the impact on clinical care using standardized videos. Perioperative Care and Operating Room Management. 2024 (Dec),37:100435
- Lobas JG. leadership in academic medicine: capabilities and conditions for organizational success. Am J Med. 2006;119(7):617-621.
- Luttrel, Marcus *Lone Survivor: The Eyewitness Account of Operation Redwing and the Lost Heroes of SEAL Team 10* (June 2006) Little, Brown and Company Hatchette Book group New York New York
- Makary MA, Sexton JB, Freischlag JA, et al. Operating room teamwork among physicians and nurses: teamwork in the eye of the beholder. *J Am Coll Surg.* 2006;202:746-752.
- Makary M, Daniel M. Medical error—The Third leading cause of death in the US. *BMJ* 2016;353 (Published 3 May 2016)
- Mazzocco K, Petitti DB, Fong KT, Bonacum D, Brookey J, Graham S, Lasky RE, Sexton JB, Thomas EJ. Surgical Team Behaviors and Patient Outcomes. *Am Jnl Surgery*. 2009; 197:678-685
- McDonald JS, Peterson S. Lethal errors in anesthesiology. *Anesthesiology*. 1985;63:A497.

- McElroy LM, Macapagal KR, Collins KM, Abecassis MM, Holl JL, Ladner DP, Gordon EG, Clinician perceptions of operating room to intensive care unit handoffs and implications for patient safety: a qualitative study. Am Journal Surgery 2015;210(4):629–635
- McGreevy JM, Otten TD. Briefing and debriefing in the operating room using fighter pilot crew resource management. *J Am Coll Surg.* 2007;205(1):169-176.
- Mlodinow L. Subliminal: How your unconscious minds rules your behavior. Vintage. Random House. NY NY. 2012.
- Molina G, Jiang W, Edmondson L, Gibbons L, Huang LC, Kiang MV, Haynes AB, **Gawande AA**, **Berry WR**, **Singer SJ**. Implementation of the Surgical Safety Checklist in South Carolina Hospitals Is Associated with Improvement in Perceived Perioperative Safety. Journal of the American College of Surgeons 2016;222(5):725–736.
- Moorthy K, Munz Y, Dosis A, Bann S, Darzi A. The effect of stress-inducing conditions on the performance of a laparoscopic task. *Surg Endosc.* 2003;17(9):1481–1484.
- Morrison M. Teamworks: Transforming Health Care's Error-Prone culture. Creative Team Publishing. San Diego CA. 2013.
- Nakhleh RE. Error reduction in surgical pathology. Arch Pathol Lab Med. 2006;130(5):630-632.
- Neily J, Mills PD, Eldridge N, Dunn EJ, Samples C, Turner JR, Revere A, DePalma RG, Bagian JP. Incorrect surgical procedures within and outside of the operating room. **Arch Surg.** 2009;144(11):1028-1034. (Veterans Affairs)
- Neily J, Mills PD, Eldridge N, Carney BT, Pepper D, Turner JR, Young-Xu Y, Gunnar W, Bagian JP. Incorrect surgical procedures within and outside of the operating room a follow up report. *JAMA Surg. 2011;146(11):1235-1239.*
- Neily J, Mills PD, Young-Xu Y, Carney BT, West P, Berger DH,et al. Association between implementation of a medical team, training program and surgical mortality. JAMA 2010; 304:1693-700.
- Nicksa G, Anderson C, Fidler R, Stewart L. Innovative Approach Using Interprofessional Simulation to Educate Surgical Residents in Technical and Nontechnical Skills in High-Risk Clinical Scenarios. *JAMA Surg.* 2015;150(3):201-207.
- **Nixon PG** . The human function curve - a paradigm for our times.Act Nerv Super (Praha). 1982;Suppl 3(Pt 1):130-3.PMID: 7183056
- **Nixon PG.** The human function curve. With special reference to cardiovascular disorders: part I. Practitioner. 1976 Nov;217(1301):765-70.PMID: 995833 No abstract available.
- **Nixon PG.** The human function curve. With special reference to cardiovascular disorders: part II. Practitioner. 1976 Dec;217(1302):935-44.PMID: 796840 Review. No abstract available.
- **Nixon PG.** Stress and the cardiovascular system. Practitioner. 1982 Sep;226(1371):1589-98.PMID: 6890677 No abstract available.
- Northouse PG. Leadership: Theory and practice. 6th ed. Los Angeles. Sage. 2013.
- NTSB: Loss of Control on Approach Colgan Air, Inc. Operating as Continental Connection Flight 3407 Bombardier DHC-8-400, N200WQ Clarence Center, New York http://www.ntsb.gov/investigations/AccidentReports/Reports/AAR1001.pdf#page=176
- NTSB: http://www.ntsb.gov/news/events/Pages/Loss_of_Control_and_Impact_with_Pacific_Ocean_Alaska_Airlines_Flight_261_McDonnell_Douglas_MD-83_N963AS_about_2.7_miles_no.aspx
- Nurok M, Czeisler CA, Lehmann S. Sleep Deprivation, Elective Surgical Procedures, and Informed Consent. N Engl J Med 2010; 363:2577-2579.
- Okray R, Lubnau T. *Crew Resource Management for the Fire Service*. Tulsa, OK: PennWell Press; 2004.
- Paul DE, Mazzia LM, Neily J, Mills PD, Turner JR, Gunnar W, Hemphill R. Errors upstream and downstream to the universal protocol associated with wrong surgery events in the Veterans Health Administration. Am Jnl Surg 2015;210(1):6-13.
- Pauley K, Flin R, Yule S, Youngson G. Surgeon's intraoperative decision making and risk management. *Am J Surg.* 2011;202(4):375-381.
- Pearce CL, Hoch JE, Jeppesen HJ, Wegge J. New forms of management. J Personnel Psychol 2010;9:151–3.
- Pearce CL, Sims HP. Vertical versus shared leadership as predictors of the effectiveness of change management teams: an examination of aversive, directive, transactional, transformational, and empowering leader behaviours. Group Dyn: Theory Res Pract 2002;6:172–97.
- Perrow, C. Normal Accidents: Living with high risk technologies. Princeton University Press. Princeton NJ 1999.
- Peterson M. The ambiguity of mental images: insights regarding the structure of shape memory and its function in creativity. In: Russkos-Ewoldson B, Intens-Peterson MJ, Anderson RE eds. *Imagery, Creativity, and Discovery: A Cognitive Perspective*. Amsterdam, AN: Elsevier Sceince Publishers B.V.; 1993.
- Phitayakorn R, Minehart RD, Hemingway MW, Pian-Smith MC, Petrusa E. Relationship between physiologic and psychological measures of autonomic activation in operating room teams during a simulated airway emergency. *Am J Surg.* 2015;209(1):86-92.
- Pizzi L, Goldfarb NI, Nash DB, Crew resource management and its applications in medicine. In: Shojania KG, Duncan BW, McDonald KM, Wachter RM, Markowitz AJ eds. *Making Health Care Safer: A Critical Analysis of Patient Safety Practices: Evidence Reports/ Technology Assessments, No. 43.* Rockville, MD: Agency for Healthcare Research and Quality; 2001. http://www.ncbi.nlm.nih.gov/books/NBK26999. Accessed December 12, 2012.
- Pollack H. Doctors, military officers, firefighters and scientists seen as among America's most prestigious occupations: Yet engineering is what the highest percentage of adults would encourage a child to pursue *The Harris Poll*September 10, 2014.

http://www.theharrispoll.com/politics/Doctors__Military_Officers__Firefighters__and_Scientists_Seen_as_Among_America_s_Most_Prestigious_Occupations.html accessed 110516

- Pronovost P. Intensive care unit safety reporting system (ICUSRS). Reported in: *Safety and Medicine*. http://ocw.jhsph.edu/courses/patientsafety/PDFs/PS_lec4_Pronovost.pdf. Accessed February 12, 2013.
- Pugh CM, DaRosa DA, Bell RH. Residents' self-reported learning needs for intraoperative knowledge: are we missing the bar? Am Journal Surgery, 2010;199(4):562-565.
- Pugh CM, Elaine R Cohen 2, Calvin Kwan 2, Janice A Cannon-Bowers 3 A comparative assessment and gap analysis of commonly used team rating scales 2014 Aug;190(2):445-50. doi: 10.1016/j.jss.2014.04.034. Epub 2014 Apr 28.
- **Pugh CM**, Law KE, Cohen ER, D'Angelo AD, Greenberg JA, Greenberg CC, Wiegmann DA. Use of **error management** theory to quantify and characterize residents' **error** recovery strategies. Am J Surg. 2020 Feb;219(2):214-220. doi: 10.1016/j.amjsurg.2019.11.013. Epub 2019 Nov 19.PMID: 31806167
- (Pugh) Law KE, Ray RD, D'Angelo AD, Cohen ER, DiMarco SM, Linsmeier E, Wiegmann DA, **Pugh CM.**J Surg Educ. Exploring Senior Residents' Intraoperative **Error Management** Strategies: A Potential Measure of Performance Improvement. 2016 Nov-Dec;73(6):e64-e70. doi: 10.1016/j.jsurg.2016.05.016. Epub 2016 Jun 29.PMID: 27372272
- (Pugh) D'Angelo AL, Cohen ER, Kwan C, Laufer S, Greenberg C, Greenberg J, Wiegmann D, **Pugh CM.** Use of decision-based simulations to assess resident readiness for operative independence. Am J Surg. 2015 Jan;209(1):132-9. doi: 10.1016/j.amjsurg.2014.10.002. Epub 2014 Oct 22.PMID: 25454962
- Rao A, Tait I, Alijani A. Systematic review and meta-analysis of the role of mental training in the acquisition of technical skills in surgery. Am Journal Surg 2015;210(3):545-553
- Rasmussen, Jens (May–June 1983). "Skills, rules, and knowledge; signals, signs, and symbols, and other distinctions in human performance models". IEEE Transactions on Systems, Man, and Cybernetics. SMC-131983 (3): 257–266. doi:10.1109/TSMC.1983.6313160. S2CID 1525146 – via IEEE Xplore.
- Rath T, Conchie B. Strengths based leadership: great leaders, teams and why people follow. New York, NY; Gallup Press. 2008
- Reason J. *Human error*. New York, NY: Cambridge University Press; 1990.
- Reason J. Understanding adverse events: human factors. *Qual Health Care*. June 1995;4(2):80-89.
- Reason J. *Managing the Risks of Organizational Accidents*. Burlington, VT: Ashgate; 1997.
- Ripley A. *The Unthinkable: Who Survives When Disaster Strikes and Why*. New York, NY: Three Rivers Press; 2000.
- Rochlin GI, LaPorte TR, and Roberts KH. 'The Self-Designing High-Reliability Organization: Aircraft Carrier Flight Operations at Sea', Naval War College Review, 1987 40(4):76–90.
- Rochlin, GI. How to hunt a very reliable organization. Journal of contingendcies and crisis management. 2011. 19(1): 14-20.
- Roehrs T; Burduvali E; Bonahoom A et al. Ethanol and sleep loss: a "dose" comparison of impairing effects. *Sleep* 2003;26(8):981-5.
- Rouse, W. B., Cannon-Bowers, J. A., & Salas, E. (1992). The role of mental models in team performance in complex systems. IEEE Transactions on Systems, Man, & Cybernetics, 22(6), 1296–1308. https://doi.org/10.1109/21.199457)
- Rowland PA, Lang NP. Communication & Professionalism Competencies: A Guide for Surgeons. Ciné-Med, Woodbury, CT2007.
- Runciman WB, Webb RK, Klepper ID, Lee R, Williamson JA, Barker L. The Australian incident monitoring study: crisis management: validation of an algorithm by analysis of 2000 incident reports. *Anaesthia Intensive Care*. 1993;21:579-592
- Runciman WB, Merry AF. Crises in clinical care: an approach to management. *Qual Saf Health Care*. 2005;14(3):156-163.
- Russ SJ, Sevdalis N, Moorthy K, Mayer EK, Rout S, Caris J, Mansell J, Davies R, Vincent C, Darzi A. A qualitative evaluation of the barriers and facilitators toward implementation of the WHO surgical safety checklist across hospitals in England: lessons from the "Surgical Checklist Implementation Project". Ann Surg. 2015 Jan;261(1):81-91
- Salas E, Wilson KA, Murphy CE, King H, Baker D. What crew resource management training will not do for patient safety: unless…?. *J Patient Saf*. 2007;3(2):1-3.
- Sami A, Waseem H, Nourah A, Areej A, Afnan A, Ghadeer A,[1] Abdulaziz A, and Arthur A.Real time observations of stressful events in the operating room. Saudi J Anaesth. 2012; 6(2):136–139.
- Savoldelli GL, Thieblemont J, Clergue F, et al. Incidence and impact of distracting events during induction of general anaesthesia for urgent surgical cases. *Eur J Anaesthesiol*. 2010;27:683–689.
- Schulman, Paul R. "Problems in the organization of organization theory: an essay in honour of Todd LaPorte." Journal of contingencies and crisis management 19, no. 1 (2011): 43-50.
- Scoggins CR, Pollock RE, Pawlik TM. Surgical Mentorship and leadership: Building for success in Academic Surgery. Springer.2018.
- Seeger MW, Sellnow TL, Ulmer RR. Communication, organization, and crisis. In: Rolff ME, ed. *Communication Yearbook*. Vol 21. Lexington, KY: U of Kentucky; 1998:231–275.
- Serfaty D, Entin E, J Johnston J. *Team coordination training* in Cannon-Bowers J and Salas E. Making Decisions Under Stress APA 1998. P 222.
- Sevdalis N, Davis R, Koutantji M, et al. Reliability of a revised NOTECHS scale for use in surgical teams. *Am J Surg*. 2008;196:184-190.
- Sevdalis N, Undre S, McDermott J, Giddie J, Diner L, Smith G. Impact of Intraoperative Distractions on Patient Safety: A Prospective Descriptive Study Using Validated Instruments. World J Surg (2014) 38:751-758.

- Sevdalis N[1], Forrest D, Undre S, Darzi A, Vincent C. Annoyances, disruptions, and interruptions in surgery: the Disruptions in Surgery Index (DiSI). World J Surg. 2008 Aug;32(8):1643-50.
- Sevdalis N, Healey AN, Vincent CA. Distracting communications in the operating theatre. *J Eval Clin Pract*. 2007;13:390–394.
- Sexton JB, Thomas EJ, Helmreich RL. Error, stress, and teamwork in medicine and aviation: cross sectional surveys. *BMJ*. March 2000;320(7237): 745–749.
- Shanafelt TD, Balch CM, Bechamps G, et al. Burnout and medical errors among American surgeons. *Ann Surg*. 2010;251(6):995-1000.
- Sharps MJ. *Processing Under Pressure: Stress, Memory and Decision-Making in Law Enforcement*. Flushing, NY: Looseleaf Law Publications; 2010
- Shipper ES, Hardaway JC. Garvey EM, Logghe H. Talking through time: trends in communication and the evolving patient-physician relationship. Bulletin ACS. 2016;101(8):19-23.
- Siddle B. *Sharpening the Warriors Edge: The Psychology and Science of Training*. 10th ed. Belleville, IL: PPCT Research publications; 2008.
- Siebert A. The survivors personality. Penguin. New York NY. 2010.
- Simone JV. Leadership lessons from Machiavelli that are not "Machiavellian". Simone's OncOpinion. Oncology Times Oct 25 2015
- Simons D, Chabris C. Gorillas in our midst: sustained inattentional blindness for dynamic events. *Perception*. 1999;28(9):1059-1074.
- Sincero SM. How does Stress Affect Performance? Feb 2012. Retrieved Mar 07, 2015 from Explorable.com: https://explorable.com/how-does-stress-affect-performance (Refernce to P Nixon)
- Spath PL. Reducing errors through work systems improvement. In: Spath PL, ed. *Error Reduction in Health Care*. San Francisco, Calif: Jossey-Bass Publisher and Chicago, Ill: AHA Press; 1999:199–234.
- Steinemann S, Berg B, Skinner A, DiTulio A, Anzelon K, Terada K, Oliver C, Ho HC, Speck C. In Situ, Multidisciplinary, Simulation-Based Teamwork Training Improves Early Trauma Care. *J. Surg Ed* 2011;68(6): 472-477.
- Stevenson J. Survive anywhere. *Backpacker*. October 2006;34(244:8):39-43.
- Sutcliffe KM, Lewton E, Rosenthal MM. Communication failures: an insidious contributor to medical mishaps. Acad Med. 2004 Feb;79(2):186-94
- Sweeney PJ, Matthews MD, Lester PB. *Leadership in Dangerous Situations*. Annapolis, MD: Naval Institute Press; 2011.
- Tan SY. http://www.acssurgerynews.com/opinions/single-view/auto-accidents-in-sleepy-medical-trainees/df2feb72ed99e926cdbb76f3d9c12d4b.html
- Ten Cate O. Entrustment as assessment: recognizing the ability, the right and the duty to act. Journal of graduate medical education. 2016;8(2):261-262.
- The survival list: 101 skills guaranteed to get you out of trouble fast. Backpacker Oct 2006;34(244:8):45-53.
- Thomas EJ, Sexton JB, Helmreich RL. Discrepant attitudes about teamwork among critical care nurses and physicians. *Crit Care Med*. 2003;31(3):956–959.
- Thompson CV, Naumann DN, Fellows JL, Bowley DM, Suggett N. Post-traumatic stress disorder amongst surgical trainees: An unrecognised risk? Surgeon. 2015 Oct 23. pii: S1479-666X(15)00099-2. doi: 10.1016/j.surge.2015.09.002.
- Tsafrir Z, Korianski J, Almog B, Many A, Wiesel O, Levin I. Effects of Fatigue on Residents' Performance in Laparoscopy Jnl Am Col Surg 2015; 221(2):564-570
- USCG. Crew resource management refresher. United States Coast Guard. 2002. http://www.uscg.mil/safety/docs/PPTs/CRM_Refresher2002.ppt. Accessed February 2, 2013.
- Venette SJ. *Risk Communication in a High Reliability Organization: APHIS PPQ's Inclusion of Risk in Decision Making*. Ann Arbor, MI: UMI Proquest Information and Learning; 2003.
- Vincent C, Moorthy K, Sarker SK, Chang A, Darzi AW. Systems approach to surgical quality and safety. *Ann Surg*. 2004;239(4):475-482.
- Vincent C. *Patient safety*. Chichester, UK: Wiley-Blackwell; 2010.
- Wachs SR. Put Conflict Resolution Skills to Work. J Oncol Pract. 2008; 4(1): 37–40. http://europepmc.org/articles/PMC2793934
- Wallace JE, Lemaire JB, Ghali WA. Physician wellness: a missing quality indicator. Lancet. 2009 Nov 14;374(9702):1714-21.
- Way LW, Stewart L, Gantert W, et al. Causes and prevention of laparoscopic bile duct injuries: analysis of 252 cases from a human factors and cognitive psychological approach. *Ann Surg*. 2003;237(4):460-469.
- Webb RK, Currie M, Morgan CA, et al. The Australian incident monitoring study: an analysis of 2000 incident reports. *Anaesthia and Intensive Care*. 1993;21:520-528.
- Weeks D: The Eight Essential Steps to Conflict Resolution: Preserving Relationships at Work, at Home, and in the Community. New York, NY, Tarcher/Putnam, 1994
- Weller, Boyd. Making a Difference Through Improving Teamwork in the Operating Room: A Systematic Review of the Evidence on What Works; Patient Safety in Anesthesia. 4:77–83, (2014);
- Weick KE, Sutcliffe KM. Managing the unexpected: resilient performance in an age of uncertainty. San Francisco CA: John Wiley; 2007.
- Weick KE. Sensemaking in organizations. Sage. Thousand Oaks. 1995.
- Weick KE. Small wins: redefining the scale of social problems. Am Psy. 1984. 39(1):40-49.

- West CP[1], Tan AD, Shanafelt TD. Association of resident fatigue and distress with occupational blood. Mayo Clin Proc. 2012 Dec;87(12):1138-44

- Wheelock A, SulimanA, Wharton R, Babu E, Hull L, Vincent C, Sevdalis N, Arora S. The Impact of Operating Room Distractions on Stress, Workload, and Teamwork. Ann Surg 2015; 261(6):1079–1084.

- Wiegmann DA, El Bardissi AW, Dearani JA, Daly RC, Sundt TM Disruptions in surgical flow and their relationship to surgical errors: an exploratory investigation. *Surgery.* 2007;142(5):658-665.

- Wiggins-Dohlvik K, Stewart RM, Babbitt RJ, Gelfond J, Zarzabal LA, Willis RE. Surgeons' performance during critical situations: competence, confidence, and composure. *Am J Surg*. 2009;198(6):817-823.

- Williams ES, Manwell LB, Konrad TR, Linzer M. The relationship of organizational culture, stress, satisfaction, and burnout with physician-reported error and suboptimal patient care: results from the MEMO study. Health Care Manage Rev. 2007 Jul-Sep;32(3):203-12.

- Williams RG[1], Silverman R, Schwind C, Fortune JB, Sutyak J, Horvath KD, Van Eaton EG, Azzie G, Potts JR 3rd, Boehler M, Dunnington GL. Surgeon information transfer and communication: factors affecting quality and efficiency of inpatient care. Ann Surg. 2007 Feb;245(2):159-69.

- Willink J, Babin Leif. Extreme Ownership: how U.S. Navy SEALS Lead and Win. St. Martin's Press. NY NY 2015.

- Woods, D. D., Dekker, S., Cook, R., & Johannesen, L. (2010). *Behind Human Error.* Burlington: Ashgate.

- Zenati MA, Maron JK. Communication and Teamwork Failure as a Barrier to Robotic Surgical Safety Proceedings of the Third Computer and Robotic Assisted Surgery (CRAS) Workshop. 2013.

- Ziewacz JE, Arriaga AF, Bader AM, et al. Crisis checklists for the operating room: development and pilot testing. *J Am Coll Surg.* 2011;213(2):212-217.

- Zilbert NR, Murnaghan L, Gallinger S, Regehr G, Moulton C. Taking a chance or playing it safe: reframing risk assessment within the surgeon's comfort zone. Ann Surg. 2015; 262(2):253-259.

- Zheng B, Martinez DV, Cassera MA, et al. A quantitative study of disruption in the operating room during laparoscopic antireflux surgery. *Surg Endosc.*2008;22:2171.

- Zhuravsky L Crisis Leadership in an Acute Clinical Setting Christchurch Hospital New Zealand ICU Experience Following the February 2011 Earthquake. *Prehosp Disaster Med*. 2015;30:1-6.

ACKNOWLEDGEMENTS:
I am eternally grateful to –
- Katherine Lipshy, My beautiful wife for her endless patience with my obsession with this guide for survival, for the past two decades
- Bradley Lipshy, for his additional drawings including the Logo for CrisisManagementLeadership
- Jarrod Lipshy, for his editing of the original and subsequent publications.
- Genesis Lipshy, for her words of wisdom, photography and Modeling skills.
- Finally to Glen Aubrey of creative team publishing for his words of wisdom and mentorship in writing, and patience in managing me, may you meet the historical figures you met in your research, in your new resting place.

In addition, I am in gratitude for the individuals listed below for their informative and encouraging conversations, phone calls, and emails leading me in the right direction during the continual revisions of this book. I am grateful for those who provided me permission to use this invaluable material in the book.

1. Benjamin Aaron, MD Chief Thoracic Surgery George Washington University Hospital 1981. (Nov 2016)
2. Jonathan S Abelson, M.D. Lahey Hospital; Past AHRQ Clinical Research Fellow Department of Surgery New York Presbyterian Hospital Weill Cornell Medical Center (Sept 2015)
3. Sonal Arora; Clinical Lecturer - Imperial College London;(Permission 2013
4. Darren M Ashcroft (& Diane Parker) BPharm MSc Ph.D., Professor of Pharmacoepidemiology, School of Pharmacy & Pharmaceutical Sciences, University of Manchester. Permission 2013
5. James William Bailey, Commander US Navy (RET) POW Vietnam 1967-1973; Former staff officer in the Office of the Chief of Naval Operations in the Pentagon. Executive Officer of the Naval ROTC unit -University of North Carolina. (May 2016)
6. Charles M. Balch, M.D., F.A.C.S.Professor of Surgery and Oncology and Dermatology Deputy Director, Johns Hopkins Institute for Clinical and Translational Research (Permission 2013)
7. John D Banja, PhD Emory University Professor Rehabilitation medicine, Medical Ethicist. The Normalization of deviance in Healthcare. (Jan 2015)
8. **Nancy Baxter, MD Deputy Dean (Research Centres) Faculty of Medicine and Health University of Sydney.** Professor of Surgery in the Department of Surgery and the Institute of Health Policy, Management and Evaluation at the University of Toronto. She is an affiliate scientist with the Li Ka Shing Knowledge Institute at St. Michael's Hospital and a Senior Adjunct Scientist in the Cancer Theme Group with the Institute for Clinical Evaluative Sciences.
9. Meredith Bell- http://www.strongforperformance.com/ "help people become stronger for work and life."
10. R. Berguer; Department of Surgery, University of California Davis, Sacramento, California and Surgical Service at Contra Costa Regional Medical Center, Martinez, California 94553, USA. (Permission 2013)
11. William Berry, MD, MPH, MPA, FACS Strategic Advisor to the Chief Medical Officer and as Co-Founder of Ariadne Labs. Chief Implementation Officer, Boston Project Director of the WHO Safe Surgery Saves Lives Program.
12. Lt Bethea, Hampton Sheriff Dept. (June 2015)
13. Bowermaster R, Eghtesady P, et al Application of the aviation black box principle.
14. Charles L Bosk. Author of *Forgive and Remember: Managing Medical Failure.* 2nd ed. Chicago, IL: University of Chicago Press; 2003
15. LD Britt, MD, FACS Chair Dept Surgery Eastern Virginia Medical School, Past President of the ACS, Member of Joint commission. (July 2016).
16. CAPT Frank K. Butler, Jr., MC USN Retired US Navy, diving medical Officer, Director of Biomedical Research for the Naval Special Warfare Command. Platoon commander Navy Underwater Demolition and SEAL (Sea/Air/Land commando) teams. Diving Medical Research Officer, Navy Experimental Diving Unit. Chief of Ophthalmology - Naval Hospital Pensacola. Naval Special Warfare Command. Ophthalmic consultant to the Divers Alert Network. *Chairman, Committee on Tactical Combat Casualty Care, Department of Defense, Joint Trauma Systems* (Feb 2015).
17. James Forrest Calland, MD, Prof Surgery UVA; Trauma/Team STEPPS. (Feb 2014).
18. Lt Gen Paul Carlton Jr. USAF Retired.
19. Raphael Chung, MD, MBA, FACS (Permission 2013)
20. Izack Cohen Industrial Engineering and Management, Technion-Israel Institute of Technology, Haifa, Israel 32000Cohen I. Improving time-critical decision making in life-threatening situations: observations and insights. *Decision Analysis.* 2008;5(2):100-110.
21. Conchie B. Rath T, Strengths based leadership: great leaders, teams and why people follow. New York, NY; Gallup Press. 2008
22. David Tom Cooke, MD, FACS, MAMSE, Professor and Founding Chief, Division of General Thoracic Surgery, Vice Chair for Faculty Development & Wellness, Physician-In-Chief, UC Davis Comprehensive Cancer Center, Immediate Past-President, Thoracic Surgery Directors Association
23. Brigetta D. Craft, RN, MSN, DNP, Contract Patient Safety Program Manager/TeamSTEPPS Healthcare Team Training, AFMOA/SGHQ, Lackland AFB, TX
24. Sayra Cristancho Scientist, Schulich Western University, Centre for Education Research & Innovation Associate Professor, Department of Surgery and Faculty of Education Faculty member, Institute for Earth and Space Exploration

25. Pat Croskerry MD, PhD, FRCP(Edin); Professor, Department of Emergency Medicine, Director, Critical Thinking Program, Division of Medical Education, Dalhousie University, Halifax, Nova Scotia, CANADA (June 2015).
26. Mihaly Csikszentmihalyi created the psychological concept of flow, a highly focused mental state. He is the Distinguished Professor of Psychology and Management at Claremont Graduate University. He is the former head of the department of psychology at the University of Chicago (Feb 2015)
27. Teo Forcht Dagi, MD served as a combat neurosurgeon and flight surgeon in the US Army; General Partner, HLM Venture Partners Distinguished Scholar and Professor at the School of Medicine, Dentistry and Biomedical Sciences, Queen's University Belfast, Northern Ireland Visiting Professor, Harvard Medical School (June 2015)
28. Robert F Dees; Major General U.S. Army Retired; Author *Resilient Warriors, Resilient Leaders* and *Resilient Nations*
29. Sidney Dekkar; - Professor in the School of Humanities at Griffith University in Brisbane, Australia; www.SidneyDekkar.com (Permission 2013):
30. Dr. Gene Deisinger, Ph.D. Deputy Chief of Police and Director of Threat Management- Virginia Tech, Blacksburg, Virginia (re VT shootinds April 16 2007 32 victims; July 2013)
31. Andrew Dennis, D.O., FACOS, FACS, DME Chair, Division of Pre Hospital and Emergency Trauma Services, RUSH Medical College; JHS Cook County Hospital Medical Director / Team Surgeon / Police Officer; Cook County Sheriff's Police Department, Emergency Services Bureau Northern Illinois Police Alarm System Emergency Services Team
32. Rorke Denver former head of basic and advanced SEAL training and author of- *DAMN FEW: making the modern day SEAL warrior. 2012. (Apr 2015)*
33. Sharmila Dissanaike MD FACS FCCM Peter C. Canizaro Chair and University Distinguished Professor at Texas Tech University Health Sciences Center in Lubbock, TX
34. Dr. Alan Diehl Ph.D. Research Psychologist and Technical Advisor United States Air Force Operational Test & Evaluation Center 1994 –2004; Senior Research Psychologist / Technical Advisor United States Air Force Inspection & Safety Center 1987 –1994; Program Scientist for Human Performance FAA 1980 –1987; Air Safety Investigator / Human Factors Specialist National Transportation Safety Board 1977 –1980; Author Air Safety Investigators: Using Science to Save Lives -- One Crash at a Time Xlibris April 2013; Silent Knights: Blowing the Whistle on Military Accidents and Their Cover-Ups Brassey's/Potomatic Books April 2002 (Mar 2014)
35. Justin Dimick, MD, FACS (Apr 2016) Chief of the Division of Minimally Invasive Surgery, and Director of the Center for Healthcare Outcomes & Policy at the University of Michigan.
36. Dietrich Dörner emeritus professor for General and Theoretical Psychology at the Institute of Theoretical Psychology at the Otto-Friedrich University in Bamberg, Germany (Permission 2013)
37. Lieutenant Colonel Joe Doty, Ph.D., U.S. Army, Retired; leadership and ethics consultant. Past deputy director of the Center for the Army Profession and Ethic.
38. Gordon Dupont, Aviation Safety Expert, CEO System Safety Services Amy C. Edmondson; Professor of Leadership and Management, HARVARD BUSINESS SCHOOL Author of Building the Future: Big Teaming for Audacious Innovation (Berrett-Koehler, 2016); Teaming: How organizations learn, innovate and compete in the knowledge economy (Jossey-Bass, 2012) (July 2016)
39. Charles Duhigg, Author of "Power of Habit" permission 2025
40. Alexander L. Eastman, MD, MPH, FACS, Lieutenant, & Medical Director Dallas Police Department (SWAT), The Trauma Center at Parkland (UT Southwestern Medical Center)
41. Amy C. Edmondson; Professor of Leadership and Management, HARVARD BUSINESS SCHOOL Author of Building the Future: Big Teaming for Audacious Innovation (Berrett-Koehler, 2016); Teaming: How organizations learn, innovate and compete in the knowledge economy (Jossey-Bass, 2012) (July 2016)
42. Pirooz Eghtesady, MD Chief, Section of Pediatric Cardiothoracic Surgery Cardiothoracic Surgeon-in-Chief, St. Louis Children's Hospital (Jan 2015)
43. Samuel Elfassy Senior Director, Corporate Safety, Environment & Quality at Air Canada. Past Chair of the North York General Foundation Board of Governors. Safety Management Systems in High Risk Environments. (July 2015)
44. Eric Elster, MD, FACS CAPT, MC, USN Professor and ChairmanThe Department of Surgery at Uniformed Services University of the Health Sciences   & the Walter Reed National Military Medical Center
45. Rani Elwy, PhD Adjunct Associate Professor health law, policy & management health psychologist, health services researcher and implementation scientist , investigator at the center for healthcare organization and implementation research (choir), a va health services research and development center of innovation, based at the boston and bedford va medical centers. at choir, health communications research focus area, and spearheaded the "disclosure technical assistance and support program
46. Randall W Engle Professor at School of Psychology at Georgia Institute of Technology found the GSU/GT Center for Advanced Brain Imaging (CABI) on the Georgia Tech campus, Adjunc Professor and Professional Fellow in the Department of Psychology at the University of Edinburgh. editor of Current Directions in Psychological Science past funding by Air Force Office of Scientific Research, and Office of Naval Research. (June 2015)
47. Anashua Rani Ghose Elwy Warren Alpert Foundation Professor of Psychiatry and Human Behavior, Professor of Behavioral and Social Sciences
48. Dr. Mica R. Endsley, PhD, PE, Chief Scientist US Air Force Pentagon

49. Amir Erez Ph.D. Huber Hurst Professor of Management Ph.D. Coordinator Warrington College of Business Administration Department of Management
50. Peter J. Fabri, MD, PhD; Surgeon and PhD in Industrial Engineering at the University of South Florida; currently faculty in Colleges of Engineering and Medicine in the new hybrid discipline of "Health Systems Engineering". (July 2016)
51. **Paula Ferrada, MD, FACS, FCCM, MAMSE** Chair, Department of Surgery – Inova Fairfax Medical Campus Medical Director, Perioperative Services – IFMC System Chief, Trauma and Acute Care Surgery – Inova Health System Professor, University of Virginia School of Medicine
52. Robin L. Feuerbacher, PhD Energy Systems Engineering Program Lead & Assistant Professor Tykeson Endowed Faculty Scholar OSU-Cascades 105A http://www.osucascades.edu/robin-feuerbacher(Permission 2013):
53. Bob Figlock, Ph.D. Navy Post Graduate School; Advanced Survey Design, LLC, Monterey, CA
54. Evie Fioratou University of Aberdeen, Aberdeen, SCT, United Kingdom   (Permission 2013):
55. Jane C.K. Fitch, MD; Past President American Society of Anesthesiologists, Past President Society of Academic Anesthesiology Associations Association of Academic Anesthesiology Chairs; John L. Plewes Professor & Chair Department of Anesthesiology
56. John Flanagan, Ranger' Apprentice Penguin (Permission 2013)
57. Mark Fleming PhD, MSc, MA CN Professor of Safety Culture Associate Professor
58. Rhona Flin; Emeritus Professor of Applied Psychology; University of Aberdeen; King's College, Old Aberdeen
59. Marc Flitter
60. Jill Fredston, "Snowstruck: In the Grip of Avalanches", 2005, Harcourt, New York/ Cindi Squire alaskaavalanche@mac.com; PUBLISHER CORRECTION: Harcourt, New York(Permission 2013):
61. Julie Freischlag, MD CEO and chief academic officer of Atrium Health Wake Forest Baptist, chief academic officer and executive vice president of Advocate Health, and executive vice president of health affairs at Wake Forest University.
62. David M. Gaba, M.D. Professor of Anesthesiology, Perioperative and Pain Medicine Stanford University; Director VA/PA Sim center (Permission 2013)
63. Atul Gawande, MD, MPH General and Endocrine Surgeon, Brigham & Women's Hospital; Professor, Harvard Chan School of Public Health; Samuel O. Thier Professor of Surgery, Harvard Medical School; Director, Ariadne Labs: a joint center for health system innovation; Founder and Chair, Lifebox; Staff Writer, The New Yorker magazine (2013, Aug 2016)
64. Darren P. Gibbs, Colonel, USAF; Chief, Readiness & Emergency Mgt Division (A7CX))
65. Lawrence Gillman, MD Canada. STARTT. Author: Gillman L., Widder S. Trauma Team Dynamics - A Trauma Crisis Resource Management Manual Springer, Switzerland 2016, 2025 (July 2015)
66. Malcolm Gladwell **HBG FAQ/Permissions Jan 2023**
67. Laurence Gonzales, Author 'Deep Survival' 3216 Otto Lane Evanston, IL 60201 www.laurencegonzales.com
68. Samuel Gorovitz ; Professor of Philosophy; former dean of Arts and Sciences, Syracuse University (Permission 2013)
69. Gordon Graham; Graham Research Consultants 6475 East Pacific Coast Highway, Suite 136, Long Beach, CA 90803 http://www.gordongraham.com/about.html (Permission 2013)
70. Caprice C. Greenberg, MD, MPH Chair in Health Services Research Vice Chair of Research, Department of Surgery Director, Wisconsin Surgical Outcomes Research Program
71. Lt. Col Dave Grossman former Ranger, paratrooper and West Point Psychology Staff; Author of *On Killing* and *On Combat*. (Apr 2015)
72. Vernon L. Grose DSc, Chairman; OMEGA SYSTEMS GROUP INCORPORATED; SMART (Systems Methodology Applied to Risk Termination) technique for managing risk. (June 2015)
73. Neil E. Grunberg, Ph.D.Director of Faculty Development, Military and Emergency Medicine Director, Leadership Research & Development Professor, Military and Emergency Medicine, School of Medicine Professor, Neuroscience, School of Medicine Professor, Graduate School of Nursing Uniformed Services University of the Health Sciences 2016 & 2025
74. Bear Grylls
75. Bob Hahn, Associate Director, School of Aviation Safety. Naval Aviation Schools Command
76. Amy L. Halverson Northwestern University Vice Chair of Education, Department of Surgery Professor
77. Robin Hemphill, MD *Chief Quality and Safety Officer Virginia Commonwealth* University *2017- present, Chief Safety and Risk Awareness Officer Director, National Center for Patient Safety 2011-2017*
78. Sarah Henrickson-Parker Assistant Professor, Virginia Tech Carilion Research Institute Assistant Professor of Biomedical Science, Virginia Tech Carilion School of Medicine Director of Human Factors Research, Carilion Clinic Research Assistant Professor of Psychology, College of Science, Virginia Tech (Feb 2016)
79. Jim Holbrook, EdD, at Crafton Hills College EMS program.
80. Robin L. Homolak RN; OR Manager VA Long Beach Medical Center
81. David B. Hoyt, MD, FACS, American College of Surgeons Executive Director (Aug 2016)
82. Joseph Ibrahim Trauma Medical Director, Level I Trauma Center Associate Program Director Orlando Regional Medical Center, (Oct 2016)
83. Institute of Medicine Katharine Bothner Associate Program Officer Deputy Executive Office Institute of Medicine
84. Kamal Itani, MD ACOS Surgery VA Boston
85. Billy Jackson; Detective, retired, Newport News, Virginia, Police Dept. 2016

86. Lenworth Jacobs Dr. Jacobs is the Professor of Surgery and Professor of Traumatology and Emergency Medicine at the University of Connecticut. He is a Trauma Surgeon at Hartford Hospital Director of Emergency Medical Services for the City of Boston and the Trauma Center at Boston City Hospital Chairman of the Hartford Consensus, Joint Committee to Increase Survival from Active Shooter and Intentional Mass Casualty Events (2016)

87. William L Johnson, retired CG Commander (O-5) Ardent Sentry / Vigilant Shield Lead Planner JS J7 Joint Training / Joint Exercise Division 2016

88. Daniel Jones, MS, MD Professor and Benjamin F. Rush, Jr. MD Chair of Surgery Assistant Dean of Simulation, Innovation & Scholarship

89. Seon Jones, MD (Lim book)

90. Richard Karl,Pilot rated to fly Boeing 737's, Captain for JetSuite, Irvine, CA,Founder Surgical Safety institute; Chairman Emeritus · Dept Surgery USF Tampa; founding Medical Director Moffitt Cancer Center; author of the book Across the Red Line: Stories from the Surgical Life. (Sept 2014)

91. Daniel Kahneman *Thinking Fast and Slow*. 2011 (2015)

92. Sean Keenan, MD FAAEM FAWM, 10th SFG(A) Surgeon, Fort Carson (Colorado Springs), Colorado

93. Major Anthony T Kern "darker shades of Blue" 1995; Convergent-knowledge.com (Permission 2013)

94. Gary Klein Cognitive Psychologist in field of cognitive Natural Decision Making. Author of *Sources of Power: How People Make Decisions* and *Seeing What Others Don't: The Remarkable Way We Gain Insights. (Mar 2016)*

95. Mary E. Klingensmith, MD Founding Director, Academy of Educators Vice Chair for Education in Surgery at Washington University School of Medicine in St. Louis, past Residency Training Program Director in General Surgery at WashU, past Associate Director for the School of Medicine Simulation Center, founding director of the medical school's Academy of Educators. Past director for the American Board of Surgery (2011–2018, Board Chair 2017-18) and of the American Board of Thoracic Surgery (2012–15). Chair of the Advisory Council for SCORE (Surgical Council on Resident Education), and oversees content for the web portal as President of SCORE,

96. Col Thomas Kolditz, author of *In Extremis Leadership: Leading As If Your Life Depended On It.* Former head of department of Behavioral Sciences and Leadership, US Military Academy, West Point. (Mar 2015)

97. Dr. Edward Kosik DO, University Oklahoma Dept Anesthesia, Simulation Center (Nov 2014)

98. Daniel Kuhn, M.D., Integrative Neuropsychiatric Services, NY

99. SreyRam Kuy, MD Baylor College of Medicine and Michael DeBakey VA Houston Tx

100. Ronda Landers DNP, RN author *"Reducing Surgical Errors: Implementing a Three-Hinge Approach to Success"* Associate Professor, Online MSN Director Rudy School of Nursing and Health Professions Cumberland University.

101. Dr. Anthony LaPorta MD, FACS Colonel Retired, US Army, Professor of Surgery, Rocky Vista University School of Medicine (Oct 2013)

102. Carter Lebares, MD, FACS, MAMSE Associate Professor of Surgery UCSF Department of Surgery Director UCSF Center for Mindfulness in Surgery

103. Terry R.Lee Environmental Psychology and Policy Research Unit, School of Psychology, University of St. Andrews, St. Andrews, Fife KY16 9JU, UK; {Malcolm Jeeves Emeritus Professor Malcolm Jeeves, C.B.E., F.Med.Sci., F.R.S.E., P.P.R.S.E. School of Psychology and Neuroscience , University of St. Andrews (Permission 2013)

104. Walter T. Lee MD MHSc Professor and Chief of Staff Department of Head and Neck Surgery & Communication Sciences Co-Director, Head and Neck Program, Duke Cancer Institute Duke Health IRB Chair Affiliate Duke Global Health Institute VAMC Staff Surgeon

105. Tim Leeuwenburg, MD -"rural proceduralist"- Kangaroo Island, Australia

106. Mark Light, IAFC CEO and Executive Director Christine A. Booth, Executive Assistant International Association of Fire Chiefs (Permission 2013)

107. Robert Bentley Lim, MD, Professor Surgery Wake Forest University, Editor Surgery During Natural Disasters, combat, terrorist attacks and crisis situations.

108. Daniel Linskey, Former Chief of Police Boston; Incident Commander during the Boston Marathon Bombing. US Marine Ret. (Mar 2016)

109. Representative Thomas Lubanau II BS JD; Wyoming State Legislature; Retired Fire Service Wyoming; Author "Crew Resource Management For the Fire Service 2002" (Sept 2013)

110. Luttrel, Marcus *Lone Survivor: The Eyewitness Account of Operation Redwing and the Lost Heroes of SEAL Team 10* (June 2006) Little, Brown and Company Hatchette Book group New York New York **HBG FAQ/Permissions Jan 2026**

111. LTC Robert L. Mabry, M.D. Director of the Military Emergency Medical Services Fellowship, the largest EMS fellowship in the nation, and the Director of Trauma Care Delivery at the Department of Defense Trauma Center of Excellence at Fort Sam Houston, TX. Prior Academic Director Department of Combat Medic Training. Battalion Surgeon and Battalion Executive Officer in the First Special Forces Group. Airborne Ranger Infantryman (1984-1987). (Feb 2015).

112. Dr. Susan E Mackinnon Minot Packer Fryer Professor of Surgery Director of the Center for Nerve Injury and Paralysis Professor of Plastic and Reconstructive Surgery Washington University School of Medicine Division of Plastic and Reconstructive Surgery

113. Amin Madani, MD Surgery Research Fellow McGill Univ. Canada; Intraoperative decision making. (Oct 2015)

114. Michael Maddaus, MD Professor and Chair, Department of surgery, Program Director of Surgery and now Life Coach for Physicians; retired thoracic Surgeon.Maier Ronald (verbal permission American College Surgeons Clinical Congress Boston MA

115. Michael D. Matthews, former law enforcement officer, professor of engineering psychology, West Point, Past president of American Psychological Asso. Society for Military Psychology. Fellow, Strategic Services Office of the Chief of Staff of the Army. (Mar 2015)

116. Sean McKay of The Asymmetric Combat Institute (ACI). Firefighter/paramedic and SWAT Rescue-Medic. Immediate Reaction Team (IRT) Methodology for high threat operator/officer extraction. (Mar 2015)

117. Karen Mazzocco, R.N., J.D for Mazzocco Ket al. Surgical Team Behaviors and Patient Outcomes. Am Jnl Surgery. 2009; 197:678-685 (Oct 2014)

118. Coach Brad McCoy. championship coach and father of University of Texas quarterback, Colt McCoy (who also provided insight); Flippen group- Sports Leadership Section (May 2016).

119. Naval Adm. William H. McRaven, Retired ninth commander of U.S. Special Operations Command* and Chancellor at The University of Texas, *May 2014 Commencement speech at the University of Texas at Austin. (* including the unit manning Operation Neptune Spear, which resulted to the killing of Osama bin Laden).*

120. Wayne Meredith, MD past Chair Department Surgery Wake Forest University

121. Thomas Mercer. RAdm, USN (retired) USS Carl Vinson; Strategic Reliability, LLC

122. CDR Mitch Morrison, PhD; Chief, Aviation Safety Division; COMDT (CG-1131); U.S. Coast Guard Headquarters (Feb 2014)

123. Carol-Anne Moulton, MBBS, Med, PhD. Hepatobiliary Surgeon University Health Network, Toronto, associate professor of Surgery at the University of Toronto. Scientist at the Wilson Centre [TGH, University of Toronto] conducting research on surgical judgment and the social psychology of surgeons. (Dec 2015)

124. Jan Newman

125. Sean Nix, DO. Trauma Surgeon Riverside Healthcare Virginia Beach VA.

126. Okray R, Lubnau T. *Crew Resource Management for the Fire Service.* Tulsa, OK: PennWell Press; 2004.

127. Chan Park, MD Director of Simulation, Veterans Affairs Durham, NC

128. Dr. Douglas E. Paull, M.D. *Clinical Adjunct Associate Professor of Medicine, Georgetown University SOM; Executive Masters in Clinical Quality and Safety Leadership (EMCQSL) Program (2018-Current), Former Co-Director of Medical Team Training (2007-2010) and Director of Patient Safety Curriculum and Medical Simulation (2010-2016) VHA National Center for Patient Safety.* (Feb 2026)

129. Keryn Pauley School of Psychology, University of Aberdeen, UK Pauley K, FlinR, Yule S, Youngson G. Surgeons intraoperative decision making and risk management. *Am J Surg.* 2011;202:375-381.131

130. Carlos A. Pellegrini, MD President American College of Surgeons (Oct 2015)

131. Charles B. Perrow emeritus professor of sociology at Yale University Professor Emeritus Sociology 493 College St, New Haven, CT 06511-8907(Permission 2013):

132. Dr. Peter J. Pronovost, MD, PhD, FCCMSr. Vice President for Patient Safety and Quality, Director of the Armstrong Institute for Patient Safety and Quality, Johns Hopkins Medicine

133. Laura Pizzi, PharmD Professor Jefferson School of Pharmacy (Permission 2013):

134. Carla M. Pugh, MD, PhD, FACS, Thomas Krummel Professor of Surgery Director of the Technology Enabled Clinical Improvement (T.E.C.I.) Center Stanford Medicine | Department of Surgery (Apr 2016 & Susan Behrens, MD, PhD)

135. Bruce Ramshaw, MD, FACS (Apr 2016) Chairman and Professor, Department of Surgery University of Tennessee - Knoxville Martin Reznek Emergency Medicine Pilot Study, U. Mass (Apr 2015)

136. Amanday Ripley Author of : "The Unthinkable: who survives when disaster strikes and why" http://www.amandaripley.com/ (Permission 2013)

137. Dale Roberts, FAA; Chief Pilot Safety and Fatigue (along with Chester Piolunek, Jr., Tom Nesthus, Aviation Safety Inspector AFS-220, Air Carrier Operations Branch and Steve Hursh) (Oct 2015)

138. Stephanie Russ University of Aberdeen, Aberdeen Behavioural Science, Developmental Psychology (July 2016)

139. William Ben Runciman, BSc (Med), MBCH, FANZCA, FJFICM, FRCA, HKCA, PhD; Professor, Patient Safety & Healthcare Human Factors | School of Psychology, Social Work & Social Policy, Sleep Research Centre - University of South Australia | Research Fellow - Australian Institute of Health Innovation – UNSW | Clinical Professor – Joanna Briggs Institute, Faculty Health Sciences - The University of Adelaide | President, Australian Patient Safety Foundation(Permission 2013):

140. Tom Russell, MD, FACS- Past Executive Director of ACS (Permission 2013)

141. Ajit K. Sachdeva, MD, FACS, FRCSC, FSACME, MAMSE Senior Vice President Academy of Master Surgeon Educators

142. Eduardo Salas, Ph.D. Pegasus & Trustee Chair Professor Department of Psychology,Institute for Simulation & Training University of Central Florida (Permission 2013)

143. Juan Sanchez, Cardiothoracic Surgeon, Chief Academic Officer at HCA Healthcare

144. Thomas Scalea, MD Chief Shock Trauma Center University of Maryland

145. Dr. Mark W. Scerbo, Ph.D., FHFES; Professor, Human Factors; Department of Psychology; Old Dominion University (Jan 2014)

146. Lt Gen Eric B. Schoomaker - United States Army lieutenant general. served as the 42nd Surgeon General of the United States Army and Commanding General, United States Army Medical Command He previously served as Commanding General, North Atlantic Regional Medical Command and Walter Reed Army Medical Center. (May 2016)

147. Dr. Matthew Seeger PhD, Professor Dean of the College of Fine, Performing and Communication Arts and Professor of Communication, Wayne State University

148. Nick Sevdalis, PhD Professor of Implementation Science & Patient Safety. Director, Centre for Implementation Science. Editor-in-Chief, BMJ Simulation & Technology Enhanced Learning. Associate Editor, Implementation Science. Health Service & Population Research Department. Institute of Psychiatry, Psychology & Neuroscience. King's College London (july 2016)

149. Tait D. Shanafelt, MD Professor of Medicine Mayo Clinic (Permission 2013)

150. Matthew J. Sharps, PhD, DABPS, FACFEI (Professor of Psychology California State University; Research Consultant, Fresno Police Department), author of Processing Under Pressure- Stress, Memory and Decision Making in Law Enforcement, Looseleaf Law Publications, Inc." (Permission 2013)

151. Bruce Siddle; CEO Human Factor Research Group; Author *Sharpening the Warrior's Edge: The Psychology and Science of Training*

152. Simons & Chabris (1999)" Professor Daniel J. Simons; http://www.dansimons.com; Professor, Department of Psychology and the Beckman Institute for Advanced Science and Technology, the University of Illinois. Co-author of 'The Invisible Gorilla', w Christopher Chabris 2010 (Permission 2013)

153. Sara Singer, PhD Professor of Health Care Management and Policy Department of Health Policy and Management, Harvard (July 2016)

154. Michael Spinks, Aircraft Safety Systems Specialist, commentator on: www.Examiner.com

155. Dr. Eric Stanley: VCU emergency medicine (Oct 2015)

156. Dimitrios Stefanidis, MD, PhD Harris B. Shumacker Jr. M.D. Professor of Surgery Professor of Surgery Vice Chair, Education Director, MIS/Bariatric Surgery Director, Department of Surgery Skills Lab

157. Lygia Stewart, MD - Nicksa G, Stewart L. Innovative Approach Using Interprofessional Simulation to Educate Surgical Residents in Technical and Nontechnical Skills in High-Risk Clinical Scenarios.

158. Daved van Stralen, M.D., F.A.A.P; Assistant Professor of Pediatrics in the Department of Pediatrics, Loma Linda University School of Medicine; Medical Director for American Medical Response, San Bernardino County, Medical Director for the San Bernardino County Fire Department (Oct 2015)

159. John Stewart, MD John H. Stewart, IV, MD, MBA, FACS. Chair, Department of Surgery and Associate Dean of Oncology Programs Department of Surgery Grady Hospital
E-mail: surgerydept@msm.edu

160. Nicksa G, Stewart L. Innovative Approach Using Interprofessional Simulation to Educate Surgical Residents in Technical and Nontechnical Skills in High-Risk Clinical Scenarios.

161. Kathleen M. Sutcliffe Bloomberg Distinguished Professor with appointments in the Carey Business School, the School of Medicine (Anesthesia and Critical Care Medicine), the School of Nursing, the Bloomberg School of Public Health, and the Armstrong Institute for Patient Safety and Quality; Sutcliffe KM, Lewton E, Rosenthal MM. Communication failures: an insidious contributor to medical mishaps. Acad Med. 2004 Feb;79(2):186-94

162. Col. Patrick Sweeney, Professor of practice of Management; executive director Allegacy Center for Leadership and Character School of Business, Wake Forest University Winston Salem. Former battalion commander in 101st airborne, former director Eisenhower Leader Development program, West Point. (Feb 2015)

163. Mr Nicholas Symons, MBChB, MSc, MRCS Chairman, London Surgical Research GroupSurgical Registrar, North East Thames Honorary Clinical Research FellowCentre for Patient Safety and Service Quality Imperial College London(Permission 2013):

164. Dana A Telem MD, MPH, Department of Surgery University of Michigan, Lazar J Greenfield M.D. Professor of Surgery Associate Chair Department of Surgery Professor of Surgery Section Head Surgery Service Chief Medical School Vice Chair Quality and patient safety, division chief minimally invasive surgery.

165. Th.J. (Olle) ten Cate, PhD Professor of medical education | Director of the Center for Research and Development of Education | University Medical Center Utrecht | Visit: Room HB 4.24, Universiteitsweg 98, 3584 CG Utrecht, The Netherlands | Postal address: P.O. Box # 85500, 3508 GA Utrecht, The Netherlands

166. Eric J. Thomas MD, MPH Professor and Associate Dean for Healthcare Quality and Griff T. Ross Professor in Humanities and Technology in Health Care Mazzocco Ket al. Surgical Team Behaviors and Patient Outcomes. Am Jnl Surgery. 2009; 197:678-685 (Oct 2014)

167. John B. Tippett Jr., CFO, MIFire Deputy Chief of Operations City of Charleston Fire Department 46 ½ Wentworth Street Charleston, SC 29401 (Permission 2013)

168. Patricia Turner, Patricia L. Turner, MD, MBA, FACS Executive Director & CEO American College of Surgeons

169. Dominique Vandijck Belgian Health Care Knowledge Center (KCE), Brussels, Belgium; (Jochen Bergs, Frank Lambrechts 1, Pascale Simons 1, Annemie Vlayen 2, Wim Marneffe 1, Johan Hellings 3, Irina Cleemput) **Barriers and facilitators related to the implementation of surgical safety checklists: a systematic review of the qualitative evidence** BMJ Qual Saf 2015 Dec;24(12):776-86. doi: 10.1136/bmjqs-2015-004021. Epub 2015 Jul 21. . PENDING BMJ noted in other communications that indirect adaptations do not require permission from BMJ

170. Lt. Gen Paul K. Van Riper, US Marine Corps Ret. Commanding General, Marine Corps Combat Development command Quantico Va. (Jan 2015)
171. George Velmahos, MD PhD, University of Massachusetts, Mass.General Hospital Chief Trauma.
172. Steven Venette, Associate Professor University of Southern Mississippi, Speech Communication
173. Professor Charles A. Vincent Faculty of Medicine, Department of Surgery & Cancer Imperial College UK (Permission 2013)
174. Stanley R. Wachs, PhD founder of Wachs Associates, a management consulting and training practice Sept 2016
175. David S. Wade, M.D., FACS, Chief Medical Officer, Federal Bureau of Investigation (Oct 2013)
176. Karl Weick (and Kathleen M. Sutcliffe); Gilbert and Ruth Whitaker Professor of Business Administration; Professor of Management and Organizations; Stephen M. Ross School of Business; Univ. Michigan (Permission 2013):
177. John A. Weigelt, MD, DVM, MMA University of South Dakota; Retired Department of Surgery, Trauma Division/ CC Medical College of Wisconsin; Editor in Chief, Journal of Surgical Education
178. Ana Wheelock, Department of Surgery and Cancer, Imperial College London, London, UK The Impact of Operating Room Distractions on Stress, Workload, and Teamwork. Ann Surg 2015; 261(6):1079–1084. (Aug 2015)
179. Jon White, MD- Chief Surgery VAMC Washington DC. (Nov 2016)
180. Jocko Willink and Lief Babin, Authors *Extreme Ownership*. MacMillian publishing Feb 2026
181. Ross Willis, PhD, Director of Surgical Education University of Texas Health Science Center San Antonio, San Antonio, TX
182. Gordon Wisbach, MD CDR USN Navy Medical Center San Diego CA
183. Linda L. Wong MD, Professor and Associate Chairman, Dept of Surgery, Univ of Hawaii, John A. Burns School of Medicine, Professor, Univ of Hawaii, Cancer Center, Director, Liver Transplant Program, Queens Medical Center
184. Stephanie Wright; Permissions Editor ; Merriam-Webster Inc.; Merriam-Webster. Com; http://www.merriam-webster.com/ ; http://www.websters-online-dictionary.org/definition (Permission 2013)
185. Steven Yule, Ph.D., Assistant Professor of Surgery Institution Brigham and Women's Hospital Department Surgery Brigham and Women's Hospital SRATUS Ctr for Medical Simulation 75 Francis St Boston MA 02115. Permission 2013
186. Jeffrey S. Young, MD, MBA, Prof.of Surgery, Director, Trauma Center, and Chief Patient Safety Officer, UVA
187. Lev Zhuravsky BA, PGCert Crit.Care, PGDip HealMgt, MHealSc (Health Management), PhD Cand. University of Otago (Feb 2015)
188. Marco Zenati, MD Chief of Cardiothoracic Surgery Harvard University. (May 2016)

I. **STEPS FOR EFFECTIVE DECISION MAKING AND COMMUNCATION PROCESSING DURING ANY SITUATION (EXCLUDING THOSE THAT DEMAND INSTANTANEOUS ENGAGEMENT BASED ON LIFE THREATENING CIRCUMSTANCES):**

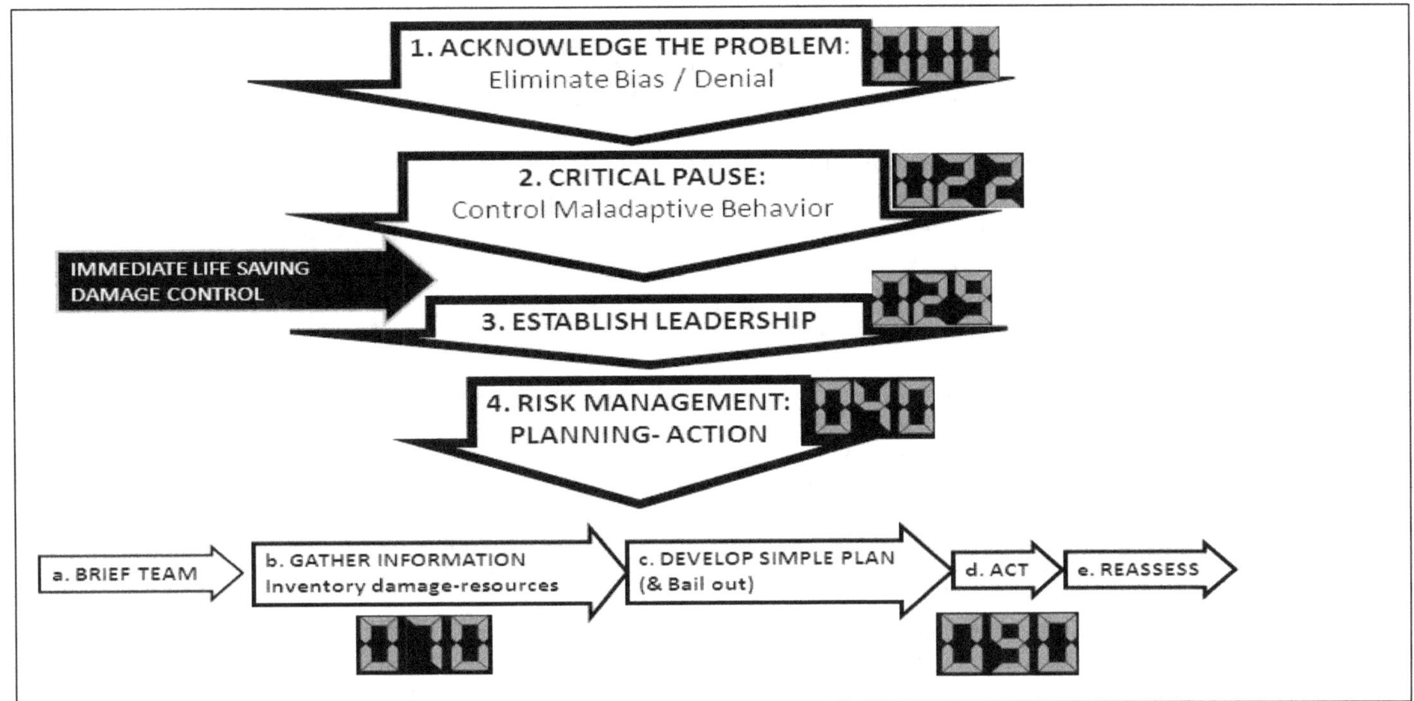

A.   **INTRODUCTION/ CRITICAL PAUSE:** Team "Leader" creates a pause in the situation to calm / quiet team members down, gain control over the communication process and introduce their intent.
EXAMPLE: *"OK everyone please stop what you are doing for a second. We need to PAUSE so we can decide what to do from this point forwards." ***

B.   **BRIEFING:** Team "leader" summarizes their personal assessment of their observation of known facts regarding the situation at hand (typically leaders propose a goal early on, but experts recommend withholding their recommendation until all the information has been gathered, thus avoiding biases or staff withholding information). *
EXAMPLE: "It looks as though our problem is……... We need to abort our original goal if that is ok with everyone else in the room. I think we have 3 minutes to discuss this and come up with a plan."

C.   **QUERY-INFORMATION GATHERING:** Team "leader" pauses the process and queries team members about their knowledge of key components of the situation at hand creating an inventory of damage, resources, obstacles, potential solutions to their dilemma and safety to proceed.
EXAMPLE: "Bob. What do you know about (your area) as it pertains to this problem? Joe. What do we know about the ability to get ……...? Jill. Do we have communication with……...? Ok.

D.   **PREDICTION, PLAN AND REASSESS:** Team members assess their knowledge base as a whole and create a series of potential solutions with expected outcomes and "bail-out" plans should their expectations not be observed. To avoid information overload, experienced leaders attempt to propose one goal/solution/plan at a time. Attempting to suggest several alternate plans can create confusion during times of stress or communication difficulties. If concern is raised an alternate can be proposed at this point. Team specifies period of time for which they will reassess the situation to determine effectiveness of current plan. **ADAPTABILITY IS KEY!**
EXAMPLE: "Based on the information we have what if we did………. (LEADERS GOAL PROPOSED)… Does anyone have a problem with that goal? No? Yes? Ok, your point is taken and I concur. So let's change our plan slightly to…...xxxx….Further questions? No. OK so this is what we are going to do. …...
*Ok. John. What do you know about our ability to…………? Jack. Do we have………? Ok. Anyone with any concerns or questions? Yes Josh. I understand that that is a concern. Let's keep watching it and Josh, let me know if you see that problem arising. Let's move on."**
"Ok, if there are no questions or facts we left out I propose that we………. John. I need you to track the progress with…. Jill. you track…... Joe. You were concerned about…. so tell us if that is an issue……… We have about 5-10 minutes to do all this so let's move. In 10 minutes if we are not close to departure…. I need you ALL to speak up if you have a barrier to get thru this to our goal of…...".
*success depends upon the use of effective communication skills described below.

II. *KEY COMPONENTS OF EFFECTIVE COMMUNICATION SKILLS:

1. **LISTENING:** Everyone should be an active listener and acknowledge comprehension.

2. **CONTROL:** Everyone should utilize controlled calm steady voices that are loud enough to be heard but without shouting.

3. **PRECISION:** The team leader shall use commands that are accurate, bold, clear, concise, and precise.

4. **EXPLICIT:** Communication shall be explicit, clear and NOT utilize implied instruction. Explicit communication does NOT assume everyone understands background information. AVOID mitigated speech - mitigated speech is an attempt to downplay our communication to be less direct, in an attempt to be polite, deferential to authority or to avoid conflict.

5. **FEEDBACK:** Communication requires continuous closed loops of communication sending and reception that requires constant feedback with open, inclusive exchange.

6. **FOCUSED:** Speakers address communication to specific staff, not global commands.

7. **AWARENESS:** All team members must recognize that perceptions, influences, situations and filters affect the message as well as the need to utilize more than one type of communication when possible (verbal, written, symbolic, non-verbal).

III.   OVERALL TEAM LEADER COMMUNICATION RESPONSIBILITIES:

•<u>Remain Respectful-</u> assertive but courteous and considerate of. Do not discount other's importance through disregard, criticism, or screaming.

•<u>Communicate clearly</u> – Remain calm. Use complete, directed communication of ideas, wants and needs. Unless impossible look directly at the person for whom the communication is being directed.

•<u>Use Open, explicit closed-loop communication</u>- before all actions closed ask if that step makes sense. Wait for concurrence response. Do not be vague. Assure purpose of communication is crystal clear. Do not assume you are understood until you are told so.

•<u>Be Inclusive</u> - include team input everyone has a personal part in the outcome of the situation. A quick solution needs to be offered followed by consensus or concise discussion of realistic alternatives. Ask for feedback. Resolve conflicts immediately.

•<u>Minimize distractions</u>.

•<u>Conduct a briefing</u>-begin with a clear statement to get everyone's attention. Explain mission, goals, team member roles, points if conflict, bailout plan. Your statement of the situation must acknowledge if the problem is real or perceived. A quick solution needs to be offered followed by consensus or concise discussion of realistic alternatives. This immediate communication needs to be succinct and clear, i.e. just "say what needs to be said."

•<u>Critical Pause</u> Take a time out before critical operation or step to query preparedness of team and safety of proceeding.

•<u>Error management</u>- Focus team on the potential for errors-

•<u>Monitoring</u>: monitor the effects of your communication and actions.

•<u>Listen</u>: be patient and listen.

•<u>Watch out for filters (See Below)</u>.

IV.   OVERALL FOLLOWER COMMUNICATION RESPONISIBILITIES.

•<u>Advocate for your team or mission</u>: Advocacy can be done in a respectful manner especially if you offer up solutions or alternate actions. If serious concerns remain do not walk away but assure that the team leader understands your concerns and communicates as such.

•<u>Provide Constructive Criticism</u>- voice concerns. Understand cues and communicate those cues in a respectful manner back to the leadership. Remember to advocate the point but Maintain respect.

•<u>Inquiry</u>: always ask for clarification if the order was not perfectly clear. Be respectful. If you need an answer to a question, ASK! Admit if you are confused or may have misunderstood direction.

V.   AVOID COMMUNICATION ERRORS:

A.   SENDER:

•Not establishing a frame of reference: receiver is not on the same page as you.

•Omitting information.

•Providing biased–weighted information.

•Forgetting that body language is important.

•Forgetting to repeat.

•Giving disrespectful communication.

B.   RECEIVER:

•Listening with bias, preconceived notions (ie not really listening).

•Thinking ahead of the sender, extrapolating the information, finishing sentences.

•Poorly prepared to receive information, not consciously ready- distracted, fatigued, complacent, reckless.

•Not requiring clarification.

•Disrespectful.

C.   FILTERS TO BE AWARE OF:

•Filters distort the information resulting in misleading or erroneous interpretations, quickly resulting in inappropriate or dangerous actions on behalf of the recipient.

•Defensive stature- Confirmation bias-resistance to change opinion, even when there is no support. Need to blame others to protect oneself.

VI. DANGERS IN COMMUNICATION:

- We need to slow down. We normally talk about 125 words a minute and think at 500-1000 words a minute.

- FAA data suggests that in over 70% of aircraft incidents, errors in the transferring of information directly contributed to the cause of that incident. In 37% of incidents, there was a failure to initiate the information transfer process- that is the information was there but not made available to those who needed it the most. In the other 37% the information was provided in a useless manner (ambiguous, garbled, incomplete, and inaccurate).

- A NTSB review of air carrier accidents from 1978-1990 revealed that 84% of the incidents were due to communication errors- usually in monitoring and challenging orders. 75% of those were due to external operational and organizational influences.

- **REALITIES IN HUMAN COMMUNICATION:** We protect ourselves when we communicate. We defend ourselves against looking ignorant. We wish to maintain consistency and support our own opinion even if we know that it may not be totally correct. We always wish to feel valued. The reality of the situation is always of secondary importance to our perception of the situation. We behave according to our perceptions. Emotions always overshadow everything. People always have their own motivation. People are afraid to ask, "Does everyone understand me?" Or say "I don't understand". 8 of 10 subordinates would not question an officer even if they suspected there might be a danger in the current conditions and orders.

COMMUNICATION REFERENCES:

Accurate Communication:	Erroneous communication: Sender	Erroneous communication: Receiver:	Filters to be aware of:
Controlled: voices should remain calm, Steady, loud enough to be heard but without shouting	not establishing a frame of reference: receiver is not on the same page as you	Listening w. bias- preconceived notions Poorly prepared to receive information, not consciously ready	Confirmation bias-resistance to change opinion, even when there is no support
Commands: need to be accurate, bold, clear, concise and precise	Omitting information	Thinking ahead of the sender, extrapolating the information,	Defensive stature
Address specific staff: not global commands	Providing biased – weighted information	finishing sentences	Blaming others
Close looped communication- need constant feedback; ask "does everyone understand me?"	forgetting body language is important	Missing non-verbal signals	Halo effect: The infallible one must be right, or I am right I am the infallible one
Open inclusive exchange	forgetting to repeat- We normally talk about 125 words a minute and think at 500-1000 words a minute.	Not requiring clarification	Odd man out"- I just don't fit in, or he does not fit in
Focus on what is right not who is right	Disrespectful communication	Disrespectful.	Fatigue, complacency, Recklessness

(*) adapted from Crew Resource in the Fire Service, Okray & Lubnau p268-269

EXTENSIVE DEBRIEFING CHECKLIST	
Ranking system (*): 1= Poorly done, ineffective and dangerous 2= Unsafe but not dangerous 3= Safe but ineffective 4= Effective but not optimal 5= Optimal.	
A. OVERALL DEBRIEFING GOALS: The team should address the following questions during a debrief:	**Rating 1-5**
Roles and responsibilities understood?	
Communication clear? Timely?	
Situation awareness maintained?	
Workload distribution equitable?	
Task assistance requested or offered?	
Were errors made or avoided?	
Availability of resources?	
What went well, what should change, what should improve?	
Modified from: TeamSTEPPS™ AHRQ called Team Strategies and>>> Tools to Enhance Performance and Patient Safety (TeamSTEPPS) Pocket Guide – 06.136 AHRQ Pub. No. 06-0 Version 06.1 Developed for the Department of Defense Patient Safety Program in collaboration with the Agency for Healthcare Research and Quality	

B. 1CRITICAL MOMENT: Moment that the overall atmosphere changed to a more tense environment due to an **UNEXPECTED CHANGE DUE TO:**	
WHAT WAS THAT CRITICAL MOMENT?	
Change in procedure/ Additional procedures not expected?	y/n
something that was supposed to happen didn't,	y/n
something that was not supposed to happen did	y/n
something simply flies in out-of-the-blue that no one could have predicted.	y/n
B2CHANGE DUE TO:	
Incremental evolution of smaller adverse events	y/n
Missing the warning signs of an impending problem	y/n
Unexpected sudden change in patient condition due to something someone on the team did or inherent patient problem, or equipment/product problem or reaction.	y/n
B3. CRISIS?	
Was this a **CRISIS**? characterized by a. **Surprise** (not expected) b. **Threat** (to the organization, team, or mission patient)c. **Rapid processing, decision times** requiring **d. transformation** (change in our current process, procedure, course of actions, etc).	y/n
B4. SEVERITY OF CONSEQUENCES: What was the overall **SEVERITY** of Event: Consequences measured in terms of degree of impact	
CATASTROPHIC - Complete mission failure, death, or loss of system.	y/n
MAJOR - Major mission degradation, severe injury, occupational illness, or major system damage.	y/n
SIGNIFICANT - Minor mission degradation, injury, minor occupational illness, or minor system damage.	y/n
MINIMAL - Less than minor mission degradation, injury, occupational illness or minor system damage.	y/n
NONE - No impact to personnel or mission outcome.	y/n

C. OVERALL TEAM MANAGEMENT:	
1. Overall Control of team	
Shock, Denial, Dissociation, Panic	acceptance planning and deliberate positive action
2. LEADERSHIP:	
Authority with Respect: assertiveness *"authority with participation, yet assertiveness with respect".*	
Respectful Clear communication:	
Inclusive of Crew- Team input: Team was aware of strategy and tactics? Team aware of upcoming actions?	
Establishing & Prioritizing Tasks Appropriately (skills and other tasks assigned)	

Managing resources - Declare emergency early on - call for help early; key players should not be leaving the room.	
Recognize and Manage conflict resolution, Team Stress & Panic using effective listening, avoiding emotions, remaining focused.	
Control non-productive hazardous emotions (Anti-authoritarian, Impulsivity, Invulnerability, Machismo, Resignation, Pressing ,"Air Show")	
Watch for and manage error: One goal-one solution error, Exclusion error, Denial	
Decision making processes / Appropriate decision style utilized with clearly defined goals	
Decisions made timely?	
Develop a model and gather information	
Prognosis/prediction and extrapolate- considered alternatives	
Planning of actions and execution	
Review effects and revision of strategy planning **– plan was monitored for success**	
3. "FOLLOWERSHIP"	
• Respect for Authority	•
• Establishment of assertiveness / Authority balance- Challenging authority with proper decorum when there are safety concerns.	•
• Personal Safety, Safety of Fellow Followers and leaders	•
• Possession of good communication skills	•
• Ego balance and check	•
• Communication to assure they have clear assignments	•
• Acceptance of direction and information as needed	•
• Reporting of any personal mistakes (This is NOT the time to hide ones errors).	•
• Constant reports of work	•
• Flexibility	•
4. SITUATIONAL AWARENESS	
SA Maintained?	y/n
If NO, then SA WAS LOST DUE TO:	i.
ii. Ambiguity: more than one interpretation of the situation is possible	y/n
iii. Distraction: Attention is being diverted from the original point of focus	y/n
iv. Fixation: see below	y/n
v. Overload: too much is happening at one time	y/n
vi. Complacency: false sense of comfort, masking impending further danger (not out of the woods yet)	y/n
vii. Improper procedure: Deviation from SOP's w/o justification	y/n
viii. Unresolved discrepancy: conflicts in communication, visual input, or conflicting conditions	y/n
ix. Lack of leadership: No one is flying the plane. (see also	y/n
5. COMMUNICATION (see details at bottom):	
Communication process was clear and timely?	
Communication clear and unhostile?	
Information and actions verified?	
Team members requested clarification on vague or ambiguous communications?	
Barriers and Filters identified and addressed?	
Clear to all that the situation had changed?	
6. TEAMWORK: Overall ranking	

D. " SYSTEMS" Issues	
Latent conditions Upper level management (Budget pressure, Staff reduction pressure, Production pressure)	
Latent conditions Middle Management (communication, training)	
Preconditions: The "Dirty Dozen": Lack of Communication, complacency, lack of knowledge, distraction, lack of teamwork, fatigue, lack of resources, pressure, lack of assertiveness, stress, lack of awareness and "the Norms" or unwritten rules everyone follows	
Defense mechanism Failures:	

E. ADDITIONAL CRITICAL EVENTS TO CONSIDER DURING A CRISIS OR SUDDEN CHANGE IN EVENTS:

1. Anesthesia:
2. Nursing:
a. FB counts- Significant change in events are moments for counts to become "off": X-ray, white board, sponge detectors.
b. Shift Change- communication in advance of shift change to allow surgeons to tailor upcoming events?
c. Equipment / Supply issues
3. Surgeons:
a. Staff- helping hands
b. Communication: surgeon to surgeon, Surgeon to anesthesia, Surgeon to Nurse.
c. Advance risk assessment and planning:

AN INTERVIEW WITH BEN AARON, MD - THE TEAM THAT SAVED RONALD REAGAN.
Washington DC March 30 1981, 2:27 pm:

On March 30 1981, 2:27 pm, John Hinckley Jr shot President Ronald Reagan using his Röhm RG-14 .22 cal blue steel revolver loaded with six "Devastator" brand cartridges (each with small aluminum and lead azide explosive charges designed to explode on contact). Until he coughed up blood, President Reagan assumed the pain in his left chest was due to rib fractures from being pushed into the limousine. Special Agent Parr thought otherwise and directed the motorcade to George Washington University Hospital. The President was in shock and the Trauma team quickly discovered a bullet entrance wound in his left axilla. Within 30 minutes, he was stabilized and transported to the O.R. where, with the assistance of Joseph M. Giordano, Chief Thoracic Surgery Benjamin L. Aaron, performed a thoracotomy. Wikipedia

An interview a few weeks later revealed the anxiety control methods both surgeons utilized when they realized they were operating on the President:

Giordano: "I looked at him and I could feel myself getting tense, which has happened to me occasionally when I do surgery. When that happens, I talk myself through it. I thought, 'O.K., calm yourself. You want this to go well. Concentrate, and do everything the way you always do it, if you expect to get good results.' But I could not divorce myself from the fact that he was the President and his wound could have been lethal."

Aaron: "He assessed the seriousness of the President's wounds, and said he too would have had 'heightened anxiety' if he had not judged that Mr. Reagan's bleeding could be controlled. Although Dr. Aaron described himself as someone who "doesn't get anxious about things," he acknowledged that he was "on edge at times." "When I couldn't feel that bullet, and I knew it should be there, I thought it might have embolized through the pulmonary veins, into the heart and gone someplace." …The bullet, it turned out, was flat. "I just couldn't feel it in that spongy lung tissue," Dr. Aaron said. "The X-ray settled me down because I realized that when I was feeling for the bullet it wasn't trapped in one place. It had room to move, and it just squirted away from my fingertips." "Then it was just a matter of hanging in there until I could find the blooming thing by passing a catheter along the bullet track. It took about five minutes of very concentrated tactile discrimination until I suddenly pinned it down and got it out."

Dr. Aaron talked with me about that experience:
"Bear in mind that all this took place 35 years ago and that it is coming from an 83 year old brain. Also, at the time, things were moving at a fast pace during which time there was not much time for reflection or organization, or to put it another way, much of the time we were "winging it" in dealing with the complexities imposed by the unique nature of the event. "

1. What leadership or crisis management experience /techniques did you discover worked well for you?

The care in the ER was flawless as regards urgent processing, mobilization of staff and systematic application of appropriate care. This was not an accident, but came about because of aggressive and thorough preparation and training of the ER staff and residents. In order to take care of the President, James Brady and Tim McCarthy (SS), the area had to be cleared of patients, the ensuing crowd screened and managed, and assignments quickly defined. No one consulted any manuals on procedures on techniques. The key was preparation and training, professionally applied.

I recall insisting, from the get-go, that everyone on my team regard the President first and foremost as a patient in trouble and to put aside any consideration of who he was or what might be swirling around beyond our perimeter of care. This kept us focused on the task at hand and help quell nervousness. You might call this the principle of putting first things first. I did not note it at the time, but have been told since that as the team leader, my calm demeanor, efficiency, decisiveness and apparent lack of nervousness did much to hold things together as this event moved along. (Jon White, MD noted that this was indeed the case- Dr. Aaron maintained a calm demeanor with no yelling and no screaming, which allowed flawless communication and the ability to resuscitate the President and rapidly transport him to the OR).

2. Consideration of changes or alterations.

One can be persuaded in such a situation that having additional professional experience at the table could be helpful and perhaps diffuse responsibility should things go wrong. I had many offers of help from fellow surgeons, but quickly put this aside in favor of a three-person team composed of me, my chief Thoracic resident and a surgical intern (just as it would be if the patient came in off the street). This seemed to me to be the simplest route to good decision making during the operation. This might be termed good management versus too many "cooks" calling the shots.

Because of the remote possibility that the bullet might have transited the dome of the left diaphragm, the ER General Surgeons strongly supported an abdominal paracentesis before opening the chest to rule out injury to the spleen, etc. I had seen no evidence of this and had reservations about taking the time to do the procedure (20 minutes or so), but as the President's condition was stable at the time, I agreed to move ahead on this even though had I found a hole in the diaphragm, I could easily have dealt with the problem through the chest. This gets down to using clinical judgment (was it safe to take the additional time) to forestall a fuss with the General Surgery group.

Putting the President, post-op, on the ICU was a management mistake, as his presence along with all of his SS entourage and visiting staff rendered the ICU unworkable. We quickly evacuated a wing of the hospital, tailored it to all the requisites and had the patient moved in 6 hours. My plan for post-op care was drastically and suddenly altered but I and my team quickly adapted to the new circumstances and moved on. Being flexible, prepared for contingencies, and able to move in different directions effectively is essential to completing the mission.

3. **What preconceptions about your skill or your medical center staffs skill proved correct? How ready were we**? Occasionally one hears that University medicine is "sterile", impersonal, isolates a patient from compassionate care and has poor inter-staff communication. Some of this may be true, but what University Medical centers do provide is well credentialed and experienced staff and first rate facilities. We were prepared for this challenge at every level of staff, management and resource availability and because of this, the event came off without a significant hitch. It was a team effort in every regard from beginning to end and a wonderful thing to be a part of.

4. **What plans or preparations proved false**? We were not prepared for the security requirements by the SS. There was a SWAT team on the roof at all times during the eleven days he was present. When he needed good quality x-rays (there was a portable machine in his suite), the halls had to be cleared and explosive sniffing dogs preceded his visit to the x-ray floor. His food supply was carefully guarded. Bullet proof glass was installed in his room (despite the fact that he was on the 3rd floor of an interior court with a window free wall opposite). ALL entrants to the 3rd floor had to undergo a SS check, each and every time they entered. Medical folk, especially doctors, are not particularly patient people by nature, so with great restraint, and resolve, we managed to work it through to a successful conclusion. The lesson here is to practice situational awareness and be willing to accept imposed restraints, always keeping the mission as our first goal.

5. **What lessons did you rehash with the residents and /or hospital staff in post scenario debriefings?**   Post mortems are standard issue for any medical event. We had many discussions after the fact, but almost all centered about things like conduct with the intrusive press (residents and especially interns, are full of false info and quite willing to share it). To relive and relieve tensions. we produced a high quality 30-minute documentary utilizing all the primary participants (doctors and nurses, etc) plus actors as the presidential party. This process brought out into the open the vital parts played by each participant and highlighted the importance of the synthesis of each performance in attaining a good outcome. On almost every count, we were satisfied with how our medical center responded to each and every challenge and this was echoed by the AMA in their commendation of our efforts.

6. **What lessons should I pass onto the young residents from your experiences**?
In our profession you can't talk the talk if you have not walked the walk. My advice is to "hunker down",that is throw your whole self into the learning process, do your homework well, and walk into each and every OR as if you own the place." You are responsible for your patient so act like it.

I hope that this insight into how our medical center and all it's integrated parts dealt with a most unusual and unexpected event will help you develop a useful syntax for your book. If you have additional questions, fire them my way and I will field them as best as I can.
Sincere regards, Ben Aaron, MD

Special thanks to Dr. Jon White, Chief Surgery VAMC Washington DC for filling in the gaps.
https://en.wikipedia.org/wiki/Attempted_assassination_of_Ronald_Reagan assessed 111316
Altman LK. THE DOCTORS WORLD. New York Times. April 21, 1981
 http://www.nytimes.com/1981/04/21/science/the-doctors-world.html assessed 111316

COMFORT ZONES AND RISK TAKING IN SURGERY

   If you have ever wondered if surgeon who appear to never sweat thru a technically challenging procedure or event have any comfort zone concerns the answer appears to be thatlikely we all have boundaries that could potentially limit us. Dr. Moulton's group from the University of Toronto interviewed 18 surgeons regarding their approach to risk-taking and comfort zones and in a personal converasation she discussed this with me.

   From these interviews it appears that even the boldest appearing surgeons likely have their breaking point. It seemed that all surveyed surgeons had a perception of where their boundary was- the place where they no longer feel comfortable. Self-assessment literature seems to indicate that we frequently do not openly acknowledge that we have a comfort zone (or may not accept that personally). As she explained, it may be that the temperamental and angry affect we see in some surgeons is actually a reflection of anxiety. It is unlikely that anyone is immune, but we simply do not discuss it. (personal communication). Conditions that create a rift in our comfort zone (push us close to, or past that boundary):

1.   <u>Alterations in the environment</u> (such as an unfamiliar hospitals (OR), change in the OR team personnel, or assistant staff can create anxiety: While the experienced surgeons have no qualms at the hospital they tend to work in daily, they seem to shy away from similar cases at other less familiar hospitals. Environment may also come into play when one is performing elective as opposed to emergent or trauma surgery. Experienced surgical oncologists reveal that the same operations they perform without hesitation in an elective circumstance would be anxiety provoking in a traumatic scene. Presence or absence of specialized surgeons on the premises can alter the surgeons comfort in performing certain procedures. Other surgeons felt more confident with certain equipment (such as certain headlamps).

2.   <u>Performance of infrequently performed procedures</u> : surgeons who do extremely complex cases on a daily basis but rarely if ever do the more mundane procedures (hernia repair) can have angst over simple cases at times.

3.   Aversion to complications based on past experiences: Some Surgeons seem to abhor complications while others accept them as a potential and mentally prepare to avoid them where they can. Anxiety about the potential harm may be due to poor past experience during the peer review process, morbidity and mortality conferences, litigation, being berated by a colleague, etc. As Dr. Kuhn related to me, there is definitely a link between our reaction to a stressful procedure and how we manage the potential for complications- we may become so anxious about doing harm it affects our care because we now take the complication very personal. This leads to a lack of tolerance for complications and potentially to limitations of the procedures we are willing to tackle. Your reaction is dependent on culture around you – a blaming culture causes you to focus on your errors… your latest nightmare affects your future case care. .. Your peer reactions to you influence future response. In addition, surgeon stereotype probably affects us. We are taught to be bold and not focus on our feelings but to push ahead in spite of the potential for a complication. So we then block out our ability to accept we have a boundary until maybe it is too late and that episode overshadows our future care. SEE NEXT SECTION.

So what do people do to avoid the anxiety of approaching or crossing that boundary and be more risk taking as opposed to risk aversive….. Preparation, preparation, and preparation seems to be the key. These surgeons gather the team and talk over the case. They may call upon experts to have them weigh in on the case. They mentally walk through the case to see where they may be at risk and develop plans to get past that potential barrier to success.

Dr. Moulton relayed that ultimately need a way to help manage people at the extremes- that is the person who is anxious about even the most minimal risk or the person who has no recognition that they have a comfort zone whatsoever. In the middle of all this is a caution on over analysis.. That is they did learn that teaching someone to overthink every single step, leads to more discomfort with a resultant impedance in performance that is intolerable. We cannot function in a setting where we have to question every step we perform. This is exactly the same thing that Pat Croskery warned me of. So, how do we teach experienced surgeons and trainees to recognize their boundaries and how to prepare themselves for the potential for risk taking? That is the ultimate question that the Toronto group is working towards. Details of that conversation are at
http://crisislead.blogspot.com/2016/10/interview-with-carol-anne-moulton.html

---

SURGEON RESILIENCY, RISK AVERSION AND PERFORMANCE CONCERNS:
As noted above prior exposure to a negative event can certainly taint your acceptance towards risk taking. Much of this relates to the physician/surgeon's resiliency. * Surgeons face stressful conditions and unpredictability on a frequent basis. In his book **Forgive and Remember**, Bosk, describes the difficulties in a Surgeon's professional life in handling failure. Essentially our patients and peers (and us) expect surgery to be a quick fix compared to medical therapy of disease. When the outcome is not perfect doubt begins to creep in. If the surgeon does not elicit help or find a solution to break the cycle, then inevitably, performance will be negatively affected. (see http://crisislead.blogspot.com/2016/08/lessons-on-resilience-and-burnoutdr.html)

Several recent studies have highlighted the risk for a Post-Traumatic Stress Disorder (PTSD) response in Trauma Surgeons and Surgical trainees. Surgical trainees have been shown to have higher rates of psychological distress than the general population (10% reported PTSD symptoms lasting more than one month) In the Journal of Trauma and Acute Care Surgery Study 40% of trauma surgeons relayed symptoms of PTSD (15% met the diagnostic criteria for PTSD). This risk was increased with the following factors:
- Male trauma surgeons operating on more than 15 cases per month
- more than seven call duties per month
- less than four hours of relaxation per day (Joseph, et al Journal of Trauma and Acute Care Surgery 2014, Thomphson et al Surgeon 2015)

Dan Kuhn* relayed the following regarding this concern:

Trauma, Training, and the Surgeon's Identity

Most surgeons believe their stress is related to a recent traumatic event. In reality, for many of us, it begins much earlier—often during training. Early experiences such as a patient death, a difficult encounter with a mentor or colleague, or a toxic training environment can leave lasting psychological imprints. How we are trained—our educational culture, expectations, and responses to error—plays a profound role in shaping how we experience and manage stress throughout our careers.

Surgeons work under extraordinary pressure and face unpredictable crises on a routine basis. They must be well informed, technically skilled, alert, and analytical at all times. When confronted with sudden uncontrolled bleeding, unexpected patient death, operative errors, or the aftermath of malpractice litigation, these experiences can have a lasting traumatic impact. Over time, unresolved trauma may give rise to negative self-concepts and emotional responses that become morbid, destructive, and self-reinforcing.

Physicians are particularly vulnerable because of the rigidity of professional identity. Being a "doctor" is not merely a role—it often becomes the core of one's sense of self. When identity is rigid and impervious, emotional numbing may develop as a defense mechanism. Appearing detached, mechanical, indifferent, or unemotional can reflect dissociation rather than resilience. In contrast, maintaining one's core sense of being—empathy, emotional awareness, and connection—allows for more adaptive responses to stress. Some clinicians cope by distancing themselves from patients or avoiding the emotional and "supratentorial" aspects of care altogether, narrowing their focus to technical performance alone.

Traumatic fixation can occur following an unexpected, overwhelming, or life-threatening event—particularly when there is a sense of loss of control. In such moments, analytical thinking may temporarily shut down as the neocortex is overridden by the limbic system's survival response. Some individuals enter a hyper-focused "fight" mode and find a solution; others freeze, becoming confused, disoriented, or dissociated. Regardless of the immediate outcome, the highly charged emotional image of the event can become fixated in memory, serving as the seed of a post-traumatic condition.

Even when the crisis is resolved quickly, the traumatic experience may already be embedded. Over time, emotionally charged memories and negative self-identities associated with the event resurface when triggered by similar situations. These responses can feel automatic and overwhelming, disrupting attention, emotional regulation, and professional functioning. Alcohol and psychotropic medications may offer temporary symptomatic relief but do not erase traumatic fixation or alter its long-term trajectory, which often becomes chronic. In many cases, traditional psychotherapy alone is insufficient to fully resolve these deeply embedded responses.

Vulnerability is heightened during periods of physical or emotional depletion—when surgeons are hungry, exhausted, jet-lagged, overworked, or burdened by external show stressors such as litigation, divorce, or fear of losing loved ones. These conditions erode resilience and increase susceptibility to traumatic reactivation.

Symptoms consistent with post-traumatic stress can include personality change, emotional withdrawal, loss of pleasure in previously enjoyed activities, dissociation, and substance use. While some individuals maintain outward function, they do so while carrying a persistent internal burden. PTSD exists along a spectrum; many highly capable surgeons continue to work effectively while experiencing chronic, unrecognized symptoms that silently shape their behavior, relationships, and well-being.

*Daniel Kuhn, M.D., Board Certified Psychiatrist, 200 West 57th Street, Suite 1205. New York, N.Y. 10019

TRAUMA DECONDITIONING: Daniel Kuhn

LEADERSHIP STYLES IN SURGERY THAT SERVE AS IDEAL MODELS FOR TRAINEES: DO WE EVEN COME CLOSE TO THE PIN?

There are many days when I look at my behavior during the day and ask myself "did I even come close to an enabling leader today or did I act in a counterproductive manner?" After reading several papers on leadership recently, I am not sure I come close to the pin.

Leadership Styles in the Operating Room: Reflections, Evidence, and Personal Growth

In 2016, I had the opportunity to interview the authors of several exceptional papers examining leadership styles in the operating room and their effects on team behavior and performance. One particularly influential study published in the **Journal of the American College of Surgeons** evaluated how different leadership styles shaped team dynamics during surgery. Using video recordings of five surgeons, the authors compared **transactional** and **transformational** leadership behaviors to better understand how specific styles elicited distinct team responses—an area that had previously received little empirical attention.

In my own observations, many surgeons appear to default toward a predominantly **transactional leadership style**—highly goal- and task-focused, with attention directed toward performance, efficiency, reward, or failure. These tendencies often overshadow **transformational leadership behaviors**, which emphasize collective mission, inspiration, intellectual engagement, and team development. This led me to question whether there is an inherent advantage—or detriment—to favoring one leadership style over the other. More specifically, does one style enhance or inhibit **psychological safety**, defined as the degree to which team members feel comfortable speaking up about concerns, uncertainties, or potential threats to patient safety?

To explore this, the Boston research group used a previously validated leadership scoring system to analyze intraoperative video recordings of five surgeons (Hu YY, Parker SH, Yule SJ, Greenberg CC, et al.). Their findings were both illuminating and personally meaningful. Surgeons who scored highly on transformational leadership consistently entered the operating room with immediate engagement—acknowledging each team member, setting a shared purpose, and fostering a collective sense of mission. Throughout the procedure, enthusiasm, support, and mutual respect were evident. Team members felt comfortable asking for clarification or raising safety concerns.

In contrast, surgeons with lower transformational scores engaged minimally with the team, even during high-tension moments. Communication was sparse, and psychological safety appeared diminished. Importantly, the study revealed that **transactional and transformational leadership are not mutually exclusive**. In fact, they are often **additive**. Surgeons can be highly task-oriented and goal-driven while simultaneously engaging, inspiring, and empowering their teams.

This realization prompted a deeply personal question: *For those of us who are inherently task-oriented, is there hope for becoming more team-oriented leaders?* I suspect I am not alone in having viewed the surgical team—at times—as a collection of tools required to accomplish a task. While perhaps uncomfortable to admit, this mindset reflects how many of us were trained.

In a prior conversation with Lt. General Paul Van Riper, we discussed the critical importance of ensuring that team members fully understand the mission's objective. Without shared understanding, individuals may execute tasks incorrectly or achieve goals at unnecessary cost—both human and operational. Clear communication, he emphasized, ultimately improves morale and effectiveness. The JACS study echoed this principle: striving to be more transformational does not negate transactional effectiveness; instead, it enhances one's ability to leverage the team to achieve objectives.

A complementary 2016 study published in the **Journal of Surgical Education** examined leadership behaviors based on how leaders utilized available team members—categorized as authoritative, explanatory, consultative, or delegative. The authors then assessed junior residents' learning preferences relative to these leadership styles.

Predictably, senior surgeons trained in earlier eras were accustomed to authoritative or explanatory leadership—being told what to do and occasionally why. In contrast, residents in this study clearly preferred **consultative and delegative styles**, where their perspectives were actively solicited and valued during intraoperative decision-making.

Personally, I recall feeling particularly engaged and motivated when an attending surgeon asked for my opinion about operative strategy. In one case, I suggested exploring a properitoneal aortic approach for patients with hostile abdomens from prior adhesions. Because my input was respected, I not only contributed meaningfully to patient care but also learned a new surgical technique. That experience reinforced a powerful lesson: **when learners feel valued, learning accelerates**.

But does leadership style truly affect patient outcomes? The answer is unequivocally yes. Poor leadership, ineffective teamwork, unnecessary distractions, and communication breakdowns have been repeatedly associated with worse outcomes, increased team stress, and reduced morale. While surgeons once claimed that such models were impractical in high-stakes surgical environments, the growing body of evidence now refutes that defense. Effective leadership models exist—and they are applicable even under extreme pressure.

After reviewing the JACS paper, several questions emerged, which the authors generously discussed with me:

1. Do transactional or transformational leadership styles improve or impede decision-making under pressure?
2. Can surgeons with dominant task-oriented personalities learn to become more transformational leaders?
3. Does transformational engagement risk distraction or complacency, particularly given evidence that irrelevant OR conversations degrade team performance?
4. Can a surgeon effectively embody both leadership styles simultaneously, or are they context-dependent?

Steven Yule, one of the study's authors, clarified that transformational leadership does not equate to unfocused or irrelevant conversation. Rather, it involves purposeful communication before, during, and after critical phases of surgery—ensuring shared understanding of goals, risks, and concerns. Irrelevant conversation, particularly during high-stress moments, is distinct and potentially harmful.

Importantly, Dr. Yule reassured me that surgeons who are already strong transactional leaders can indeed learn transformational behaviors. Transformational leadership enhances team function and resident education, making it an essential skill set rather than an optional one.

In follow-up conversations with Caprice Greenberg, her work on communication and performance improvement further reinforced these findings. She emphasized that transactional leadership forms the foundation of surgical practice, while transformational leadership is layered atop it. Surgeons who established rapport early, shared decision-making, and actively engaged all team members—including learning names and roles—were consistently more effective.

This perspective challenges the common belief that it is the hospital's responsibility to provide a consistent team. In reality, high-performing organizations leverage staff rotation to promote fresh perspectives and prevent complacency. Teams that work together continuously may assume too much and communicate too little. New team members ask questions—and those questions often prevent errors.

Hu YY, Parker S, Yule SJ, Greenberg CC Henrickson. and al; Kissable-lee NA, Yule, Pozner and al; w permission Dr Yule & Greenberg

INTERVIEWS FROM CHAPTER IV.

FATIGUE AND PERFORMANCE REDUCTION VS INVINCIBILITY.

Sleep Deprivation, Fatigue, and Performance in High-Risk Professions

The effort to understand the effects of sleep deprivation on fatigue and performance in high-risk professions has been ongoing for decades. A landmark 1997 article published in **Nature** demonstrated that after 17 hours of sustained wakefulness, cognitive psychomotor performance—measured using computer-based eye–hand coordination tasks—declined to a level equivalent to impairment at a blood alcohol concentration (BAC) of 0.05%. After 24 hours of sustained wakefulness, performance deteriorated further, reaching an impairment equivalent to a BAC of approximately 0.10% (Dawson et al.). Subsequent authors have echoed these findings, warning that the loss of even a single night's sleep (approximately 25 hours of wakefulness) may be functionally equivalent to legal intoxication—a comparison highlighted by Lt. Col. Dave Grossman in *On Combat*.

These findings raised particular concern among human-factors experts studying aviation and medicine. Helmreich, for example, examined beliefs about fatigue among pilots and surgeons. In a 2000 survey conducted by Sexton and Helmreich, respondents were asked whether they agreed with the statement: *"Even when fatigued, I perform effectively during critical times."* While only 26% of pilots agreed, a striking 70% of surgeons endorsed this belief—highlighting a profound cultural difference in how fatigue is perceived and acknowledged within these two safety-critical professions.

In 2010, the **Federal Aviation Administration** released a formal statement on pilot fatigue following the crash of Colgan Air Flight 3407 in February 2009. Although the FAA had already initiated efforts to revise fatigue-related policies—as evidenced by its 2008 conference on pilot fatigue—the accident accelerated public and regulatory scrutiny. The **National Transportation Safety Board** determined that the crash resulted, in part, from the pilots' failure to appropriately respond to stall warnings associated with dangerously low airspeed. The investigation noted that the captain had spent the night prior to the accident sleeping in the company crew room, obtaining at best eight hours of interrupted sleep. The NTSB chairperson emphasized that "fatigue-impaired performance is not unlike alcohol-impaired performance," citing a 2003 study published in *Sleep* in which sleep-deprived individuals performed worse on certain tasks than those who were legally intoxicated.

In August 2015, the **American College of Surgeons** reissued a consensus statement on *Addressing Surgeon Fatigue and Sleep Deprivation*. Then–ACS President Dr. Carlos Pellegrini acknowledged that the evidence linking sleep deprivation to adverse outcomes in health care remained equivocal, but nonetheless urged a balanced and reasonable approach. He emphasized the importance of collaboration between surgeons and healthcare institutions to develop practical solutions grounded in professional judgment—solutions that ensure adequate surgical coverage while also supporting surgeons who recognize and report fatigue.

In personal discussions, Dr. Pellegrini highlighted a critical methodological challenge: accurately measuring sleep deprivation in surgeons. Unlike pilots on regulated duty schedules, surgeons who are not on call may theoretically obtain adequate sleep, yet still experience significant fatigue due to stressors such as litigation, administrative burden, emotional strain, or disrupted sleep architecture. These confounders make objective assessment particularly difficult.

Also in August 2015, Dr. Baxter's group in Toronto published a controversial study in the **New England Journal of Medicine** examining surgeons who provided patient care between midnight and 7 a.m. and then performed major elective operations the following day. The authors reported no significant increase in short-term postoperative complications compared with surgeons who had not worked overnight. Their conclusion—that sleep loss from overnight medical care did not measurably affect short-term outcomes—was accompanied by a recommendation that broad-based policy changes regarding duty hours may not be necessary.

In subsequent discussions, Dr. Baxter emphasized that her group explicitly acknowledged important limitations. They noted that the effects of **profound sleep loss** warranted further study and stressed the importance of critically assessing *all* sources of fatigue before implementing blanket policies. The study's focus on short-term outcomes left unanswered questions regarding longer-term consequences of fatigue, including oncologic outcomes, complication recurrence, and cumulative cognitive strain.

Dr. Pellegrini cautioned strongly against interpreting these findings as reassurance that sleep deprivation is benign. He emphasized that fatigue will eventually degrade concentration and technical skill in any profession. He further noted that studies suggesting minimal impact often focus narrowly on short-term endpoints, while the potential influence of fatigue on long-term outcomes remains largely unexplored. Given what is already known about the dangers of distraction in the operating room, ignoring the possible contribution of sleep deprivation and fatigue would be irresponsible—even if we have yet to define these constructs with precision.

In discussions with the FAA Pilot Sleep Deprivation Program, I learned that aviation fatigue policy evolved over decades through a deliberate process of "rest management." Rather than unilateral regulation, policies emerged through consensus among the Aviation Rulemaking Committee, airline management, and pilot labor unions. This process began in 2008 and culminated in finalized regulations in 2013. Their experience underscores the value of collaborative, evidence-informed policymaking and suggests that aviation partners may offer valuable guidance as surgery continues to grapple with fatigue, safety, and professional responsibility.

Core Insight

Fatigue-related impairment is real, measurable, and culturally mediated. While evidence in surgery remains complex and at times contradictory, the parallels with aviation are instructive. A thoughtful, collaborative approach—grounded in human factors science, professional accountability, and institutional partnership—offers the most promising path forward.
W permission Dr Pellegrini

Resiliency-Lessons on Leadership through the eyes of Daniel Linskey, Boston Police Chief and Incident Commander during the 2013 Boston Marathon Bombing-

Daniel Linskey, a retired Marine, was gracious to talk to me about his role and response during the Boston Marathon Bombing April 15 2013 as Chief of Police Boston and Incident Commander.

His greatest advice to me was "realize you **WILL** be overwhelmed… learn how to control yourself quickly, take in cues, so you can open your file cabinet and then control the team." He said that you have to understand that under extreme duress the amygdala response will "hijack you". Police Chief Linskey's conversation reminded me that it takes an abundance of training to achieve that degree of resilience. Very few humans can withstand that degree of pressure and maintain focus without significant training. Even then, you just do not know what your response will be.

Former Boston Police Chief **Daniel Linskey** recalled that on the day of the 2013 Boston Marathon bombing, he felt prepared—but alert. By that time, he had already led multiple full-scale, citywide disaster rehearsals known as *Boston Urban Shield*. Yet, as he later reflected, nothing could truly prepare him for what he was about to face.

Chief Linskey was a "boots-on-the-ground" leader that day, positioned in the field rather than operating from a command center. Not far from where he had just been standing in casual conversation, the first bomb detonated. He witnessed an eight-year-old child torn apart by the blast.

In that instant, a realization struck him with devastating force. Earlier, he had noticed backpacks in the area and felt uneasy, sensing something was wrong. He now understood that distraction—an innocent conversation—had interrupted his vigilance. As he tried desperately to stop the child's exsanguination, his mind fixated on one thought: *I missed the backpack.* He felt personally responsible for the boy's death.

Guilt quickly compounded the horror. He became overwhelmed, acutely aware that he was the city's top police officer—and yet had no control. He described hyperventilating, shaking, and feeling increasingly unmoored. His analytical capacity collapsed under the weight of emotion and shock.

Instinct eventually took over. He began responding directly to those in need, tending to victims alongside first responders. This helped him regain some control over his fight-or-flight response and restore clarity of thought. Yet rather than stepping into the role of strategic leader, he defaulted to task-oriented action. In later reflection, he realized that subconsciously it was easier *not* to lead. He felt overwhelmed and hoped—perhaps without realizing it—that someone else would take charge.

What felt like an eternity passed before a State Trooper he knew well physically grabbed him and began yelling. The trooper told him bluntly that he needed to regain control and take command of the scene.

That moment triggered something profound. Chief Linskey described a wave of realization washing over him. Almost instantly, he became calm—deeply, unmistakably calm. He knew exactly what he was going to say before he said it. Years of training and experience seemed to unlock simultaneously, as if an internal library had opened. Everything became clear: what to do, what not to do, and how to proceed.

Order began to emerge from chaos. He re-established command, issued calm and deliberate instructions, and allowed rehearsed sequences to guide his actions. The situation stabilized—not because the horror had ended, but because leadership had reasserted itself.

At the conclusion of our conversation, Chief Linskey shared several lessons that he felt were critical for leaders in any high-risk profession:

1. **You can never be fully ready for catastrophe.**
   No amount of rehearsal can replicate the emotional shock of a true disaster. Even with simulation, people will freeze or falter when fear takes over. Training must be as realistic as possible and must emphasize resilience and survivorship—not just procedures.

2. **Self-doubt is inevitable—lead anyway.**
   At the moment a crisis hits, confidence is irrelevant. What matters is whether your team believes *you* are in control. You must project calmness. Guilt—whether deserved or not—must be set aside immediately. Others are relying on you.

3. **Limit priorities.**
   Never give people more than four or five priorities. Beyond that, cognitive overload sets in and performance degrades.

4. **Manage information ruthlessly.**
   In a crisis, information is often incomplete, outdated, or wrong. Leaders must rapidly assess:
   - Who provided the information?
   - What exactly was said?
   - When did it arise in the timeline?
   - How was it obtained?
   - Will it help or worsen the situation?

Accepting information blindly—or rejecting it reflexively—can be equally dangerous.

5. **In crisis, solutions matter more than procedures.**
   Overreliance on rules or fear of protocol violations can cause fatal delays. Excessive information and rigid adherence to process can be deadly.

6. **People do not behave in crisis as they do in rehearsal.**
   One example was tourniquet use. Despite prior training, many responders hesitated because they had been conditioned earlier in their careers *not* to use tourniquets. Even when holding lifesaving equipment, they failed to act. Training must explicitly address these cognitive barriers.

7. **Emotional decompression is not optional.**
   Leaders must recognize when and how to discharge emotional load. Sometimes this happens in seconds—stepping away to breathe, cry, or release tension. Afterward, structured psychological support is essential. In law enforcement, critical incident stress management teams are deployed immediately. Comparable systems remain rare in medicine.

Translational Insight for Medicine

Chief Linskey's experience underscores a reality deeply relevant to surgeons and physician leaders: **training prepares the mind, but catastrophe overwhelms the nervous system.** Leadership under extreme stress is not about perfection—it is about reclaiming control, projecting calm, managing information, and caring for both the team and oneself after the event.

Shared with permission by **Daniel Linskey**, former Chief of Police, Boston; Incident Commander during the 2013 Boston Marathon bombing; U.S. Marine (Ret.).

TEAM ORGANIZATION IN TRAUMA IN AN AUSTERE ENVIRONMENT: TRAUMA AND EMERGENCY SURGERY IN UNUSUAL SITUATION.

Seon Jones and Gordon Wisbach wrote a chapter on *"Trauma in an Austere Environment: Trauma and Emergency Surgery in Unusual situation"* in COL Robert B. Lim, MD, U.S. Army, text **Surgery during natural disasters, combat, terrorist attacks, and crisis situation.**

Checklists, Speed, and Survival in Life-Threatening Situations

In personal communications, I posed the following question to the authors:

I frequently hear surgeons argue that checklists and teamwork principles have no place in emergency or life-threatening situations. When the World Health Organization Surgical Safety Checklist or similar principles are discussed, a common refrain is: "The patient is dying—checklists waste valuable time and are unnecessary." Yet your work suggests the opposite in managing teams under austere, high-risk conditions. Have you had success promoting these principles in civilian settings? If so, how do you convince others that moving fast without direction and rehearsal may actually slow us down?

Seon Jones's Response

A major source of resistance to checklists, Jones explained, is **poor checklist design.** Long, rigid, generic, and all-inclusive checklists are often burdensome and may be irrelevant—or even harmful—in emergency settings. Checklists intended for life-threatening crises must be fundamentally different from those designed for controlled, deliberate environments.

He offered an aviation analogy. Preflight checklists are intentionally slow and methodical, ensuring that no safety step is missed. In contrast, **in-flight emergency checklists** are concise, prioritized, and executed rapidly—often within seconds. To an untrained observer, it may appear that pulling out a checklist would delay action and lead to disaster. In reality, pilots use these tools precisely because they **accelerate correct action under stress.**

Emergency checklists work because they are **practiced and drilled repeatedly.** Every critical step is embedded in memory and executed in a specific sequence without hesitation. This principle, Jones noted, is one that medicine has historically resisted applying to major trauma resuscitation—even though we already accept it in other domains.

In fact, clinicians routinely use checklists in **Advanced Cardiac Life Support (ACLS)** and **Basic Life Support (BLS).** We rehearse these algorithms using printed cognitive aids, yet most providers can recite the initial steps from memory:

1. Open the airway
2. Provide breaths
3. If no pulse, begin compressions
4. Assess rhythm when the AED arrives
5. Defibrillate or administer medications as indicated

These are checklists—accepted, trusted, and lifesaving.

Jones emphasized that **emergency checklists must be designed with the cognitive state of the clinician in mind.** Trauma, fear, time pressure, and cognitive overload fundamentally change how people think and act. Once developed, these checklists must be deliberately practiced and stress-tested. The first time a team encounters a checklist should never be during an actual emergency. Rehearsal also reveals flaws—steps that are impractical, counterproductive, or irrelevant—and allows refinement before lives are on the line.

Addressing the concern that "moving fast without direction may actually slow you down," Jones encouraged skeptics to reflect on their own experiences. Nearly every clinician can recall jumping into an urgent procedure only to realize—too late—that essential elements were missing:

- The patient was not fully prepped
- The chest tube or scalpel was not in the room
- No sedation or paralytics were drawn up
- The oxygen tank was empty
- The laryngoscope light was not checked
- A difficult airway plan had not been considered
- No bougie, LMA, fiberoptic scope, or surgical airway kit was available

What begins as urgency quickly devolves into chaos. Time is lost—not saved—because preparation and sequencing were neglected.

Core Insight

Speed without structure is an illusion. In high-risk, time-critical environments, well-designed, well-rehearsed emergency checklists do not slow teams down—they prevent catastrophic delays, reduce cognitive overload, and enable coordinated action when it matters most.

W permission Wisbach and Lim

IN AN ENCOUNTER WITH A NOVEL SITUATION WHICH ONE WINS:
FLUID INTELLIGENCE, CRYSTALIZED INTELLIGENCE OR WORKING MEMORY?

Fluid Intelligence, Working Memory, and Crisis Performance

An area that increasingly emerges in discussions of crisis management is the interplay between **fluid intelligence, working memory,** and **crystallized intelligence**—concepts well described in cognitive psychology and reflected in performance patterns observed in the **Wechsler Adult Intelligence Scale (WAIS)** verbal and performance scores across the lifespan.

I was fortunate to discuss these constructs with a leading expert in the field, **Randall Engle.** Fluid intelligence refers to our capacity to confront **novel, previously unencountered situations** and engage in rapid problem-solving—the cognitive "MacGyver" skill set that allows us to navigate *"Oh my God, how do we get through this?"* scenarios. In contrast, **crystallized intelligence** reflects the accumulated knowledge we acquire over time—our growing repository of experience that allows us to manage situations that are familiar or structurally similar to those we have encountered before.

Working memory is the mental workspace that allows us to hold, manipulate, and prioritize information at any given moment. It is the cognitive system we rely on for reasoning, comprehension, learning, and—critically—attention control under stress.

Dr. Engle has emphasized that **crystallized intelligence continues to grow throughout life.** As we age, we accumulate knowledge, vocabulary, and experience, and we become increasingly adept at pattern recognition and adaptation. Fluid intelligence, however, follows a different trajectory. It tends to peak in early adulthood (approximately age 22), plateau through midlife (around age 42), and then gradually—but progressively—declines thereafter.

One particularly important insight from this work relates to how individuals **discard faulty or unhelpful information** during problem-solving. People with lower fluid intelligence often demonstrate a phenomenon known as *resampling*: after correctly determining that a hypothesis or solution is not viable, they later return to it—wasting time and cognitive resources. High fluid intelligence performers, by contrast, actively inhibit that information once it has been disproven and move on. They do not revisit dead ends.

This distinction has profound implications for crisis leadership. In high-stakes situations, **the ability to abandon information that is unhelpful in that specific context**—even if it is generally valid in other situations—is essential. Leaders must learn not only how to acquire and apply information, but also how to **let go of it when it no longer serves the problem at hand**.

Another key point Dr. Engle emphasized is the relationship between **working memory capacity and impulse control**. Individuals with higher working memory are better able to regulate impulses, suppress distractions, and maintain goal-directed behavior. While this may seem intuitive, what is often overlooked is how **sleep deprivation degrades working memory capacity**, leading to impaired inhibition, impulsivity, and diminished cognitive control. Importantly, sleep loss simultaneously reduces fluid intelligence—further compounding the risk of poor decision-making under pressure.

Translational Insight for Crisis Leadership

Crisis performance is not merely a function of experience or intelligence in the traditional sense. It depends on:

- The ability to **solve novel problems** (fluid intelligence),
- The capacity to **manage cognitive load and impulses** (working memory),
- And the wisdom to **apply experience selectively** (crystallized intelligence).

Fatigue, stress, and overload erode all three—particularly fluid intelligence and working memory—precisely when they are needed most.

http://examinedexistence.com/wp-content/uploads/2013/12/crystallized-fluid.jpg Horn JL. Age differences in fluid and crystallized intelligence. Acta Psychologica. 1967;26:107–129

And personal Conversation Randle Engle

INTERVIEWS FROM CHAPTER V. CONCLUSION:

VULNERABILITY AND RESILIENCY- A LESSON ON HUMANITY FROM TIM LEEUWENBURG ("rural proceduralist"- Kangaroo Island, Australia).

Vulnerability, Error, and the Myth of the Unbreakable Physician

This may be familiar to some, but a few months ago I watched a profoundly moving video from a presentation given by **Tim Leeuwenburg** at the 2015 **SMACC Chicago** (Social Media and Critical Care Conference). His talk—*"All Alone on Kangaroo Island"*—explores what happens when physicians confront their deepest vulnerabilities.

Without revealing the entire presentation, Dr. Leeuwenburg recounts a period of intense anguish and shame following a misdiagnosis that led to a patient developing sepsis and subsequently becoming paralyzed. The emotional injury deepened when he later learned that a nurse at the receiving facility had told the patient's wife she should sue him. What followed was a two-year ordeal marked by alcohol use, suicidal ideation, and profound isolation. Ultimately, he was able to reconcile with both the patient and his wife. That reconciliation—and the suffering that preceded it—fundamentally altered how he viewed life, empathy, and compassion.

Notably, he received what many of us recognize as the *typical* support offered to physicians after catastrophic outcomes related to error: minimal, fragmented, and largely symbolic.

Watching this talk brought back memories of earlier **American College of Surgeons** publications highlighting burnout among surgeons and its strong association with medical errors, distraction, cascading mistakes, substance use, and suicide. Around the same time, the **American Society of Anesthesiologists** published a 2012 paper noting how rare it was for anesthesiologists to take time off after witnessing tragedy in the operating room.

More recently, a CRNA shared with me a story of caring for a young mother who died from hemorrhage after a delivery complication—only to be expected to proceed directly to the next case. This is a scenario most clinicians recognize all too well. By contrast, a conversation I had last year with a local sheriff's deputy—formerly a state trooper—offered a stark comparison. He described being called at 2 a.m. on a bitterly cold January night to the scene of a wrong-way collision involving an intoxicated driver and a car carrying four college students. Despite years of experience, nothing prepared him for what he encountered. Even a decade later, he recalled with vivid clarity the steam rising from bodies severed by seatbelts.

When I asked whether he had to return to duty immediately—much like physicians often do—he surprised me. A police counselor had responded directly to the scene to assess whether officers were fit for duty. He was not. A replacement was found, and he was relieved.

I later asked **Daniel Linskey**, former Boston Police Chief and incident commander during the Boston Marathon bombing, about this practice. He confirmed that on-scene mental health professionals are routinely deployed to assess readiness, provide immediate support, and determine who needs time away. First responder services, it seems, often take better care of their professionals than medicine does.

Returning to Dr. Leeuwenburg's talk, he reminds us that vulnerability is universal. Shame and guilt are occupational hazards in medicine. They surface when we encounter medical error, administrative frustration, unmet expectations, moral distress, and work–life imbalance. We enter the profession idealizing perfection—and are deeply unsettled by the inevitability of "good enough." The gap between expectation and reality breeds disappointment, self-reproach, and isolation.

His lessons were simple but profound:

- **Resilience is not a solo pursuit**—it is built with others.
- **We are not alone**, even when it feels that way.

- • **Kindness and empathy toward colleagues matter**, especially when we cannot see their struggles.
- • **Exposing our own vulnerability** — carefully and courageously — can help both ourselves and others heal.

He closes by describing his care of a firefighter with unsurvivable injuries, focusing not on heroic intervention but on humane presence. The lasting memory was not a procedure, but a conversation with the firefighter's wife — one grounded in compassion rather than control.

When I asked Dr. Leeuwenburg why he chose this topic for SMACC Chicago, he admitted he was nervous. He was deliberately stepping away from the familiar narratives of heroic resuscitation to address topics we rarely discuss openly: burnout, depression, shame, and PTSD. It was a bold choice — and a necessary one.

Core Insight

Medicine remains deeply uncomfortable with vulnerability, yet unaddressed vulnerability is one of the greatest threats to clinician well-being, patient safety, and professional longevity. Other high-risk professions have recognized this reality and built systems of immediate psychological support. It is time for medicine to do the same.

W permission Dr Leeuwenburg

CHAPTER V. CULTURES

*Organizational culture, Mistakes, endurance/grit, willpower, burnout…. what do these have to do with the development of Habits? Borrowed from Charles Duhig: **Power of Habits***

Routines, Culture, and the Architecture of Behavior
What Is a Routine?

A routine is a habitual, automatic process by which the brain converts a sequence of actions into an efficient, unconscious pattern — a phenomenon often referred to as chunking. Routines allow the brain to conserve cognitive resources by reducing the need for continuous conscious decision-making. They are the primary mechanism through which humans achieve efficiency.

The Benefits and Risks of Routines
Benefits

Once a routine is established, conscious oversight is no longer required. This allows attention and cognitive capacity to be redirected elsewhere. Adults can perform hundreds of complex routines — walking, driving, operating equipment — effortlessly and without deliberation. This efficiency reduces stress and mental fatigue.

Risks

The danger arises when consciousness disengages at the wrong moment. Failure to interrupt a routine when conditions change can lead to errors — ranging from minor (missing a turn while driving) to catastrophic (inadvertently injuring the common bile duct or ureter during surgery).

Fortunately, humans possess innate protective mechanisms that can interrupt routines — but only if appropriate cues are recognized.

Why Do We Develop Routines?

Most routines are triggered by cues, proceed through an automatic sequence, and conclude with some form of reward. Understanding these cues and rewards allows us to understand not only individual habits, but also organizational culture. Routines may be simple or extraordinarily complex. Driving to work, for example, is cognitively demanding yet largely subconscious. The "reward" is freedom to plan the day or listen to music. The danger emerges when attention is diverted (e.g., phone use). If no hazard occurs, the routine continues uninterrupted. If conditions change suddenly — such as a car stopping abruptly — automaticity may delay corrective action.

The same phenomenon occurs in the operating room. During routine procedures, surgeons often function in automated mode. Environmental cues — noise, interruptions, distractions — may or may not penetrate awareness. While routines reduce stress and cognitive load, they also require cognitive forcing strategies: deliberately designed triggers that "wake us up" during high-risk moments we might otherwise miss.

Organizational Culture as Collective Routine
How Do Routines Shape Culture?

Organizational culture is largely a reflection of ingrained routines and habits, not formal strategic plans. These behaviors are learned — not genetic — and arise in response to prior stimuli, incentives, and rewards. Like individual habits (smoking, exercising, reading), organizational routines develop because they solve a problem or reduce stress at some point in time.

In The Power of Habit, Charles Duhigg describes how many organizational routines emerge from competition, conflict, and mistrust rather than collaboration. Departments learn to protect themselves, often at the expense of the broader mission. While conflict can be productive, it becomes destructive when it undermines shared purpose.

Changing Bad Routines and Cultures

Breaking a habit — or changing a culture — requires interrupting automatic behavior. As described by Tony Dungy, high-performing teams succeed when players react instinctively in the right way. However, to change dysfunctional habits, teams must temporarily overthink their behavior.

The process involves:

1. Identifying triggers
2. Recognizing rewards
3. Replacing the old behavior with a new one that preserves familiarity while producing a better outcome

This process—often called awareness training—is foundational in rehabilitation and behavior change. Avoiding triggers may work short-term, but durable change requires modifying responses.

Automaticity only develops when individuals trust that the new behavior reliably produces the desired outcome. Without trust, people revert to old habits.

Individual Behavior and Cultural Drift

Cultures often degrade through small individual deviations. One person arrives late; others follow. Over time, lateness becomes normalized. The "reward" is reduced stress—no one stands out. Accountability dissolves.

Attempts to correct this by pressuring one group fail unless the system is perceived as fair. Without consistent reinforcement or shared belief in the purpose of change, teams lose faith and revert to old habits.

As Dungy observed, teams without conviction are not truly teams—just people working together. Sustainable change requires belief in a greater purpose beyond superficial rewards.

Changing Culture Takes Time

Effective leaders understand that entrenched cultures cannot be changed overnight. Duhigg refers to keystone habits—small but influential routines that trigger broader behavioral cascades. Leaders must identify and target these first.

Routines form from layered habits accumulated over time, often without conscious awareness. Workers may struggle to articulate why they behave as they do. That is why culture change requires patience, analysis, and sustained effort.

Small wins matter. In Small Wins, Karl Weick showed that people become overwhelmed by large problems and disengage. Breaking problems into manageable parts—and celebrating incremental progress—builds momentum.

However, small wins alone are insufficient. Without continued reinforcement and resource allocation, momentum fades.

Where Success Typically Comes From

Ironically, many organizational success stories arise after disasters. Effective leaders harness crises as catalysts for learning. Preparedness breeds resilience, but long-term change occurs only when the group itself embraces the need for change.

Few enduring transformations are driven by leaders alone. They occur when collective belief aligns with action. Changing a habit requires deciding that change is necessary—and that decision requires willpower.

Willpower, Self-Discipline, and Grit

What if people "just don't have the willpower"?

In their seminal paper, Angela Duckworth and Martin Seligman demonstrated that self-discipline predicts academic success better than IQ (Self Discipline Outdoes IQ). Self-regulated individuals are better able to sustain focus and enact change.

However, willpower is finite. Like a muscle, it fatigues. Effective leaders understand this and prioritize tasks requiring willpower while minimizing energy spent on low-value distractions. Impulse regulation—not raw endurance—may be the key to sustaining discipline.

One method to strengthen willpower is anticipatory rehearsal: mentally and physically practicing responses to stressful or uncomfortable scenarios. This transforms threats into anticipated challenges and creates positive habit loops. Role-playing may feel awkward, but it is a proven mechanism for behavioral readiness.

Finally, organizations can support habit change by:

- Setting achievable goals
- Clearly communicating expectations
- Recognizing success authentically
- Minimizing incivility, which rapidly depletes willpower
- Providing individuals a sense of control and agency

Core Insight

Routines shape individuals. Individuals shape culture. Culture determines outcomes.

Lasting change requires awareness, belief, discipline, and time—and leaders who understand how human behavior actually works.

Routines, Culture, and the Architecture of Behavior

What Is a Routine?

A **routine** is a habitual, automatic process by which the brain converts a sequence of actions into an efficient, unconscious pattern—a phenomenon often referred to as **chunking**. Routines allow the brain to conserve cognitive resources by reducing the need for continuous conscious decision-making. They are the primary mechanism through which humans achieve efficiency.

The Benefits and Risks of Routines

Benefits

Once a routine is established, conscious oversight is no longer required. This allows attention and cognitive capacity to be redirected elsewhere. Adults can perform hundreds of complex routines—walking, driving, operating equipment—effortlessly and without deliberation. This efficiency reduces stress and mental fatigue.

Risks

The danger arises when consciousness disengages at the wrong moment. Failure to interrupt a routine when conditions change can lead to errors—ranging from minor (missing a turn while driving) to catastrophic (inadvertently injuring the common bile duct or ureter during surgery).

Fortunately, humans possess innate protective mechanisms that can interrupt routines—but only if appropriate cues are recognized.

Why Do We Develop Routines?

Most routines are triggered by **cues**, proceed through an automatic sequence, and conclude with some form of **reward**. Understanding these cues and rewards allows us to understand not only individual habits, but also **organizational culture**. Routines may be simple or extraordinarily complex. Driving to work, for example, is cognitively demanding yet largely subconscious. The "reward" is freedom to plan the day or listen to music. The danger emerges when attention is diverted (e.g., phone use). If no hazard occurs, the routine continues uninterrupted. If conditions change suddenly—such as a car stopping abruptly—automaticity may delay corrective action.

The same phenomenon occurs in the operating room. During routine procedures, surgeons often function in automated mode. Environmental cues—noise, interruptions, distractions—may or may not penetrate awareness. While routines reduce stress and cognitive load, they also require **cognitive forcing strategies**: deliberately designed triggers that "wake us up" during high-risk moments we might otherwise miss.

Organizational Culture as Collective Routine

How Do Routines Shape Culture?

Organizational culture is largely a reflection of **ingrained routines and habits**, not formal strategic plans. These behaviors are learned—not genetic—and arise in response to prior stimuli, incentives, and rewards. Like individual habits (smoking, exercising, reading), organizational routines develop because they solve a problem or reduce stress at some point in time.

In The Power of Habit, **Charles Duhigg** describes how many organizational routines emerge from competition, conflict, and mistrust rather than collaboration. Departments learn to protect themselves, often at the expense of the broader mission. While conflict can be productive, it becomes destructive when it undermines shared purpose.

Changing Bad Routines and Cultures

Breaking a habit—or changing a culture—requires **interrupting automatic behavior**. As described by **Tony Dungy**, high-performing teams succeed when players react instinctively in the right way. However, to change dysfunctional habits, teams must temporarily overthink their behavior.

The process involves:

1. Identifying triggers
2. Recognizing rewards
3. Replacing the old behavior with a new one that preserves familiarity while producing a better outcome

This process—often called **awareness training**—is foundational in rehabilitation and behavior change. Avoiding triggers may work short-term, but durable change requires modifying responses.

Automaticity only develops when individuals trust that the new behavior reliably produces the desired outcome. Without trust, people revert to old habits.

Individual Behavior and Cultural Drift

Cultures often degrade through **small individual deviations**. One person arrives late; others follow. Over time, lateness becomes normalized. The "reward" is reduced stress—no one stands out. Accountability dissolves.

Attempts to correct this by pressuring one group fail unless the system is perceived as fair. Without consistent reinforcement or shared belief in the purpose of change, teams lose faith and revert to old habits.

As Dungy observed, teams without conviction are not truly teams—just people working together. Sustainable change requires belief in a **greater purpose** beyond superficial rewards.

Changing Culture Takes Time

Effective leaders understand that entrenched cultures cannot be changed overnight. Duhigg refers to **keystone habits**—small but influential routines that trigger broader behavioral cascades. Leaders must identify and target these first.

Routines form from layered habits accumulated over time, often without conscious awareness. Workers may struggle to articulate why they behave as they do. That is why culture change requires patience, analysis, and sustained effort.

Small wins matter. In Small Wins, **Karl Weick** showed that people become overwhelmed by large problems and disengage. Breaking problems into manageable parts—and celebrating incremental progress—builds momentum.

However, small wins alone are insufficient. Without continued reinforcement and resource allocation, momentum fades.

Where Success Typically Comes From

Ironically, many organizational success stories arise after disasters. Effective leaders harness crises as catalysts for learning. Preparedness breeds resilience, but long-term change occurs only when **the group itself embraces the need for change**. Few enduring transformations are driven by leaders alone. They occur when collective belief aligns with action. Changing a habit requires deciding that change is necessary — and that decision requires willpower.

Willpower, Self-Discipline, and Grit

What if people "just don't have the willpower"?

In their seminal paper, **Angela Duckworth** and **Martin Seligman** demonstrated that **self-discipline predicts academic success better than IQ** (Self Discipline Outdoes IQ). Self-regulated individuals are better able to sustain focus and enact change. However, willpower is **finite**. Like a muscle, it fatigues. Effective leaders understand this and prioritize tasks requiring willpower while minimizing energy spent on low-value distractions. Impulse regulation — not raw endurance — may be the key to sustaining discipline.

One method to strengthen willpower is **anticipatory rehearsal**: mentally and physically practicing responses to stressful or uncomfortable scenarios. This transforms threats into anticipated challenges and creates positive habit loops. Role-playing may feel awkward, but it is a proven mechanism for behavioral readiness.

Finally, organizations can support habit change by:

- Setting achievable goals
- Clearly communicating expectations
- Recognizing success authentically
- Minimizing incivility, which rapidly depletes willpower
- Providing individuals a sense of control and agency

Core Insight

Routines shape individuals. Individuals shape culture. Culture determines outcomes.

Lasting change requires awareness, belief, discipline, and time — and leaders who understand how human behavior actually works.

W permission Charles Duhig

- Paths To Resiliency w Lipshy Lebares Schoomacher Mackinnon Narrated ONLINE VERSION 122523 https://youtu.be/y4Ktt3fHERg
- Effective leadership against all odds Lt Gen Paul Carlton USAF Ret By KEN LIPSHY 111023 https://youtu.be/ShyPmijvr_M
- Wayne Meredith Wake Forest Approach to Maintaining Surgical Team Effectiveness and Resiliency 081923 https://youtu.be/pwiA5nVn2GM
- Crisis Management Leadership: AN INTERVIEW WITH BEN AARON, MD - THE TEAM THAT SAVED RONALD REAGAN (crisislead.blogspot.com) https://crisislead.blogspot.com/2024/01/
- Crisis Management Leadership: FIRESIDE CHAT WITH WAYNE MEREDITH, MD: THE FIFTEEN YEAR WAKE FOREST APPROACH TO ESTABLISHING AND MAINTAINING TEAM EFFECTIVENESS AND RESILIENCY. August 2023 (crisislead.blogspot.com) https://crisislead.blogspot.com/2023/
- Crisis Management Leadership: WHY AM I A DREAMER AND OTHERS INNOVATORS? (crisislead.blogspot.com)
- Dana Telem; FAILING FORWARD- ALLOWING MENTORSHIP TO HELP YOU GROW Crisis Management Leadership: September 2020 (crisislead.blogspot.com) https://crisislead.blogspot.com/2020/09/failing-forward-allowing-mentorship-to.html
- JOSEPH IBRAHIM RECALLS THEIR RESPONSE TO THE JUNE 2016 ORLANDO PULSE NIGHTCLUB MASSACRE. Crisis Management Leadership: December 2016 (crisislead.blogspot.com)
- "POLICE OFFICER USES A TOURNIQUET TO SAVE A LIFE!" -THE COOPERATIVE EFFORTS BETWEEN SURGEONS AND POLICE FORCES TO IMPLEMENT STRATEGIES TO PREVENT NEEDLESS DEATHS FROM EXSANGUINATION- INTERVIEWS WITH LENWORTH JACOBS, ALEXANDER EASTMAN, FRANK BUTLER, DANIEL LINSKEY. http://crisislead.blogspot.com/2016/11/police-officer-uses-tourniquet-to-save.html
- Daniel Kuhn Interview: surgeons, PTSD, Stress and Comfort zones http://crisislead.blogspot.com/2016/11/daniel-kuhn-interview-surgeons-ptsd.html Stress and Comfort zones- with Dan Kuhn http://crisislead.blogspot.com/2016/10/stress-and-comfort-zones-with-dan-kuhn.html
- INTERVIEW WITH Carol-Anne Moulton COMFORT ZONES AND RISK TAKING IN SURGERY http://crisislead.blogspot.com/2016/10/interview-with-carol-anne-moulton.html

- "THE SOUTH CAROLINA SAFE SURGERY 2015 INITIATIVE" ADJUNCTS AND BARRIERS TO IMPLEMENTING A STATEWIDE SURGICAL SAFETY CHECKLIST FU Interview with William Berry http://crisislead.blogspot.com/2016/09/the-south-carolina-safe-surgery-2015.html
- THE SOUTH CAROLINA SAFE SURGERY 2015 INITIATIVE- ADJUNCTS AND BARRIERS TO IMPLEMENTING A STATEWIDE SURGICAL SAFETY CHECKLIST (conversation with the Harvard and SCHA groups). http://crisislead.blogspot.com/2016/08/the-south-carolina-safe-surgery-2015.html
- LESSONS ON RESILIENCE AND BURNOUT:DR. WAYNE SOTILE PHD AT THE ANNUAL FEAGIN LEADERSHIP CONFERENCE DUKE UNIVERSITY. http://crisislead.blogspot.com/2016/08/lessons-on-resilience-and-burnoutdr.html
- SURGEONS' DISCLOSURE OF CLINICAL ADVERSE EVENTS- INTERVIEW WITH THE BOSTON VA STUDY GROUP http://crisislead.blogspot.com/2016/08/surgeons-disclosure-of-clinical-adverse_21.html
- COMFORT ZONES AND RISK TAKING IN SURGERY- A Discussion with Dr. Moulton Dec 2015 http://crisislead.blogspot.com/2016/08/comfort-zones-and-risk-taking-in.html
- 'TEAMING' A DYNAMIC CONCEPT DISCUSSED WITH AMY EDMONDSON. http://crisislead.blogspot.com/2016/08/teaming-dynamic-concept-discussed-with_8.html
- "HUMAN ERROR, NOT COMMUNICATION AND SYSTEMS, UNDERLIES SURGICAL COMPLICATIONS": A FOLLOWUP CONVERSATION WITH PETER FABRI MD. http://crisislead.blogspot.com/2016/06/human-error-not-communication-and_29.html
- IMPACT OF INCIVILITY ON TEAM PERFORMANCE- CONVERSATION WITH AMIR EREZ REGARDING THEIR RESEARCH ON RUDENESS http://crisislead.blogspot.com/2016/06/impact-of-incivility-on-team_17.html
- INTRAOPERATIVE LEADERSHIP SKILLS: follow up conversation with Sarah Henrickson Parker PhD http://crisislead.blogspot.com/2016/06/intraoperative-leadership-skills-follow.html
- LESSONS ON RESILIENCY IN LEADERSHIP BY ERIC B. SCHOOMAKER MD, PhD, (Lieutenant General, US Army (retired) FORMER SURGEON GENERAL OF THE U.S. ARMY & COMANDING GENERAL, US ARMY MEDICAL COMMAND)–MINDFULNESS, MEDITATION AND LIVING IN THE MOMENT AS A LEADERSHIP STRENGTH. http://crisislead.blogspot.com/2016/06/lessons-on-resiliency-in-leadership-by.html
- THE AFFECTIVE ASPECT OF SITUATIONAL AWARENESS AND LEADERSHIP- with Jim Holbrook http://crisislead.blogspot.com/2016/06/the-affective-aspect-of-situational.html
- RESILIENCE AND BURNOUT: DR. WAYNE SOTILE PHD ANSWERS OUR QUESTIONS ABOUT LIFESTYLE CHANGES http://crisislead.blogspot.com/2016/06/resilience-and-burnout-dr-wayne-sotile.html
- RESILIENCE AND BURNOUT: LESSONS FROM DR. WAYNE SOTILE PHD AT THE ANNUAL FEAGIN LEADERSHIP CONFERENCE DUKE UNIVERSITY.http://crisislead.blogspot.com/2016/05/resilience-and-burnout-lessons-from-dr.html
- LESSONS ON LEADERSHIP AND RESILIENCY LEARNED IN THE HANOI HILTON POW CAMP FROM JIM BAILEY, POW SURVIVOR. http://crisislead.blogspot.com/2016/06/lessons-on-leadership-and-resiliency.html
- COMMUNICATION AND TEAMWORK FAILURE AS A BARRIER TO ROBOTIC SURGICAL SAFETY- A call with MARCO A. ZENATI http://crisislead.blogspot.com/2016/06/communication-and-teamwork-failure-as.html
- IMPLEMENTING VALUE-BASED CLINICAL QUALITY IMPROVEMENT IN HEALTHCARE- A DISCUSSION WITH BRUCE RAMSHAW http://crisislead.blogspot.com/2016/05/implementing-value-based-clinical.html
- INNOVATIVE STRATEGIES FOR IMPROVING SURGICAL PERFORMANCE - DISCUSSION WITH JUSTIN DIMICK http://crisislead.blogspot.com/2016/05/innovative-strategies-for-improving.html
- RESILIENCY-LESSONS ON LEADERSHIP THROUGH THE EYES OF DANIEL LINSKEY, BOSTON POLICE CHIEF AND INCIDENT COMMANDER DURING THE 2013 BOSTON MARATHON BOMBING- http://crisislead.blogspot.com/2016/05/resiliency-lessons-on-leadership.html
- VULNERABILITY AND RESILIENCY- A LESSON ON HUMANITY FROM TIM LEEUWENBURG. http://crisislead.blogspot.com/2016/04/vulnerability-and-resiliency-lesson-on.html
- ERRORS OF OMMISSION OR COMMISSION- a call with Carla Pugh http://crisislead.blogspot.com/2016/04/errors-of-ommission-or-commission.html

- LEADERSHIP STYLES IN SURGERY THAT SERVE AS IDEAL MODELS FOR TRAINEES: DO WE EVEN COME CLOSE TO THE PIN? http://crisislead.blogspot.com/2016/03/leadership-styles-in-surgery-that-serve.html
- Leadership Styles and Team Behavior -FU conversation with Caprice Greenberg and Steven Yule http://crisislead.blogspot.com/2016/03/leadership-styles-and-team-behavior-fu.html
- Surgical Trainee Response Patterns to Catastrophic Events, are we failing as parental models? http://crisislead.blogspot.com/2016/03/surgical-trainee-response-patterns-to.html
- Myth or Reality: 1. Operating Room Distractions http://crisislead.blogspot.com/2016/03/myth-or-reality-1-operating-room.html
- MYTH OR REALITY: 2. FATIGUE AND PERFORMANCE REDUCTION VS INVINCIBILITY. http://crisislead.blogspot.com/2016/03/myth-or-reality-2-fatigue-and.html
- Natural Decision Making under duress: a Conversation with Gary Klein http://crisislead.blogspot.com/2016/03/natural-decision-making-under-duress.html
- Pattern Recognition and Critical thinking- A Call with Leading Critical Thinker, Pat Croskerry http://crisislead.blogspot.com/2016/03/pattern-recognition-and-critical.html
- Breakfast with Ret. Marine Commander, Lt Gen Van Riper - Immediate Engagement vs Holding back and acquiring pertinent information before acting - when do you know you are savvy enough for one or the other? http://crisislead.blogspot.com/2016/03/breakfast-with-ret-marine-commander-lt.html
- DECISION MAKING DURING INTRAOPERATIVE CHALLENGES- THE CALGARY STUDIES http://crisislead.blogspot.com/2016/03/decision-making-during-intraoperative.html
- SPEAKING UP: Are we enabling our trainees or hindering them? http://crisislead.blogspot.com/2016/03/speaking-up-are-we-enabling-our.html
- Self Awareness- Can this be modified? http://crisislead.blogspot.com/2016/03/self-awareness-can-this-be-modified.html
- "Preoccupation with Failure" http://crisislead.blogspot.com/2016/03/preoccupation-with-failure.html
- Risk Tolerance http://crisislead.blogspot.com/2016/03/risk-tolerance.html
- Healthy Organizational Climate: Conversation with Patrick Sweeney http://crisislead.blogspot.com/2016/03/healthy-organizational-climate.html
- "Calm Is Contagious" Lessons from Rorke Denver http://crisislead.blogspot.com/2016/03/calm-is-contagious-lessons-from-rorke.html
- Military Theology on Crisis Training- Conversation with Rorke Denver and Dave Grossman http://crisislead.blogspot.com/2016/03/military-theology-on-crisis-training.html
- "What the OR Can learn from the Cockpit" A Chat with Richard Karl http://crisislead.blogspot.com/2016/03/what-or-can-learn-from-cockpit-chat.html
- Lessons from Sam Elfassy, Senior Director, Corporate Safety- Air Canada. http://crisislead.blogspot.com/2016/03/lessons-from-sam-elfassy-senior.html
- West Point Leadership Authors (REPOSTED TO GENERATE INTEREST FOR NEXT YEARS APDS) http://crisislead.blogspot.com/2016/03/west-point-leadership-authors-reposted.html
- Fluid Intelligence: Are we already doomed by the time we finish Surgery Residency? http://crisislead.blogspot.com/2016/03/fluid-intelligence-are-we-already.html
- "Errors upstream and downstream to the universal protocol associated with wrong surgery events" Douglas Paul http://crisislead.blogspot.com/2016/03/errors-upstream-and-downstream-to.html
- STATE OF FLOW VS REMAINING ON-GUARD - LESSONS FROM MIHALY CSIKSZENTMIHALYI AND DANIEL KAHNEMAN http://crisislead.blogspot.com/2016/03/state-of-flow-vs-remaining-on-guard.html
- Burnout in Medicine - Dr Freischlag advice on thriving and surviving in medicine http://crisislead.blogspot.com/2016/03/burnout-in-medicine-dr-freischlag.html
- Robert Lim Editor Surgery During Natural Disasters, combat, terrorist attacks and crisis situations.Blogspot.crisislead

Statement of Declaration Regarding Use of ChatGPT
I affirm that I utilized ChatGPT solely as an editorial assistance tool for the purposes of grammar refinement, organizational improvement, and consolidation of existing content.
All original ideas, interpretations, analyses, and substantive content are entirely my own intellectual work. ChatGPT was not used to generate new concepts, arguments, data, or scholarly insights. Rather, it functioned strictly as a writing support resource to enhance clarity, coherence, and readability.
I take full responsibility for the accuracy, integrity, and originality of the final submitted document.

Kenneth A. Lipshy, MD FACS is an undergraduate from the University of Texas at Austin, Medical School Graduate at UTHSC Houston, Surgical Intern from Baylor College of Medicine Houson Texas, Surgery Resident from Marshal University Huntington WV, Surgery Oncology Fellow From Medical College of Virginia Richmod Virginia, past Chair of the American College of Surgeons Committee on Trauma Region 13 VA state, Advanced Trauma Life Support Instructor, VA Stop The Bleed Coordinator, Adjunct Associate Professor Surgery at Uniformed Services University HS Bethesda, Adjunct Professor Surgery Wake Forest University Winston Salem NC, Adjunct Associate Professor Surgery Campbell University and Chief of Staff Surgery.
In developing the Crisis Management Leadership Guides, Kenneth Lipshy, MD has interviewed hundreds of experts from dozens of fields, on topics ranging from Leadership, Survivorship, Patient Safety, Teamwork, Human error, etc. Most of those interviews can be found at http://crisislead.blogspot.com. For more information visit http://www.crisismanagementleadership.com/.

CRISIS MANAGEMENT LEADERSHIP: TEAM TRAINING TO SURVIVE THE CRITICAL MOMENT 5th Edition is the next addition in a series of books centered on the development of leadership skills that can be utilized in effective management during a crisis. While originally aimed a Health Professionals, the guide has proven useful for many professions. The ongoing work has been the result of collaboration with over two decades as a leader with insight from ingerviews of over 200 professionals in multiple fields who are experts in leadership, crisis management, human error, patient safety and the like.